Meta-analysis in Infectious Diseases

Guest Editor

MATTHEW E. FALAGAS, MD, MSc, DSc

INFECTIOUS DISEASE CLINICS OF NORTH AMERICA

www.id.theclinics.com

Consulting Editor
ROBERT C. MOELLERING, Jr, MD

June 2009 • Volume 23 • Number 2

SAUNDERS an imprint of ELSEVIER, Inc.

W.B. SAUNDERS COMPANY

A Division of Elsevier Inc.

1600 John F. Kennedy Blvd., Suite 1800, Philadelphia, PA 19103-2899.

http://www.theclinics.com

INFECTIOUS DISEASE CLINICS OF NORTH AMERICA Volume 23, Number 2

June 2009 ISSN 0891–5520, ISBN-10: 1-4377-0492-1, ISBN-13: 978-1-4377-0492-1

Editor: Barbara Cohen-Kligerman

Infectious Disease Clinics of North America (ISSN 0891–5520) is published in March, June, September, and December (For Post Office use only: volume 23 issue 2 of 4) by Elsevier Inc., 360 Park Avenue South, New York, NY 10010-1710. Business and Editorial Offices: 1600 John F. Kennedy Blvd., Suite 1800, Philadelphia, PA 19103-2899. Customer Service Office: 6277 Sea Harbor Drive, Orlando, FL 32887-4800. Periodicals postage paid at New York, NY and additional mailing offices. Subscription prices are $218.00 per year for US individuals, $366.00 per year for US institutions, $109.00 per year for US students, $257.00 per year for Canadian individuals, $453.00 per year for Canadian institutions, $307.00 per year for international individuals, $453.00 per year for international institutions, and $151.00 per year for Canadian and international students. To receive student rate, orders must be accompanied by name of affiliated institution, date of term, and the *signature* of program/residency coordinator on institution letterhead. Orders will be billed at individual rate until proof of status is received. Foreign air speed delivery is included in all *Clinics* subscription prices. All prices are subject to change without notice. **POSTMASTER**: Send address changes to *Infectious Disease Clinics of North America*, Elsevier Periodicals Customer Service, 11830 Westline Industrial Drive, St. Louis, MO 63146. **Customer Service: 1-800-654-2452 (US). From outside of the US, call 1-314-453-7041. Fax: 1-314-453-5170. E-mail: JournalsCustomerService-usa@elsevier.com (print support) or JournalsOnlineSupport-usa@elsevier.com (online support).**

Infectious Disease Clinics of North America is also published in Spanish by Editorial Inter-Médica, Junin 917, 1ᵉʳ A 1113, Buenos Aires, Argentina.

Reprints. For copies of 100 or more, of articles in this publication, please contact the Commercial Reprints Department, Elsevier Inc., 360 Park Avenue South, New York, New York 10010-1710. Tel. (212) 633-3812, Fax: (212) 462-1935, E-mail: reprints@elsevier.com.

Infectious Disease Clinics of North America is covered in *MEDLINE/PubMed (Index Medicus), Current Contents/Clinical Medicine, Science Citation Alert, SCISEARCH,* and *Research Alert.*

Printed and bound by CPI Group (UK) Ltd, Croydon, CR0 4YY

Transferred to Digital Print 2011

Contributors

GUEST EDITOR

MATTHEW E. FALAGAS, MD, MSc, DSc
Adjunct Associate Professor of Medicine, Tufts University School of Medicine, Boston, Massachusetts; Director, Alfa Institute of Biomedical Sciences (AIBS); and Director, Infectious Diseases Clinic, "Henry Dunant" Hospital, Athens, Greece

AUTHORS

MICHAEL BARZA, MD
Department of Medicine, Caritas Carney Hospital; and School of Medicine, Tufts University, Boston, Massachusetts

MARIA A. CATALDO, MD, PhD
Infectious Diseases Consultant, Department of Infectious Diseases, Università Cattolica Sacro Cuore, Roma, Italy

JONATHAN C. CRAIG, MBChB, DCh, MM (Clin Epi), PhD, FRACP
School of Public Health, University of Sydney, Sydney, New South Wales, Australia

MARIO CRUCIANI, MD
Center of Preventive Medicine & HIV Outpatient Clinic; Consultant in Infectious Diseases, G. Fracastoro Hospital, San Bonifacio, Verona; and Adjunct Professor, Infectious Diseases Specialty School, University of Padua, Padua, Italy

GEORGE DIMOPOULOS, MD
Lecturer in Medicine, Alfa Institute of Biomedical Sciences (AIBS), Marousi; and Critical Care Department, Attikon University Hospital, Athens, Greece

MATTHEW E. FALAGAS, MD, MSc, DSc
Adjunct Associate Professor of Medicine, Tufts University School of Medicine, Boston, Massachusetts; Director, Alfa Institute of Biomedical Sciences (AIBS); and Director, Infectious Diseases Clinic, "Henry Dunant" Hospital, Athens, Greece

PAUL GARNER, MB, BS, MD, FFPHM
Liverpool School of Tropical Medicine, Liverpool, United Kingdom

HELLEN GELBAND, MHS
Resources for the Future, Washington, DC

CHRISTIAN GLUUD, MD, DrMedSc
Cochrane Hepato-Biliary Group, Copenhagen Trial Unit, Centre for Clinical Intervention Research, Rigshospitalet, Copenhagen University Hospital, Copenhagen, Denmark

LISE L. GLUUD, MD, DrMedSc
Cochrane Hepato-Biliary Group, Copenhagen Trial Unit, Centre for Clinical Intervention Research, Rigshospitalet, Copenhagen University Hospital; and Department of Internal Medicine, Gentofte University Hospital, Copenhagen, Denmark

ALEXANDROS P. GRAMMATIKOS, MD, MSc
Alfa Institute of Biomedical Sciences (AIBS), Athens; and Department of Medicine, "G. Gennimatas" Hospital, Thessaloniki, Greece

PATRICIA GRAVES, MSPH, PhD
The Carter Center, Atlanta, Georgia

DAVIDSON H. HAMER, MD
Associate Professor of International Health and Medicine, Boston University Schools of Public Health and Medicine, Center for International Health & Development, Boston, Massachusetts

KATHARINE JONES, MBChB, MRCGP, DTM&H
Liverpool School of Tropical Medicine, Liverpool, United Kingdom

JOSEPH LAU, MD
School of Medicine, Tufts University; and Center for Clinical Evidence Synthesis, Institute for Clinical Research and Health Policy Studies, Tufts Medical Center, Boston, Massachusetts

LEONARD LEIBOVICI, MD
Head, Department of Medicine E, Beilinson Campus, Rabin Medical Center, Petah-Tiqva; and Professor of Medicine, Sackler Faculty of Medicine, Tel-Aviv University, Tel-Aviv, Israel

HARRIET MACLEHOSE, BSc, PhD, MA
Liverpool School of Tropical Medicine, Liverpool, United Kingdom

ELPIS MANTADAKIS, MD, PhD
Department of Pediatrics, University District Hospital of Alexandroupolis and Democritus University of Thrace, Alexandroupolis, Thrace, Greece

PHILIP MASSON, MBChB, BA (Hons), MA (Oxon), MRCP (UK)
Department of Renal Medicine, Royal Infirmary of Edinburgh, Scotland, United Kingdom

SANDRA MATHESON, BSc (Hons), MPH
Centre for Kidney Research, The Children's Hospital, Westmead, New South Wales, Australia

DIMITRIOS K. MATTHAIOU, MD
Alfa Institute of Biomedical Sciences (AIBS), Marousi, Athens; Department of Medicine, "G. Gennimatas" General Hospital, Thessaloniki, Greece

CARLO MENGOLI, MD
Associate Professor of Infectious Diseases, Department of Histology, Microbiology and Medical Biotechnology, University of Padua, Padua, Italy

PIERO OLLIARO, MD, PhD
United Nations Children's Fund/UNDP/World Bank/World Health Organization Special
Program on Research & Training in Tropical Diseases

MICAL PAUL, MD
Unit of Infectious Diseases, Rabin Medical Center, Beilinson Campus, Petah Tikva; and
Senior Lecturer, Sackler Faculty of Medicine, Tel-Aviv University, Petah Tikva, Israel

GEORGE PEPPAS, MD, PhD
Alfa Institute of Biomedical Sciences (AIBS), Marousi; Department of Surgery, Henry
Dunant Hospital, Athens, Greece

ANASTASIOS I. PITSOUNIS, MD
Alfa Institute of Biomedical Sciences, Athens, Greece

PETROS I. RAFAILIDIS, MD, MSc, MRCP
Alfa Institute of Biomedical Sciences, Athens, Greece

ILIAS I. SIEMPOS, MD
Alfa Institute of Biomedical Sciences (AIBS), Marousi, Athens, Greece

EVELINA TACCONELLI, MD, PhD
Assistant Professor of Infectious Diseases, Department of Infectious Diseases, Università
Cattolica Sacro Cuore, Roma, Italy

THOMAS A. TRIKALINOS, MD
School of Medicine, Tufts University; and Center for Clinical Evidence Synthesis, Institute
for Clinical Research and Health Policy Studies, Tufts Medical Center, Boston,
Massachusetts

PASCHALIS I. VERGIDIS, MD
Infectious Diseases Fellow, Boston Medical Center, Department of Medicine, Section of
Infectious Diseases, Boston, Massachusetts

ANGELA C. WEBSTER, MBBS, MM (Clin Epi), PhD, MRCP (UK)
School of Public Health, University of Sydney, Sydney, New South Wales, Australia

Contents

Preface   xiii

Matthew E. Falagas

Systematic Reviews and Meta-analyses in Infectious Diseases: How areThey Done
and What are Their Strengths and Limitations?   181

Leonard Leibovici and Matthew E. Falagas

In systematic reviews data from original research are assembled in their
entirety, critically appraised, and sometimes combined through meta-
analysis to answer a clear clinical question. In infectious diseases, as in
other domains, systematic reviews and meta-analyses are the type of
research most easily translated into clinical practice. Practitioners should
familiarize themselves with the methodology of systematic reviews and
meta-analyses, their interpretation, and their limitations.

Statistical Considerations in Meta-analysis   195

Michael Barza, Thomas A. Trikalinos, and Joseph Lau

Systematic reviews and meta-analyses have recently emerged as key
sources of evidence to inform clinical care, from bedside individualized
decisions to policy making. This article discusses the principles behind
statistical methods for quantitative evidence synthesis, including meta-
analysis and meta-regression. The authors present pertinent concepts in
an intuitive and nonmathematical fashion by use of examples from the
infectious diseases literature.

Identifying Risk Factors for Infections: The Role of Meta-analyses   211

Evelina Tacconelli and Maria A. Cataldo

Systemic reviews and meta-analyses of risk factors for infections are assuming greater importance in influencing policy makers worldwide.
Meta-analyses of risk factors for infections should strictly follow guidelines
for meta-analysis of observational studies. A study protocol should be
written in advance, completed literature searches should be performed,
and studies selected in a reproducible and objective fashion. Biologic
plausibility should be addressed. Reported findings should be interpreted
with caution, taking into account the limitations of methodologic aspects
of risk factors studies.

An Overview of Meta-analyses of Diagnostic Tests in Infectious Diseases   225

Mario Cruciani and Carlo Mengoli

This review summarizes meta-analyses evaluating the accuracy of diagnostic tests for infectious diseases. Systematic searches identified 55

meta-analyses that satisfied inclusion criteria of reporting diagnostic accuracy of an index test compared with a reference test. All reviews were assessed for methods and reporting. The overall assessment underlined problems in several key steps: reporting detailed information from primary studies about the study design and patient characteristics, reference and index tests characteristics, and review methods. The execution and reporting of systematic reviews of diagnostic tests need to be improved.

Meta-analyses on the Optimization of the Duration of Antimicrobial Treatment for Various Infections   **269**

Petros I. Rafailidis, Anastasios I. Pitsounis, and Matthew E. Falagas

A mainstay of antibiotic treatment is its optimal duration for the management of infections. Many randomized control trials have been conducted on these issues during the last years. The results from these randomized control trials have been analyzed by various meta-analyses. To address the role of meta-analyses that compared a short-duration with a long-duration of the same antibiotic treatment for various infections a search was made in PubMed, Scopus, and Cochrane databases for relevant meta-analyses.

Combination Antimicrobial Treatment Versus Monotherapy: The Contribution of Meta-analyses   **277**

Mical Paul and Leonard Leibovici

Interactions between antibiotic combinations predicted by in vitro studies are not consistently reflected in clinical trials. Beta-lactam–aminoglycoside combinations, synergistic in vitro, do not confer improved survival or cure and do not prevent breakthrough infections. These conclusions are derived from recent systematic reviews and meta-analyses of randomized, controlled trials. Often, pertinent clinical outcomes could not be assessed meaningfully in individual randomized trials, but their compilation leads to strong conclusions relating to outcomes that affect the individual patient. Systematic reviews have made possible the evidence-based use of antibiotic combinations.

Meta-analytical Studies on the Epidemiology, Prevention, and Treatment of Human Immunodeficiency Virus Infection   **295**

Paschalis I. Vergidis, Matthew E. Falagas, and Davidson H. Hamer

HIV/AIDS remains a global health problem of unprecedented dimensions. An abundance of studies have been conducted on the epidemiology of HIV infection, therapeutic options, and outcomes. Original research data have been combined and critically appraised through meta-analyses. In this article we review several meta-analyses published on HIV infection/AIDS since the year 2000 with a focus on risk factors for HIV acquisition, epidemiology, mother-to-child transmission, antiretroviral therapy, and efficacy of vaccinations in HIV-positive individuals.

Meta-analyses on Behavioral Interventions to Reduce the Risk of Transmission of HIV   309

Paschalis I. Vergidis and Matthew E. Falagas

Several behavioral interventions focused in safe sex practices have been implemented in an attempt to reduce the risk of HIV transmission. In this article we review relevant meta-analyses based on studies conducted in heterosexual adults and adolescents, in minority populations, in men who have sex with men, in injection drug users, and in HIV-infected individuals. We discuss the effectiveness of behavioral interventions implemented in the individual, group, and community levels.

Meta-analyses on Viral Hepatitis   315

Lise L. Gluud and Christian Gluud

This article summarizes meta-analyses on interventions for acute and chronic viral hepatitis. The primary focus is on interventions assessed in systematic reviews and meta-analyses of randomized trials. The interventions assessed include active and passive immunization for hepatitis A and B and treatments for hepatitis B and C. The results of meta-analyses on conventional interferon-alpha, pegylated interferon alpha, lamivudine, adefovir, and interferon plus ribavirin are summarized.

Meta-analyses on the Prevention and Treatment of Respiratory Tract Infections   331

Ilias I. Siempos, George Dimopoulos, and Matthew E. Falagas

This article evaluates published meta-analyses dealing with the prevention and/or treatment of respiratory tract infections of bacterial origin in adult immunocompetent patients. The infections studied were otitis, sinusitis, tonsillitis/tonsillopharyngitis, acute exacerbations of chronic obstructive pulmonary disease, community-acquired pneumonia, and nosocomial pneumonia (including ventilator-associated pneumonia).

Meta-analyses in Prevention and Treatment of Urinary Tract Infections   335

Philip Masson, Sandra Matheson, Angela C. Webster, and Jonathan C. Craig

Urinary tract infections (UTI) are common, and complications result in significant morbidity and mortality and also consume resources. This overview summarizes the current evidence for the prevention and treatment of UTI in adults and children from meta-analyses. The quality and applicability of this evidence in clinical practice for different patient groups is discussed. Suggestions are made for future research, because it is apparent that there are evidence gaps for particular subgroups of people.

Systematic Reviews in Malaria: Global Policies Need Global Reviews   387

Paul Garner, Hellen Gelband, Patricia Graves, Katherine Jones, Harriet MacLehose, Piero Olliaro, on behalf of the Editorial Board, Cochrane Infectious Diseases Group

This article highlights systematic reviews of malaria research and what has been learned about applying methods of research synthesis in this particular infectious disease over the last 15 years. It illustrates how systematic reviews have been used to guide policy, shows what has been learned about synthesizing research in this area, and reflects on how best to maximize their uptake in policy and practice.

Meta-analysis on Surgical Infections   405

Dimitrios K. Matthaiou, George Peppas, and Matthew E. Falagas

Surgical infections include surgical site infections and other infections requiring surgical intervention to resolve along with antibiotic treatment. The authors sought to conduct a review focusing on the application of the technique of meta-analyses in the study of surgical infections. Ninety meta-analyses were included in the review, which mainly focus on the use of antimicrobial prophylaxis and on the comparison of different techniques and procedures or therapeutic regimens for the treatment of surgical infections. The majority concern surgical infections in the field of abdominal surgery. Although surgical site infection rates or clinical efficacy are reported in all meta-analyses, mortality is reported as primary outcome in only a few. Meta-analyses focusing exclusively on surgical infections, reporting data on mortality as a primary outcome, and comparing different antibiotic regimens for the treatment of surgical infections may help the clinician with decision making.

Meta-analyses on Pediatric Infections and Vaccines   431

Alexandros P. Grammatikos, Elpis Mantadakis, and Matthew E. Falagas

More than 200 meta-analyses have been published about immunizations and pediatric infections. This extraordinary number reflects the huge amount of research related to these two important scientific fields. This interest is not surprising for two reasons: (1) pediatric infections continue to represent one of the most significant causes of mortality in children worldwide, accounting for approximately 60% of childhood deaths; and (2) vaccines are among the most effective means of preventive medicine available today, having helped humanity achieve substantial victories against numerous infectious threats. Meta-analyses have contributed immensely to research into both immunizations and pediatric infections by enabling us to investigate current practices and to develop strategies to improve them. Even more important is the contribution of meta-analyses to highlighting those areas of research regarding pediatric infections and vaccines where more studies are urgently needed.

Index   459

FORTHCOMING ISSUES

September 2009
Infections in the Intensive Care Unit
Marin H. Kollef, MD, and
Scott T. Micek, PharmD,
Guest Editors

December 2009
Antibacterial Therapy and Newer Agents
Donald Kaye, MD, and
Keith Kaye, MD, *Guest Editors*

March 2010
Atypical Pneumonias
Burke A. Cunha, MD,
Guest Editor

RECENT ISSUES

March 2009
Staphylococcal Infections
Rachel J. Gorwitz, MD, MPH, and
John A. Jernigan, MD, MS,
Guest Editors

December 2008
Infectious Diseases in Women
Lisa M. Hollier, MD, and
George D. Wendel, Jr, MD,
Guest Editors

September 2008
Tick-borne Diseases, Part II:
Other Tick-borne Diseases
Jonathan A. Edlow, MD, *Guest Editor*

ISSUES OF RELATED INTEREST

Medical Clinics of North America November 2008 (Vol. 92, No. 6)
New and Emerging Infectious Diseases
Mary Elizabeth Wilson, *Guest Editor*
Available at: http://www.medical.theclinics.com/

Surgical Clinics of North America February 2009 (Vol 89, No. 1)
Surgical Infections
J. Mazuski, *Guest Editor*
Available at: http://www.surgical.theclinics.com/

VISIT THE CLINICS ONLINE!

Access your subscription at:
www.theclinics.com

FORTHCOMING ISSUES

September 2009
Infections in the Intensive Care Unit
Marin H. Kollef, MD, and
Scott T. Micek, PharmD,
Guest Editors

December 2009
Antibacterial Therapy and New Agents
Donald Kaye, MD, and
Keith Kaye, MD, Guest Editors

March 2010
Atypical Pneumonias
Burke A. Cunha, MD,
Guest Editor

RECENT ISSUES

March 2009
Staphylococcal Infections
Rachel J. Gorwitz, MD, MPH, and
John A. Jernigan, MD, MS,
Guest Editors

December 2008
Infectious Diseases in Women
Lisa M. Hollier, MD, and
George D. Wendel, Jr, MD,
Guest Editors

September 2008
Tick-borne Diseases, Part II:
Other Tick-borne Diseases
Jonathan A. Edlow, MD, Guest Editor

ISSUES OF RELATED INTEREST:

Medical Clinics of North America November 2008 (Vol 92, No. 6)
New and Emerging Infectious Diseases
Mary Elizabeth Wilson, Guest Editor
Available at: http://www.medical.theclinics.com

Preface

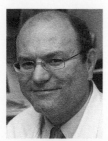

Matthew E. Falagas, MD, MSc, DSc
Guest Editor

The increasing body of research data in clinical medicine has led to the need for evidence synthesis studies. Thus, a considerable number of systematic reviews and meta-analyses have been published dealing with important issues in various fields of clinical medicine. In this issue of *Infectious Diseases Clinics of North America* experts in performing meta-analyses and authorities in infectious diseases have contributed 14 articles summarizing published evidence synthesis studies in infectious diseases.

In the introductory article, the strengths and limitations of systematic reviews and meta-analyses are reviewed. In the following article the main statistical considerations of meta-analyses are thoroughly discussed. The contribution of meta-analyses in the identification of risk factors for infections and the comparison of diagnostic tests is reviewed in the subsequent two articles. Also, two articles are devoted to important clinical therapeutic questions in infectious diseases: the optimal duration of antimicrobial treatment and the comparison of combination antimicrobial treatment with monotherapy. Six articles summarize the contribution of meta-analyses to various hot clinical questions for specific infections: HIV-AIDS, viral hepatitis, respiratory tract infections, urinary tract infections, and malaria. Finally, the last two articles deal with the role of meta-analyses in advancing knowledge regarding the management of infections in two special populations: surgical patients and pediatric patients.

Matthew E. Falagas, MD, MSc, DSc
Alfa Institute of Biomedical Sciences
9 Neapoleos Street
151 23 Marousi, Athens, Greece

Tufts University School of Medicine
145 Harrison Street
Boston, MA 02111, USA

E-mail address:
m.falagas@aibs.gr

Infect Dis Clin N Am 23 (2009) xiii
doi:10.1016/j.idc.2009.02.002
0891-5520/09/$ – see front matter © 2009 Elsevier Inc. All rights reserved.

id.theclinics.com

Systematic Reviews and Meta-analyses in Infectious Diseases: How are They Done and What are Their Strengths and Limitations?

Leonard Leibovici, MD[a,b,*], Matthew E. Falagas, MD, MSC, DSC[c,d]

KEYWORDS

- Systematic reviews • Meta-analysis
- Evidence-based medicine • Randomized controlled trials

In a systematic review, data from original research (research already done and, in most cases, already published) are assembled in their entirety, are appraised critically according to a predefined protocol, and sometimes are combined through meta-analysis, to answer a clear clinical question.

A helpful systematic review starts with a clinical question (usually about treatment or diagnosis) that is relevant to patients and clinicians. Classical, narrative reviews, in contrast, examine a medical domain in its entity, often without asking exact questions about management (**Table 1**). Systematic reviews also are distinguished from original research, because clinical studies often seek to explain and understand a phenomenon or are done to promote the use of a drug, without a clear clinical need. For example, a clinician might perform a systematic review to determine whether antibiotic drugs should be prescribed for acute sinusitis[1,2] (for most patients, antibiotics should not be prescribed). If antibiotics are needed, the next question is whether one drug is more efficient than others. Many clinical trials addressing patients who have sinusitis have compared a new drug with another to show equivalence. Because most patients will improve without antibiotic treatment, it is easy to show equivalence and support the use of new drug.

[a] Department of Medicine E, Beilinson Campus, Rabin Medical Center, Petah-Tiqva 49100, Israel
[b] Sackler Faculty of Medicine, Tel-Aviv University, Tel-Aviv, Israel
[c] Alfa Institute of Biomedical Sciences (AIBS), 9 Neapoleos Street, 151 23 Marousi, Athens, Greece
[d] Tufts University Schoool of Medicine, Boston, Massachusetts, USA.
* Corresponding author. Department of Medicine E, Beilinson Campus, Rabin Medical Center, Petah-Tiqva 49100, Israel.
E-mail address: leibovic@post.tau.ac.il (L. Leibovici).

Infect Dis Clin N Am 23 (2009) 181–194
doi:10.1016/j.idc.2009.01.002
0891-5520/09/$ – see front matter
id.theclinics.com

Table 1
Comparison of classical, narrative reviews and systematic reviews

Characteristic	Narrative Review	Systematic Review
Focus	Usually wide (eg, what is new about this disorder?)	Focused (eg, is this treatment effective for the disorder? What is the sensitivity and specificity of this test?)
Predefined study protocol	Uncommon	Common
Defined clinical question	Often absent	Intervention (or test), population, and outcomes sharply defined
Inclusion and exclusion criteria for studies	Uncommon	Defined a priori; nonarbitrary (eg, studies in languages other than English are not excluded)
Explicit search strategy (search phrase/s and databases or other sources for identifying studies)	Uncommon	Required
Description of studies	Arbitrary	Relevant details on studies and patients are extracted and presented in a uniform format
Methodologic qualities of included studies	Arbitrarily described	Extracted systematically and used to test whether weaker methodology was associated with an exaggerated effect
Data extraction	Variable	Often performed independently by more than one reviewer
Summary of results in meta-analysis	Uncommon	Performed if possible
Sensitivity analysis, analysis of subgroups, and meta-regression	Uncommon	Performed if possible, mainly as an attempt to test whether the treatment is more successful in certain subgroups of patients
Description of treatment effects	Haphazard	Usually a clear distinction is made between relative measures of effectiveness (eg, relative risk) and absolute risk reduction, which should influence clinical decisions
Conclusions in face of unavailable data	Valuable, if the review is authoritative and well-informed: using clinical experience, pathophysiological insight, analogies, and other appropriate data	Unusual

From Leibovici L, Reeves D. Systematic reviews and meta-analyses in the *Journal of Antimicrobial Chemotherapy.* J Antimicrob Chemother 2005;56(5):804; with permission.

Biases can influence the results of research. Biases are more likely than not to work in favor of the new drug or intervention.[3] Researchers believe in their own research, as indeed they should. Clinicians asked to participate in a trial of a new drug probably tend to think that the new drug will offer some advantage. (If the new and the old are exactly at equipoise, with an equal chance that the new drug would do good or harm compared with the old, then why should a clinician enroll patients?). Drug companies depend on large returns created by the marketing of a successful drug. If a chink is created in the wall that protects against bias, the chance is that bias will influence results in favor of the new drug.

It is common knowledge that not only is the subconscious at work but that sometimes manipulations are done knowingly to influence the interpretation of results of clinical research.[4] In a systematic review, efforts are made to remove, as much as possible, the effects of bias on the results.

Questions of interest often are addressed by a number of clinical studies. It is only natural that clinicians remember the most influential, that is, those published in prestigious journals or showing a significant effect. Negative results, however, might have been published in less prestigious journals or in languages other than English (the *lingua franca* of today) or might not have been published at all. Large, industry-funded studies have a better chance of being completed and published than researcher-driven studies. A systematic review assembles all the relevant research done on the subject, trying to avoid the bias of the most influential publications: if a study is methodologically correct, it should be included in the review. Finally, where appropriate, meta-analysis is used to combine the results of all the studies that were included in the review to offer a summary result and a measure of the confidence merited by this result.

This article describes the formulation of the clinical question; examines the strategies that are used to avoid bias; and looks at the efforts made in a systematic review to assemble all the relevant research and combine it, if possible. It also considers how results can be interpreted more easily in local terms. It reviews the weaknesses and strengths of systematic reviews and meta-analyses with special reference to infectious diseases. The goal is to offer the reader a guide on how to recognize good, helpful systematic reviews and how to interpret their results.

THE CLINICAL QUESTION

Guided by the methodology of evidence-based medicine, a systematic review starts with a clinical question that has three components: does the defined intervention improve the predefined outcome in a given population? A protocol is written for each systematic review and meta-analysis. To avoid post hoc and multiple comparisons, the protocol should be followed closely.

The Clinical Question: Intervention

The definition of intervention might be broad (eg, drugs with activity against methicillin resistant *Staphylococcus aureus*) or very narrow (eg, the use of 2 g of vancomycin daily). Both ways are legitimate. With a broader definition, one might have difficulty applying the results in clinical practice for specific patients. With the narrow definition, one might find only a few studies to include and miss a general effect.

The Clinical Question: Population

The definition of the population should have a clinical coherence. For example, a review might define its population as "patients who have a complicated urinary tract infection"; in clinical practice, however, the difference between a patient who has prostatitis and a pregnant young woman who has pyelonephritis is so large that it makes no sense to try and look for a similar effect in both groups of patients. Nonetheless, there is nothing wrong in using systematic reviews and meta-analyses to look for broader phenomena (eg, whether a combination of a β-lactam drug and an aminoglycoside is synergistic in treating gram-negative infections or in preventing emergence of resistance).[5-7] The answer will improve understanding but may be less helpful for guiding practice.

A second tension between explanatory and pragmatic definitions of the population exists in infectious diseases. What matters to the clinician is a definition of the population as close as possible to clinical reality (eg, is the new antibiotic better than the old one in women who have dysuria and pyuria?). To explore efficacy and mechanisms of action, the population of interest is women who have dysuria, pyuria, and significant growth of bacteria in the urine (and this is the definition often sought by the regulatory authorities). For the patient and clinician, however, the pragmatic definition of patient population is what matters.

The Clinical Question: Outcomes

Definition of outcomes is crucial. The main outcome should be one that matters to the patient. For example, in treating severe bacterial infections that have a fatality rate of 5% to 10% or more, the main outcome of interest to the patient probably is survival (given that bacterial infections are acute diseases, and resolution is relatively fast and uneventful). Then the patient might ask about major adverse events (eg, the need for tracheal intubation, hemodialysis, or operation). An early return to former functional capacity and daily activity are important to most patients, and a reduction in hospital stay probably is important as well. These outcomes should be the main outcomes in protocols of systematic reviews of severe bacterial infections.

The problems are evident: almost no randomized, controlled trial assigns fatality as the primary outcome, mainly because the sample size needed to show a difference in fatality is very large and may turn the trial into very expensive, sometimes unpractical, endeavor. (A cynic also might claim that all-cause mortality is an outcome that is very difficult to manipulate.) The time to true recovery is seldom reported.

The outcomes actually used in trials on the treatment of severe infections are problematic: they are of less interest to patients and are prone to manipulation. A composite outcome often is used to define "clinical success" in treating infections. Usually clinical success is defined as a combination of improvement in the signs and symptoms of sepsis and a lack of complications on a given day. Often, however, it also includes "no change in antibiotic treatment," a component that is of no real interest to patients. (If the patient improves, does it matter much to the patient if another drug was prescribed on the second or third day?) In unblinded studies comparing a new antibiotic drug with old ones, physicians probably will change treatment more readily in patients given the old drug than in patients given the new, presumably promising antibiotic.

In two large, systematic reviews addressing severe infections[5,6] (ie, infections with overall mortality rates of about 8%), the authors found no correlation between the rate of clinical success reported in the original trials and the fatality rate, and they could not show that the direction of the intervention effect was similar looking at the success rate and at the all-cause fatality rate. In a systematic review and meta-analysis on the effectiveness and efficacy of cefepime,[8] the authors found a significant increase in the rate of all-cause fatality in patients given cefepime as compared with patients treated with other β-lactam antibiotics; however, there was no difference whatsoever in the success rate.

Infection-related death is another outcome that should be de-emphasized. In the absence of post mortem findings, the attribution of death to one cause is arguable and might be biased. What matters to patients is whether a drug prevents death, not infection-related deaths.

In infections that cause discomfort but no major complications or death, resolution of discomfort should be selected as the main outcome; that is, what probably matters to women who have cystitis is early improvement of dysuria.

It is not by chance that the authors here are stressing the main outcome. To avoid multiple comparisons and fishing for significance, the conclusions of a systematic review should be based chiefly on the main outcome that matters to patients and that has been prespecified in the protocol as such.[9]

Secondary efficacy outcomes are important. They may be explanatory outcomes (eg, eradication of infection proven by negative cultures). Equally important are the outcomes that look at possible harm done by the study medication. In treating patients who have HIV, for example, the efficacy of many antiretroviral regimens is similar, and the choice between them is based on their adverse events. Adverse events often are poorly reported in the original studies, and the poor reporting is associated with bias.[10] In a systematic review one should extract the methods by which adverse events were collected from the original reports, examine the methods of reporting, and distinguish between adverse events that matter little to patients and those that are associated with harm. An asymptomatic and completely reversible rise in liver enzymes or creatinine level, even if common, matters little to patients. The need for hemodialysis or grave vestibular damage matters. Lumping together patients who have a rise in creatinine of more than 0.5 mg/dL and patients who needed hemodialysis under the heading of "nephrotoxicity" is misleading. Thus the protocol of a systematic review should plan separate collection of data on severe adverse events and on milder, less significant ones.

A topic specific to antibiotic treatment is induction or selection of resistance. Most systematic reviews on interventions include only randomized, controlled trials. The time scale of trials is ill fitted to address change in resistance. If two antibiotic drugs are compared, however, and resistance occurs much frequently in one arm of the trial than in the other arm, the reader should be informed. The authors advise collecting data on the isolation of resistant strains during the trials. Data often are available and are important.[11]

AVOIDING BIAS

In systematic reviews attempts are made both to neutralize bias that might be inherent in the original research and to reduce to a minimum bias that might be introduced through the workings of the review.

Selection of Studies for Inclusion in the Review

Most systematic reviews on interventions include only randomized, controlled trials. It is logical to assume that true randomization (equivalent to the toss of a fair coin) ensures that the only intentional difference between the study groups is the intervention and that other differences are small and directed by chance only. When the treatment effect in randomized, controlled trials and nonrandomized comparative studies is compared, it generally is larger in nonrandomized studies,[12] suggesting that nonrandomized studies carry a larger risk for bias and that bias usually favors the new drug or treatment. Thus in most systematic reviews the main defense against bias exaggerating the treatment effect in the original studies is to include only randomized, controlled trials.

Problematic inclusion criteria are language (eg, including only studies published in English) and status of publication (eg, including only studies published in a journal but not those presented at a conference or those not published at all). Both studies published in languages other than English and studies published in formats other than a journal tend to be smaller and to have less methodological rigor but also to show smaller treatment effects.[13,14] The authors think the readers of systematic reviews are better served by the presentation of the entirety of the research that was done (and not only the research published) addressing the question of the review. The difference in methodological rigor between studies can be addressed within the systematic review. Often, however, authors of systematic reviews and meta-analyses do not receive the additional data needed for evidence synthesis when they request them from the investigators of unpublished studies.

The date of completion or publication is another limit sometimes imposed on inclusion of studies (eg, including only studies completed or published in the last 2 decades). If used, the time limit should not be arbitrary. The time limit suggests that conditions (eg, patterns of pathogens or resistance; the intensiveness of chemotherapy) have changed so much in recent times that studies performed a long time ago no longer are relevant for current practice.

Assessment of the Methodological Quality of the Original Studies

In a seminal paper, Schulz and colleagues[15] showed the treatment effect was exaggerated in randomized, controlled trials that scored badly on the methodological aspects of allocation concealment and the blinding and exclusion of participants from analysis after randomization. Inappropriate or unreported allocation concealment was associated with a greater degree of exaggeration. Allocation concealment is considered adequate if the researcher had no way of knowing, before the enrollment of the participant, the arm of the treatment the participant to would be allocated. Central randomization (ie, the participant fits inclusion criteria, is offered participation, and agrees to participate by signing consent; and only then the researcher contacts a central point and is informed of the allocation to one of the study arms) and the use of closed, opaque envelopes (the participant fits inclusion criteria, is offered participation and agrees to participate by signing consent; and then the envelope is opened) are counted as adequate allocation concealment. Blinding of the participants, researchers, and outcome assessors is discussed in depth by Schulz and colleagues.[16]

Whether flawed methodology is universally and uniformly related to the exaggeration of treatment effects is debatable. For example, it might lead to bias in measuring subjective outcomes but not in measuring objective outcomes, such as death of any cause.[17] The authors believe that the methodological strength of trials included in a systematic review should be assessed. If the results are combined using meta-analysis, one can separate the studies with adequate methodology from the others and ask whether the treatment effect is similar. If it is not, one should use the results of the methodologically correct studies.

Amassing All Evidence

To show that a serious effort was made to identify and locate all trials that were performed on the subject, the search phrase should be comprehensive and sensitive. More than one computerized database should be searched. The usual databases used are PubMed (http://www.ncbi.nlm.nih.gov/sites/entrez%3Fdb%3Dpubmed); the

Cochrane Central Register of Controlled Trials (http://www.mrw.interscience.wiley.com/cochrane); and Embase (http://www.embase.com). Journals in Spanish, Japanese, and Chinese are not always represented in these databases, however, and trials might be located by searching databases dedicated to publications in these languages (eg, LILACS, http://bvsmodelo.bvsalud.org/site/lilacs/I/homepage.htm).

Additional data and studies that were not published can be located on the Food and Drug Administration Website (New Drug Applications). Authors often provide supplementary data, not included in the original publications, and point to unpublished studies. The authors and others investigators[18] often have been frustrated by research data that are on record only with the drug companies and are not available to the first author of the published report.

Controlling Bias in the Workings of the Systematic Review

Two main mechanisms guard against that bias in the working of the systematic review: loyalty to the original protocol and decisions on inclusion and exclusion of studies and data extraction made independently by two or more researchers.

META-ANALYSIS

Meta-analysis is a statistical combination of treatment effects from separate studies. It is not a mathematical addition of numbers, because that would involve direct comparison of patients from one study with those in another. The treatment effect (expressed, for example, as the relative risk [RR]) usually is weighted by the variance of the study. Besides the combination of treatment effects, the principles and statistical methods of meta-analysis may be used for evidence pooling in various types of studies, including the diagnostic performance of tests.

Combining Studies

Deciding whether studies are similar enough to combine in meta-analysis is not always straightforward. For example, combining the results of randomized, controlled trials comparing oral teicoplanin to oral vancomycin for *Clostridium difficile* diarrhea is straightforward,[19] but the decision to combine the effects of probiotics to prevent *Clostridium difficile* diarrhea is not a trivial decision.[20] Doing so assumes that the mechanism of action of probiotics (if, indeed, such a mechanism exists) is basically similar enough to overcome the differences in the type, quantity, and vehicle of the micro-organisms that were used.

The authors thought that the question of the effectiveness of the combination of β-lactam/aminoglycoside combination could be addressed by combining the results of studies using different drugs.[5-7] This assumption was criticized, and critics argued that this question should be investigated in selected pairs of drugs only.

Gøtzsche and Johansen[21] have combined in a meta-analysis prophylactic and empiric antifungal treatment versus placebo in patients with neutropenia. They probably assumed that in this setting prophylaxis is difficult to distinguish from treatment (when prophylaxis is started, a fungal infection already might have commenced, and antifungal treatment for persistent fever in neutropenic patients might act as prophylaxis in many cases). The present authors thought the two approaches should not be combined, because the clinical decisions are needed at different points in time. The mechanism of action for the two approaches differs. When new approaches were tried, the evidence for antifungal prophylaxis in high-risk neutropenic patients was excellent;[22] but evidence for empiric treatment of persistent fever was almost nonexistent.[23]

It is difficult to offer a rule on the combination of results of different studies in meta-analysis. Every combination (except the simplest) has underlying assumptions. The reader of a meta-analysis should formulate these assumptions explicitly, even if the author did not do so. To adopt the results of the meta-analysis, the reader must agree with its assumptions.

Heterogeneity

Exploring heterogeneity in a meta-analysis should start, both for the authors and for the reader, before reaching results (for the authors, at the stage of the protocol). One should ask a priori which factors are likely to influence the treatment effect. For example, in analyzing antibiotic prophylaxis in patients who have neutropenic fever, the obvious factor to address is the drug used for prophylaxis. The authors would like to see a separate analysis for absorbable and nonabsorbable drugs and separate analyses for different absorbable drugs (eg, fluoroquinolones and trimethoprim/sulfamethoxazole). Other factors likely to influence results are the type of infection, susceptibility to antibiotics, grade of severity, and underlying disorders. Aspects of methodological rigor should be used to explore heterogeneity, asking whether methodologically weaker studies exaggerated the treatment effect.

The second time heterogeneity should be inspected is when the results of the meta-analysis are available. A visual inspection of the meta-analysis plots will show whether the results of different studies show the same overall direction of the treatment effect. If they do not, one should question the source of the difference in the treatment effects (eg, different drugs, different populations, or a difference in the definition of outcome). One should place less confidence in meta-analyses that have discordant treatment effects for the various studies and no explanation of the variance. For example in a meta-analysis of treatments for brucellosis,[24] the relapse rate for tetracycline-rifampicin was significantly higher than for tetracycline-streptomycin, with an RR of 2.86 and a 95% confidence interval (CI), 1.84 to 4.43. This summary RR was obtained from combining 12 studies in a forest plot (**Fig. 1**). On inspecting the plot, tetracycline-streptomycin had a lower relapse rate in all studies, without exception; thus, there was no heterogeneity to explain, and confidence in the result can be high. In the same article, however, a comparison was made between treatments for *Brucella* that contain quinolones versus treatments that do not. The summary RR for five trials that were included was 1.83 (95% CI, 1.11–3.02), showing a higher failure rate with regimens including quinolones (**Fig. 2**). In inspecting the figure, three studies show no difference between regimens, and the significant overall result is caused almost entirely by one study with very high rates of failure in the quinolone arm. Clearly the treatment effect was not homogenous across trials, and the confidence that can be put on this result (although it reached statistical significance) is less than that shown in the analysis in **Fig. 1**.

Two points should be emphasized here: (1) the author and reader should inspect the results for heterogeneity; and (2) unless the plots and data for the meta-analysis are provided for the reader, the ability to judge the results is limited.

Most meta-analyses provide formal measurements of statistical heterogeneity. The χ^2 test for heterogeneity assesses whether the trials combined in the meta-analysis had approximately the same, fixed, treatment effect so that the difference between them can be assign to chance alone, or whether the treatment effect differs so much among trials that the difference cannot be blamed only on chance. The χ^2 test is not sensitive to detect heterogeneity when, as happens often, only a few studies are included. I^2 is a measure of inconsistency across studies and is less susceptible to the number of studies. A helpful description is provided in the *Cochrane Handbook*.[25]

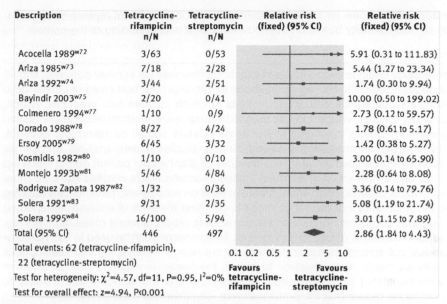

Description	Tetracycline-rifampicin n/N	Tetracycline-streptomycin n/N	Relative risk (fixed) (95% CI)	Relative risk (fixed) (95% CI)
Acocella 1989[w72]	3/63	0/53		5.91 (0.31 to 111.83)
Ariza 1985[w73]	7/18	2/28		5.44 (1.27 to 23.34)
Ariza 1992[w74]	3/44	2/51		1.74 (0.30 to 9.94)
Bayindir 2003[w75]	2/20	0/41		10.00 (0.50 to 199.02)
Colmenero 1994[w77]	1/10	0/9		2.73 (0.12 to 59.57)
Dorado 1988[w78]	8/27	4/24		1.78 (0.61 to 5.17)
Ersoy 2005[w79]	6/45	3/32		1.42 (0.38 to 5.27)
Kosmidis 1982[w80]	1/10	0/10		3.00 (0.14 to 65.90)
Montejo 1993b[w81]	5/46	4/84		2.28 (0.64 to 8.08)
Rodriguez Zapata 1987[w82]	1/32	0/36		3.36 (0.14 to 79.76)
Solera 1991[w83]	9/31	2/35		5.08 (1.19 to 21.74)
Solera 1995[w84]	16/100	5/94		3.01 (1.15 to 7.89)
Total (95% CI)	446	497		2.86 (1.84 to 4.43)

Total events: 62 (tetracycline-rifampicin),
22 (tetracycline-streptomycin)

Test for heterogeneity: $\chi^2=4.57$, df=11, P=0.95, I^2=0%

Test for overall effect: z=4.94, P<0.001

0.1 0.2 0.5 1   2   5   10

Favours tetracycline-rifampicin   Favours tetracycline-streptomycin

Fig. 1. Relapse of brucellosis with tetracycline-rifampicin versus tetracycline-streptomycin. (*From* Skalsky K, Yahav D, Bishara J, et al. Treatment of human brucellosis: systematic review and meta-analysis of randomized controlled trials. BMJ 2008;336(7646):702; with permission.)

In the first example (**Fig. 1**), the formal tests detect no heterogeneity ($P = .95$ for the χ^2 test, $I^2 = 0$%). In the second example, the heterogeneity that was detected on inspection is found on the formal tests as well: $P = .1$, $I^2 = 43$%.

The usual methods for combining results in meta-analysis assume a fixed treatment effect and cannot be used when statistical heterogeneity exists. The practice then is to use a random-effect model, which does not assume a fixed value for the treatment effect but rather assumes a distribution for it (usually a normal one). The random-effect model usually provides more conservative predictions but involves assumptions that are not easier to prove than those of the fixed-effect model. The use of the

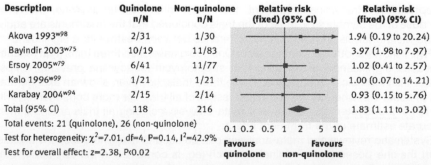

Description	Quinolone n/N	Non-quinolone n/N	Relative risk (fixed) (95% CI)	Relative risk (fixed) (95% CI)
Akova 1993[w98]	2/31	1/30		1.94 (0.19 to 20.24)
Bayindir 2003[w75]	10/19	11/83		3.97 (1.98 to 7.97)
Ersoy 2005[w79]	6/41	11/77		1.02 (0.41 to 2.57)
Kalo 1996[w99]	1/21	1/21		1.00 (0.07 to 14.21)
Karabay 2004[w94]	2/15	2/14		0.93 (0.15 to 5.76)
Total (95% CI)	118	216		1.83 (1.11 to 3.02)

Total events: 21 (quinolone), 26 (non-quinolone)

Test for heterogeneity: $\chi^2=7.01$, df=4, P=0.14, I^2=42.9%

Test for overall effect: z=2.38, P<0.02

0.1 0.2 0.5 1   2   5   10

Favours quinolone   Favours non-quinolone

Fig. 2. Overall failure for treatment of brucellosis with or without quinolones. (*From* Skalsky K, Yahav D, Bishara J, et al. Treatment of human brucellosis: systematic review and meta-analysis of randomized controlled trials. BMJ 2008;336(7646):701–4; with permission.)

random-effect model (or any other statistical method) should not replace the exploration of heterogeneity based on the knowledge and understanding of the domain.

Problems

Some study designs encountered in infectious diseases (as in other domains) should
not be analyzed using the regular methods for dichotomous outcomes or difference in
means for continuous outcomes. In trials in which clusters (eg, practices, wards,
hospitals, classes, villages) rather than individuals were randomized, the correlation
between individuals belonging to the same clusters should be taken into account,
both in the original analysis and in combining the studies in meta-analysis. Sometimes
outcomes are counted as rates (eg, episodes of diarrhea per patient during follow-up
in trials on the prevention of diarrhea). Patients sometimes are enrolled into trials more
than once (a situation often encountered in trials on neutropenic patients), invalidating
the assumption of independence made in counting the units of analysis. In reporting
continuous outcomes, studies on the same topic report different measurements (eg,
means, medians, or differences in means). Meta-analysis can be used in such circum-
stances, but special statistical techniques are needed, and additional assumptions
usually are made. It is unrealistic to expect the reader to examine critically whether
the methods that were used are adequate, and it is the author's responsibility to
convince the reader that the problems were identified and dealt with properly.

STRENGTHS

Many of the strengths of systematic reviews and meta-analyses have been addressed
in the previous sections, but they merit additional emphasis. A systematic review asks
a clinical question that is relevant to patients and clinicians and is free of other considerations. The outcome is one that matters to patients. Efforts are made to avoid bias
by including all relevant research, correcting for possible bias in the original research,
and eliminating bias that might be created through the workings of the systematic
review.

Meta-analysis makes it possible to look at events that were too rare in the original
studies to show a statistically significant difference. For example, a systematic review
and meta-analysis found that antibiotic prophylaxis reduces mortality in high-risk neutropenic patients (RR 0.67, 95% CI, 0.55–0.81).[26] To be powered to show such a reduction in mortality (assuming a mortality rate of about 5%), a single trial would have to
recruit about 3000 patients, a very difficult task to manage. **Fig. 1** is an excellent visual
demonstration of this point. In all 12 trials, relapse of brucellosis was less common with
streptomycin-tetracycline treatment than with rifampicin-tetracycline; however,
because of the sample size, most of the trials concluded that the treatments are equivalent. Meta-analysis showed that the difference between treatments is significant.

Fig. 1 shows another advantage also. One could have cited three trials (that reached
statistical significance) as showing that streptomycin-tetracycline prevents relapse
better then rifampicin-tetracycline. These three trials, however, show an exaggerated
RR of about 4.2, whereas the combined results of all trials are more conservative, with
an RR of 2.9. Systematic review and meta-analysis including all trials attains a more
accurate estimate of the treatment effect.

Systematic reviews and meta-analyses can be used to examine questions broader
than the one posed in the original research (eg, is combination therapy better than
monotherapy? What is the influence of the length of antibiotic treatment on development of resistance?). They can point at areas where research evidence is sorely
needed but lacking.[27]

LIMITATIONS

The preference for randomized, controlled trials affords systematic reviews rigor and diminishes bias but is also one of their main weaknesses. For a given question a systematic review might miss examining common practice. For example, a combination of a β-lactam drug and a macrolide often is prescribed for community-acquired pneumonia. A legitimate question is whether a β-lactam is equivalent to the combination, in all patients or in subgroups. This question, however, was not addressed in any randomized, controlled trial and therefore will be ignored in a systematic review limited to randomized, controlled trials. The reader should keep this limitation in mind (see **Table 1**).

Authors of systematic reviews sometimes are accused of ignorance of the medical domain (an easy way to test that possible flaw is to see whether the authors have published previously on the subject.[28]) The present authors strongly advise authors of systematic reviews to enroll researchers who are active in the domain and practitioners dealing with the questions in clinical practice. The important decisions in a systematic review often are based on an understanding of the medical domain and not on methodology.

In this article, the authors have emphasized the importance of outcomes that matter to patients. These outcomes might not have been collected in the original research or might not have been published. The reader should be aware that the outcomes reported in a systematic review might originate from only a part of the original trials.

Regrettably, authors sometimes sin against the commandments of good systematic reviews and meta-analyses. Searches are conducted only in one database or include only articles in English; outcomes that make little sense are selected and emphasized; counts are added arithmetically. The methods of the systematic review should be taken into account when one is seeking to employ its results.

INTERPRETING RESULTS

To apply the results of systematic reviews, clinicians should be convinced that the results are relevant to their patients. For example, systematic reviews including mainly older studies may not be relevant to practice today. Susceptibility to antibiotics, supportive treatment, or chemotherapy regimens might have changed to a degree that makes the results of older studies (and their compilation) irrelevant. Effect treatment may be different in different regions. For example, iron supplementation probably is beneficial in iron-deficient children, but it is unclear if this benefit is maintained in malaria-rich areas.[29]

The logic underlying meta-analysis is that relative measurements from different studies (eg, RR or odds ratio) are similar to a degree that allows combination. For the clinician and patient, however, it is the reduction in absolute risk that matters. The clinician should translate the relative measures provided in systematic reviews into absolute risk reduction or numbers needed to treat. To do so, the clinician should know (or guess) the baseline proportion of the outcome in the local group of patients.

Even knowing that research shows a clear benefit for an intervention, patients might elect not to choose this intervention. For example, although streptomycin-tetracycline prevents relapse of brucellosis better than rifampicin-tetracycline, patients might prefer the oral regimen and avoid injections.[30] The duty of the clinician is to offer the data and evidence to patients, including the balance between benefit and harm or inconvenience.

In infectious diseases, future resistance to antibiotics is a major consideration. Randomized, controlled trials are not conducted on a time scale that allows the influence of different regimens on resistance to be elucidated. Nevertheless, this consideration should be taken into account. For example, opponents of antibiotic prophylaxis in neutropenic patients cite the risk of future resistance, although prophylaxis has been shown to reduce mortality.

Evidence is not the only consideration for practice. To adopt an intervention, decision makers must make decisions based on cost-effectiveness and often on cost alone. The threshold of evidence for a favorable balance between benefit and harm should be reached first, however, and this determination is the role of systematic reviews and meta-analyses.

THE COCHRANE COLLABORATION

The Cochrane Collaboration (www.cochrane.org) relies on volunteers to support the writing and dissemination of systematic reviews. It does not accept funding from the drug industry or from other sources that might have vested interests. The support takes the form of researching and formulating rules for performing systematic reviews and meta-analyses. These rules (much more comprehensive than those given in this article) are detailed in the *Cochrane Handbook*,[25] a source highly recommended to researchers intending to perform systematic reviews and to readers. The Cochrane Collaboration works through review groups dedicated to specific subjects. A major advantage of writing Cochrane reviews is that the protocol of the review, as well as the completed review, is subject to peer review. Cochrane reviews are collected in the Cochrane Library. At present the Cochrane Library contains about 330 systematic reviews on antibiotic treatment, 53 systematic reviews on managing or preventing malaria, and about 230 reviews on HIV-infected or AIDS patients as well as on other topics in infectious diseases.

SUMMARY

In infectious diseases, as in other domains, systematic reviews and meta-analyses are the type of research most easily translated into clinical practice. Practitioners should familiarize themselves with the methodology of systematic reviews and meta-analyses, their interpretation, and their limitations.

REFERENCES

1. Falagas ME, Giannopoulou KP, Vardakas KZ, et al. Comparison of antibiotics with placebo for treatment of acute sinusitis: a meta-analysis of randomised controlled trials. Lancet Infect Dis 2008;8(9):543–52.
2. Ahovuo-Saloranta A, Borisenko OV, Kovanen N, et al. Antibiotics for acute maxillary sinusitis. Cochrane Database Syst Rev 2008;(2):CD000243.
3. Chalmers I, Matthews R. What are the implications of optimism bias in clinical research? Lancet 2006;367(9509):449–50.
4. Waxman HA. The lessons of Vioxx—drug safety and sales. N Engl J Med 2005; 352(25):2576–8.
5. Paul M, Benuri-Silbiger I, Soares-Weiser K, et al. Beta lactam monotherapy versus beta lactam-aminoglycoside combination therapy for sepsis in immunocompetent patients: systematic review and meta-analysis of randomised trials. BMJ 2004; 328(7441):668–72.
6. Paul M, Soares-Weiser K, Leibovici L. Beta lactam monotherapy versus beta lactam-aminoglycoside combination therapy for fever with neutropenia: systematic review and meta-analysis. BMJ 2003;326(7399):1111–5.

7. Bliziotis IA, Samonis G, Vardakas KZ, et al. Effect of aminoglycoside and beta-lactam combination therapy versus beta-lactam monotherapy on the emergence of antimicrobial resistance: a meta-analysis of randomized, controlled trials. Clin Infect Dis 2005;41(2):149–58.

8. Yahav D, Paul M, Fraser A, et al. Efficacy and safety of cefepime: a systematic review and meta-analysis. Lancet Infect Dis 2007;7(5):338–48.

9. Dwan K, Altman DG, Arnaiz JA, et al. Systematic review of the empirical evidence of study publication bias and outcome reporting bias. PLoS ONE 2008;3(8):e3081.

10. Chowers M, Gottesman B, Paul M, et al. Safety reporting in randomised clinical trials of HAART: systematic review. Barcelona, Spain: 18th European Congress of Clinical Microbiology and Infectious Diseases (ECCMID); 2008. p.19–22.

11. Leibovici L, Soares-Weiser K, Paul M, et al. Considering resistance in systematic reviews of antibiotic treatment. J Antimicrob Chemother 2003;52(4):564–71.

12. Ioannidis JP, Haidich AB, Pappa M, et al. Comparison of evidence of treatment effects in randomized and nonrandomized studies. JAMA 2001;286(7):821–30.

13. Jüni P, Holenstein F, Sterne J, et al. Direction and impact of language bias in meta-analyses of controlled trials: empirical study. Int J Epidemiol 2002;31(1):115–23.

14. Hopewell S, McDonald S, Clarke M, et al. Grey literature in meta-analyses of randomized trials of health care interventions. Cochrane Database Syst Rev. 2007;(2):MR000010.

15. Schulz KF, Chalmers I, Hayes RJ, et al. Empirical evidence of bias. Dimensions of methodological quality associated with estimates of treatment effects in controlled trials. JAMA 1995;273(5):408–12.

16. Schulz KF, Chalmers I, Altman DG. The landscape and lexicon of blinding in randomized trials. Ann Intern Med. 2002;136(3):254–9.

17. Wood L, Egger M, Gluud LL, et al. Empirical evidence of bias in treatment effect estimates in controlled trials with different interventions and outcomes: meta-epidemiological study. BMJ 2008;336(7644):601–5.

18. Johansen HK, Gotzsche PC. Problems in the design and reporting of trials of anti-fungal agents encountered during meta-analysis. JAMA 1999;282(18):1752–9.

19. Nelson R. Antibiotic treatment for *Clostridium difficile*-associated diarrhea in adults. Cochrane Database Syst Rev. 2007;(3):CD004610.

20. McFarland LV. Meta-analysis of probiotics for the prevention of antibiotic associated diarrhea and the treatment of *Clostridium difficile* disease. Am J Gastroenterol 2006;101(4):812–22.

21. Gøtzsche PC, Johansen HK. Meta-analysis of prophylactic or empirical antifungal treatment versus placebo or no treatment in patients with cancer complicated by neutropenia. BMJ 1997;314(7089):1238–44.

22. Robenshtok E, Gafter-Gvili A, Goldberg E, et al. Antifungal prophylaxis in cancer patients after chemotherapy or hematopoietic stem-cell transplantation: systematic review and meta-analysis. J Clin Oncol. 2007;25(34):5471–89.

23. Goldberg E, Gafter-Gvili A, Robenshtok E, et al. Empirical antifungal therapy for patients with neutropenia and persistent fever: systematic review and meta-analysis. Eur J Cancer 2008;44:2192–203.

24. Skalsky K, Yahav D, Bishara J, et al. Treatment of human brucellosis: systematic review and meta-analysis of randomized controlled trials. BMJ 2008;336(7646):701–4.

25. Higgins JPT, Green S, editors. Cochrane handbook for systematic reviews of interventions version 5.0.0 [updated February 2008]. Available at. www.cochrane-handbook.org; 2008. The Cochrane Collaboration. Accessed February, 2009.

26. Gafter-Gvili A, Fraser A, Paul M, et al. Meta-analysis: antibiotic prophylaxis reduces mortality in neutropenic patients. Ann Intern Med 2005;142(12 Pt 1): 979–95.
27. Fraser A, Paul M, Attamna A, et al. Drugs for preventing tuberculosis in people at risk of multiple-drug-resistant pulmonary tuberculosis. Cochrane Database Syst Rev 2006;(2):CD005435.
28. Farr1 BM, Jarvis WR. Methicillin-resistant *Staphylococcus aureus*: misinterpretation and misrepresentation of active detection and isolation. Clin Infect Dis 2008; 47:1238–9.
29. Iannotti LL, Tielsch JM, Black MM, et al. Iron supplementation in early childhood: health benefits and risks. Am J Clin Nutr 2006;84(6):1261–76.
30. Pappas G, Siozopoulou V, Akritidis N, et al. Doxycycline-rifampicin: physicians' inferior choice in brucellosis or how convenience reigns over science. J Infect 2007;54:459–62.

Statistical Considerations in Meta-analysis

Michael Barza, MD[a,b], Thomas A. Trikalinos, MD[b,c], Joseph Lau, MD[b,c,*]

KEYWORDS

- Systematic review • Meta-analysis • Meta-regression
- Quantitative synthesis • Pooling

The explosive growth of biomedical publications has produced a voluminous literature that is beyond the ability of any practicing physician to master. Clinicians seeking answers to specific questions commonly find a plethora of material of varying quality and conflicting results that make clinical decision-making difficult. Often, there are multiple small studies of an issue, with none reaching statistical significance and with no useful conclusion.

One way to harmonize a discordant literature is by meta-analysis: a statistical method of combining the results of multiple studies. The term "meta-analysis" was coined in 1976 in the social science literature.[1] The term is derived from the Greek "meta," or "end" analysis, signifying a form of summing up or final reckoning. However, as we shall see, evidence is never static:[2] new studies are continually being published and their results may agree or disagree with older studies. Not infrequently, this can result in changes in the conclusions of meta-analyses.[3,4]

The first meta-analysis (although it was not called such) has generally been credited to the statistician Karl Pearson, who in 1904 published an analysis that combined several sets of data on the effects of enteric fever (typhoid) inoculation used in several British army expeditions.[5] His aim was to overcome the problem of indefinite conclusions from several small studies. However, he noted that the data came from heterogeneous populations and settings and the results were so discrepant that he wondered about the credibility of the combined analyses. His observations are themes that would recur in many subsequent meta-analyses, and these issues have been the basis for criticisms of meta-analysis, as well as for research conducted to address

[a] Department of Medicine, Caritas Carney Hospital, Boston, MA, USA
[b] School of Medicine, Tufts University, Boston, MA, USA
[c] Center for Clinical Evidence Synthesis, Institute for Clinical Research and Health Policy Studies, Tufts Medical Center, 800 Washington Street, Box #63, Boston, MA 02111, USA
* Corresponding author. Center for Clinical Evidence Synthesis, Institute for Clinical Research and Health Policy Studies, Tufts Medical Center, 800 Washington Street, Box #63, Boston, MA 02111.
E-mail address: jlau1@tuftsmedicalcenter.org (J. Lau).

Infect Dis Clin N Am 23 (2009) 195–210
doi:10.1016/j.idc.2009.01.003
0891-5520/09/$ – see front matter © 2009 Elsevier Inc. All rights reserved.
id.theclinics.com

those criticisms. Meta-analysis did not begin to appear regularly in the medical litera-ture until the late 1970s.[6] Since then, thousands of meta-analyses have been pub-lished in virtually all fields of medicine and biomedical research, numerous advances have been made in the analytical techniques for meta-analysis, and many empiric evaluations of meta-analyses have provided insights on how best to interpret their results.

This article describes the steps in conducting a systematic review and the principles of the statistical methods commonly used in meta-analyses, to help readers to appre-ciate the papers and articles that follow. The authors focus on the concepts rather than the mathematical details, and alert the reader to potential pitfalls and limitations in meta-analyses.

SYSTEMATIC REVIEW AND META-ANALYSIS

A meta-analysis is generally preceded by a systematic review. As opposed to the traditional narrative review, which is often wide-ranging, selective in its citations, and potentially biased in its conclusions, a systematic review addresses a specific question, is comprehensive in its retrieval of literature, and uses rigorous methods to minimize bias in its analysis and conclusions. Meta-analyses are often contained within systematic reviews. A meta-analysis uses statistical procedures to combine data addressing a specific question from multiple studies that meet the eligibility criteria. As a result, meta-analyses can answer questions that single trials lack the power to address.[7] Moreover, by providing estimates of the magnitude of the effects of an intervention, meta-analysis provides useful information for comparison of alter-natives and for decision and cost-effectiveness analyses.[8]

Most meta-analyses involve randomized controlled trials (RCTs) of interventions, but there are also many meta-analyses that assess the relationships of risks and health outcomes and evaluate the accuracy of diagnostic tests. In addition to RCTs, meta-analyses can also be applied to cohort studies, case-controlled studies, non-comparative or retrospective studies, genetic studies, and even case reports.[9] RCTs of interventions have been a favorite target because they are the most likely to yield reliable results that can be applied directly to patient care.

Steps in Conducting a Systematic Review

Table 1 summarizes the steps to be followed to perform a systematic review.

The first step is to formulate clear focused key questions for the systematic review.[10] In practice, this means that one has to define the population, intervention (or exposure), comparators, outcomes, and study designs of interest, a set of charac-teristics typically referred to as "PICOD." Essentially, the PICOD characteristics dictate the eligibility criteria for studies that will be included in the systematic review (and the meta-analysis, by extension). There is a tradeoff between the stringency of PICOD definitions and the number of potentially eligible studies and the generaliz-ability of the review findings. Inappropriately lenient definitions can allow the inclusion of studies so dissimilar they have uncertain applicability to the population of interest. In contrast, overly narrowing the PICOD scope can result in too few studies to allow for meaningful quantitative analyses. Framing the key questions and the PICOD charac-teristics is typically an iterative process.[10]

The protocol should also specify the information sources to be accessed, the criteria for determining which studies will be included in the meta-analysis, the data to be extracted, and the analytical approaches for combining the data, as discussed below.

Table 1	
Steps to perform a systematic review	
Step	**Description**
1. Formulate the question and develop protocol	Refine the key questions of the review. Specify the PICOD items for study eligibility. Develop the protocol for the review.
2. Systematic literature search and screening	Develop search strategies and query electronic databases. Screen returned titles/abstracts for eligibility.
3. Critical appraisal of eligible studies and data extraction	Appraise the susceptibility of studies to biases Evaluate their applicability to the target population and setting. Extract numerical and other information.
4. Quantitative analyses	Perform meta-analysis, meta-regression or other analyses, as applicable. Perform sensitivity and exploratory analyses.
5. Interpretation	Put the findings into context. What do these results suggest for current practice and for future research?

Identifying relevant literature relies mostly on searches of structured electronic databases. MEDLINE, the most commonly used database, can be accessed through the free Pubmed (www.ncbi.nlm.nih.gov/sites/entrez) portal. Other electronic databases exist and they can cover publications not indexed in MEDLINE. However, for most research questions, querying non-MEDLINE sources yields few, if any additional relevant articles. Databases are queried using search strategies, combinations of pertinent terms describing the population, intervention, and study design of interest. The exact contents and syntax of search strategies vary by example. Search strategies are not directly transferable across databases or across different portals for the same database: a search strategy developed for Pubmed MEDLINE cannot work unmodified on OVID MEDLINE or in EMBASE (another general database). Finally, hand searching, perusal of reference lists of relevant papers and past systematic reviews, and searching of additional resources such as the National Library of Medicine's ClinicalTrials.gov Web site (a prospective registry of clinical trials) can also be used. After the searches, the systematic reviewers screen titles and abstracts of the yielded citations and the full text of all potentially eligible articles using the prespecified criteria, and determine which are eligible for analysis.

Critically appraising the quality of studies is a prerequisite for deciding whether they have avoided serious biases, so that their inclusion in the analysis will provide reliable results. However, which deficiencies are most prone to introduce bias and how these biases affect the results is difficult to determine. Some empiric research suggests that poor concealment of allocation and inadequacy of randomization are the most important deficiencies and tend to lead to an exaggeration of the benefits of treatment.[11] Empiric assessments of the several dozens of proposed approaches to derive "quality scores" to assess study design and conduct have yielded conflicting results.[12] Instead of using quality scores, many investigators now use individual components of quality assessment (eg, blinding, adequacy of random allocation) as part of the sensitivity analyses: that is, they assess the effect on the overall result of excluding trials that do not meet specified quality standards.

The remainder of this article discusses commonly used metrics to describe intervention effects, quantitative methods to calculate a grand mean (an overall summary estimate) of the effect, as well as methods to identify, explore and explain the between-study variability.[13]

EFFECT METRICS IN PRIMARY STUDIES

Before describing methods for the quantitative synthesis of information from several studies, one needs to briefly review metrics typically used to describe the effects of interventions or the strength of associations in the medical domain (**Table 2**).

Binary outcomes (such as the proportion of people with an event at a given time point) are naturally presented as a contingency table. The risk difference is the difference in the proportion of events between the compared groups, and expresses difference in the absolute risk for an event. For example, if an event occurs in 10% (say 10 out of 100) in the control group but in 6% (12 out of 200) in the intervention group, the risk difference is 4% (10% − 6%). The risk ratio and the odds ratio are multiplicative measures of risk; they express how many times the risk and odds for the outcome of interest differ across the compared groups. The risk ratio for the event in the intervention group in the preceding example is 60% (6%/10%). The odds ratio

Table 2
Metrics describing intervention effects or strength of association

Examples and Sufficient Statistics				Metric and Definition	
Binary outcomes					
For example, number (or proportion) with:				Risk difference	$(x_1/N_1) - (x_2/N_2)$
Meningitis				Risk ratio	$(x_1/N_1)/(x_2/N_2)$
Dead					
Without symptomatic improvement				Odds ratio	$(x_1/r_1)/(x_2/r_2)$
	Events	*No events*	*Total*		
Group 1	x_1	r_1	N_1		
Group 2	x_2	r_2	N_2		
Continuous outcomes					
For example, mean:				Mean difference	$m_1 - m_2$
Number of days with symptoms					
Visual analog pain score				Standardized	$(m_1 - m_2)/s'$
	Mean	*SD*	*Total*	mean difference	
Group 1	m_1	s_1	N_1		
Group 2	m_2	s_2	N_2		

Binary outcomes: In case-controlled studies one can meaningfully calculate only the odds ratio, which can be interpreted as an approximation of the risk ratio for a relatively rare event in the general population. In RCTs (and prospective cohort studies) one can also calculate the risk ratio, which is easier to interpret than the odds ratio (change in risk versus change in odds, respectively). Continuous outcomes: The standardized mean difference expresses the mean difference relative to its standard deviation (S'). Alternative standardized mean difference metrics differ in the exact formula for S'. Standardized mean differences are used to bring some continuous metrics to the same scale, so as to facilitate their synthesis (eg, pain scores with different instruments). A popular interpretation is that a standardized mean difference expresses the average percentile standing of the average person in Group 1, relative to the average person in Group 2: that is, when it is 0 (no difference), the mean of Group 1 is at the 50th percentile in Group 2.
Abbreviation: SD, standard deviation.

is 12/188 divided by 10/90 = 0.57. The multiplicative effects measures are most often used in meta-analysis, because risk differences can differ dramatically across studies with varying event rates in the comparator or control group.

For continuous outcomes, a commonly used metric is the mean difference; a standardized version of it is often used when one needs to bring together measurements in different scales (eg, pain scores measured with different instruments). For example, if the mean blood pressure (systolic/diastolic) in the control group is 135/85 mm Hg and in the intervention group is 125/80 mm Hg, the mean difference is 10/5 mm Hg. Details on the different metrics and their interpretation can be found elsewhere.[14,15]

Other types of outcomes analyses are also examined in primary studies (eg, time-to-event outcomes in survival analyses), but these are not discussed in this article.

QUANTITATIVE SYNTHESIS—WHY NOT SIMPLY POOL DATA?

Meta-analysis is based on statistically rigorous methods, explicitly developed to synthesize information from different studies. Simply pooling numerical data across all studies, as if they were identical strata of a single study, can lead to misleading results.[16–18] Briefly consider the fictitious example of **Table 3**, where simple pooling yields a grossly misleading summary, inconsistent with the constituent studies. (As shall be shown later in this article, the results indicate marked heterogeneity between the studies in the incidence of the event.) Even if the point estimate of the simple pooling approach happened to be correct, the width of the accompanying confidence interval would be improperly narrow: this naive approach ignores the fact that data are obtained from different studies and systematically underestimates the variance of the summary effect estimate.

FIXED-EFFECTS AND RANDOM-EFFECTS META-ANALYSIS

Meta-analysis provides a summary estimate by weighting each study's effect in inverse proportion to its variance. This makes intuitive sense: more precise studies with smaller variance (usually the larger ones) receive more weight than less precise ones (that have larger variance and usually smaller sample size).

There are several approaches to meta-analysis, but a most important distinction is between fixed- and random-effects methods.

Table 3
Fictitious example illustrating Simpson's paradox

Study or Summary	Intervention A		Intervention B		Risk Ratio (95% CI)
	Events	Total	Events	Total	
Study 1	32	608	64	1216	1.00 (0.66, 1.51)
Study 2	120	240	80	160	1.00 (0.82, 1.22)
Simple pooling (wrong)	152	848	124	1,376	1.98 (1.59, 2.47)
Meta-analysis (correct)[a]	—	—	—	—	1.00 (0.84, 1.20)

Meta-analysis synthesizes the risk ratio of each study to obtain the summary effect (see text). Note that the meta-analysis summary effect has narrower confidence intervals (CI) than each of studies 1 or 2.
[a] Inverse variance fixed effects method.

Fixed Effects Meta-analysis

Fixed effects meta-analysis assumes that all studies are sampled from the same population (**Fig. 1**). Put differently, all studies estimate a single true effect, and the observed between-study variability is attributed solely to chance (sampling variability). It is as if one had a basket full of white and red balls and, with eyes closed, picked small batches of balls at random, then studied each batch to determine the proportion of balls of each color before combining the results in a meta-analysis. The summary effect of the meta-analysis (the grand mean) estimates the (unobserved) "truth." The inverse-variance method, an often-used fixed-effects method, obtains the summary estimate by weighting the effect of each study inversely proportionally to its variance. This general method can be used to combine any metric, provided that it is approximately normally distributed and that its variance is known (or can be calculated from the data). Especially for binary outcomes, fixed effects meta-analysis alternatives include the Mantel-Haenszel method[19] and the Peto method[20] (only for the odds-ratio metric).

To determine if a fixed-effects model is appropriate, one must assess the degree of heterogeneity (dissimilarity) among the studies. The Q statistic[21] is the most common approach to test for the presence of statistical heterogeneity in the results of studies in the meta-analysis. When the Q statistic is excessively large (as compared with a χ^2 distribution with $k-1$ degrees of freedom, with k being the number of studies), it suggests that the fixed-effects model assumption does not hold for the data. Because it is a relatively insensitive statistic, it is typically considered significant if $P<.10$.[21,22]

Random-Effects Meta-analysis

Random-effects approaches allow for between-study variability (heterogeneity) and incorporate it in the calculations. Here, it is assumed that there is no single true effect, but rather a range (a distribution) of study-specific true effects (**Fig. 2**). This situation might arise if there were some underlying differences, identified or not, between the populations in different studies. The study-specific true effects are distributed around an overall "grand mean." In the random-effects model, between-study dissimilarities are reflected in the spread of the distribution of the study-specific true effects around their grand mean. The variance of this distribution, τ^2, is also known as heterogeneity. The more dissimilar the study effects, the broader their distribution and the larger the

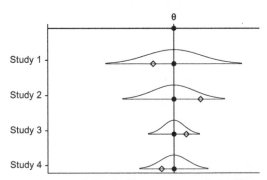

Fig. 1. Schematic representation of fixed-effects meta-analysis. Shown is a hypothetical meta-analysis of four studies, represented by four normal distributions. The fixed-effects model assumes that the true (unobserved) effect in all four studies (*circles*) is the same and equal to a common effect θ. The observed effect in each study (*diamond*) deviates from the common effect θ because of chance.

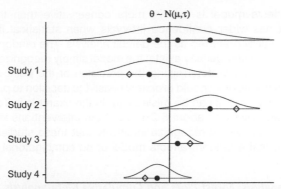

Fig. 2. Schematic representation of random-effects meta-analysis. The figure shows a hypo-thetical meta-analysis of four studies, each with its own normal distribution. The random-effects model assumes that the study-specific true effects (*circles*) can differ somewhat among the studies, probably reflecting some differences in the populations, the interventions, or some other factor, but that these true effects are distributed around a common grand mean μ with variance τ^2. Note that the observed effect in each study (*diamond*) deviates from its own underlying true effect (*circle*) and from the grand mean μ, as shown in the figure.

heterogeneity. If study effects are very similar, τ^2 becomes small or even 0. There are many methods[23] to estimate τ^2, but the most commonly used is the DerSimonian and Laird moments-based method.[24]

In the random-effects model, the estimates of the study effects receive weights that are inversely proportional to the sum of their variance and the heterogeneity param-eter. Random-effects methods tend to weigh studies more democratically than fixed-effects meta-analysis: In the extreme case that τ^2 is much larger than the vari-ances of the individual study estimates, all studies in the meta-analysis would receive approximately the same weight ($\approx 1/\tau^2$). Conversely, if there is no between-study heterogeneity ($\tau^2 = 0$), then the random-effects weights will be identical to the fixed-effects weights and both approaches will yield the same results.

Q is fairly insensitive in detecting genuine heterogeneity when there are relatively few studies, and may over-interpret unimportant heterogeneity when there are many studies.[22] Alternative approaches quantify the extent of heterogeneity using metrics that are less dependent on the number of synthesized studies and can be compared across meta-analyses.[18] One such metric, I^2, expresses the percentage of between-study variability that is attributable to heterogeneity rather than chance. It ranges between 0% and 100%, and increasing values imply more extensive between-study heterogeneity. Values over 75% denote extreme heterogeneity.[18] The estimates of Q, τ^2, and I^2 are unstable when only few studies are combined.[25]

Which Model Should One Choose, Fixed or Random Effects?

Between-study heterogeneity in the broader context may refer to differences in the design and conduct of the various combined studies, study populations, interventions, comparators, outcome definitions, or other factors. There may be obvious differences that explain any observed between-study heterogeneity (eg, differences in dosing schedules, length of observation, populations tested) or the explanation may not be apparent.

The random-effects model is usually more conservative than the fixed-effects model; that is, it has wider confidence intervals when statistical heterogeneity is non-zero, and is usually preferred as the default analysis. The random-effects model does not explain why heterogeneity exists: the model simply recognizes heterogeneity and takes it into account in determining the precision of the point estimate. When heterogeneity is extreme, one should probably revisit the decision to provide an overall summary, because the result can be misleading. In the example in **Table 3**, in which the incidence of an event was about 5.2% with both interventions in study one and 50% in study two, one would recognize intuitively that these studies show marked heterogeneity and that a random-effects model or no combinatorial method should be used.

Graphs in Meta-analysis: Forest Plots and Cumulative Meta-analysis

A typical way to present a meta-analysis is a forest plot, where each study is shown with its effect size and 95% confidence interval (**Fig. 3**, *left panel*); the summary effect

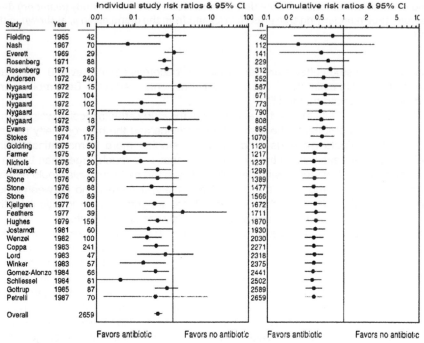

Fig. 3. Typical meta-analysis plots. The figure shows a meta-analysis addressing the use of antibiotic prophylaxis versus no treatment in colon surgery. The outcome is wound infection. There are 32 trials, ordered chronologically. The risk ratio was chosen as a metric of the effect size. The left panel is a typical meta-analysis "forest plot" with a random effects summary. Each study is represented by a filled circle (denoting its risk ratio estimate) and a horizontal line (denoting the corresponding 95% confidence interval). The right panel is a cumulative meta-analysis, where the summary risk ratio (by random effects modeling) is re-estimated each time a study is added as time progresses. Note that the effectiveness of antibiotics could have been identified as early as 1971 after five studies in approximately 300 patients. *n*: Sample size (*left*) or cumulative number of patients (*right*). (*From* Ioannidis JP, Lau J. State of the evidence: current status and prospects of meta-analysis in infectious diseases. Clin Infect Dis 1999;29:1179; with permission.)

and 95% confidence interval is also shown ("Overall," *bottom of left panel*). Another common graphic presentation is a cumulative meta-analysis plot, where studies are placed in chronologic order and the summary estimate and 95% confidence interval is plotted as studies are sequentially added to the calculations (see **Fig. 3**, *right panel*).[26,27] In other words, each point is a summary estimate (with confidence intervals) of studies up to that time. Cumulative meta-analysis is a compelling way to examine trends in the evolution of the summary-effect size, and to assess the impact of a specific study on the overall conclusions (see **Fig. 3**).[26] The figure shows that many studies were performed long after cumulative meta-analysis would have shown a significant beneficial effect of antibiotic prophylaxis in colon surgery.

EXPLORING REASONS FOR STATISTICAL HETEROGENEITY

One of the main uses of meta-analysis is to quantify and explain between-study heterogeneity. In reality, clinical and methodologic variability is abundant in any collection of studies. Often, this variability translates to statistical heterogeneity across study results.[28,29] The exploration of heterogeneity can yield insights into the mechanisms of treatment effects (eg, differences in regimens or duration of observation might explain the differences in outcomes) and identify populations more or less likely to benefit from the treatment. These inferences may not be apparent from individual studies.

There are several ways to investigate the reasons for heterogeneity; among them are subgroup analysis and meta-regression. The subgroup analysis approach, a variation on those described above, groups categories of subjects (eg, by age, sex) to compare effect sizes. The meta-regression approach uses regression analysis to determine the influence of selected variables (the independent variables) on the effect size (the dependent variable). In a meta-regression studies are regarded as if they were individual patients, but their effects are properly weighted to account for their different variances.[7]

Meta-regression is a very useful framework for exploring and understanding heterogeneity.[30,31] For example, in patients infected with HIV type 1, zidovudine monotherapy has time-limited effectiveness: trials in the late 1980s and early 1990s showed large and statistically significant effects favoring zidovudine monotherapy over placebo or no treatment for delaying the progression to advanced disease, as well as favorable effects on mortality.[32] However, larger trials with longer follow-up showed no difference in the long term (>3 years). In this case, a grand mean from a meta-analysis would be highly misleading because it would combine studies of varying duration; the most appropriate presentation of the analysis is through meta-regression (**Fig. 4**).[13]

Study-Level Versus Patient-Level Covariates

Note that there are two distinct types of characteristics of each study that can be considered in subgroup and meta-regression analyses. First, there are study-level factors that apply equally to all patients in a study, such as the duration of follow up (see **Fig. 4**) or definitions of outcome. Second, there are patient-level summary statistics that may obscure the effect of variations within the study, as for example, mean age or percentage of diabetics.[13,33] It could be that outcomes are different for younger patients or those with diabetes, but these important influences may not be apparent in aggregate data. Meta-regression is accurate and most useful in the first case. It is usually not helpful in the second case because the aggregate data embrace a range of values (eg, varying ages) and the relation between the outcome and the value of interest is generally not provided in publications. However, meta-analysis

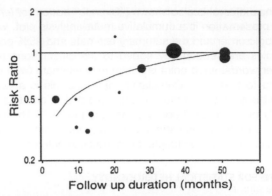

Fig. 4. Meta-regression of the risk ratio for mortality against follow-up duration in random-ized trials of zidovudine monotherapy versus placebo or no treatment. Trials are repre-sented as filled circles with size proportional to their weight in a meta-regression. The solid curve is the meta-regression line summarizing the relationship between the effects of zidovudine monotherapy and the duration of follow-up. The meta-regression supports the notion of time-limited effectiveness for the intervention: trials with shorter follow-up duration show larger effects, whereas trials with longer follow-up show no effect. The hori-zontal line at risk ratio 1.00 is the line of no effect. (*Data from* Ioannidis JP, Cappelleri JC, Sacks HS, et al. The relationship between-study design, results, and reporting of randomized clinical trials of HIV infection. Control Clin Trials 1997;18:431–44.)

can be used in the second case if one can gain access to the individual patient data. For example, in a meta-analysis of individual patient data from eight randomized trials of high-dose acyclovir in patients with HIV infection versus placebo, it was found that a higher CD4 cell count at baseline is associated with a lower hazard for mortality (hazard ratio for square root transformed CD4 cell count 0.89 [95% CI: 0.87, 0.91]). In contrast, a meta-regression of aggregate data (using the [square root] mean base-line CD4 cell count in each trial as the explanatory variable) would not reach the same conclusion (the corresponding effect would be 0.98 [95% CI: 0.93, 1.04]; calculations from data reported in the same article). Simply put, the average baseline CD4 cell count is not the baseline CD4 cell count of the average patient.

The example above makes the important point that meta-regression on summaries of patient level data can yield very misleading results, even in the opposite direction from the more correct individual patient data analyses.[33,34] The example illustrates the concept of ecological fallacy, a phenomenon in which associations apparently present at the aggregate (group) level are not necessarily true at the individual-patient level.

Exploring the Event Rate in the Control Group

Variation in control rate across studies may reflect differences in patient populations, in the underlying baseline risk of patients, or in study characteristics, such as length of follow-up, intervention delivery, or methods of outcome ascertainment. Patients at different baseline risks may experience different benefits and harms from an interven-tion.[35] When between-study heterogeneity exists but the reasons are not evident or information on patient and study characteristics is too skimpy to allow for exploration, the rate of events in the control group may serve as a useful indicator of heterogeneity.[36]

If there are marked differences between studies in the event rate in controls and an association is found between treatment effects and the control rate, then a single combined estimate is not the best estimate for individual patients. It is likely that some subgroups of patients respond better to the intervention under examination.[36] Formal approaches to this problem include hierarchical and Bayesian meta-regression models.[36–38]

Two recent examples in which control event rates may have played a role in heterogeneity in the field of infectious diseases are worth noting. In a meta-analysis of the efficacy of various treatment regimens for malaria in African children, there was no overall difference between two regimens.[39] However, there was marked heterogeneity among the trials. There was even heterogeneity in outcomes among sites within the same trial. Amodiaquine plus sulfadoxine/pyrimethamine showed greater efficacy than amodiaquine plus artesunate in areas with high-transmission rates of malaria.[39] This analysis suggested that the baseline rate of transmission was an important determinant of relative efficacy.

In a meta-analysis of the efficacy of *Haemophilus influenzae* type b immunization of children, a study done in Alaska yielded results different from the others. The investigators suggested that a higher intensity of exposure to the pathogen in Alaska may have diminished the apparent efficacy of the vaccine.[40] In this case, as in the preceding one, differences in event rates (exposures) correlated with differences in the seeming efficacy of interventions.

Most often, one would expect a higher event rate to show a greater benefit of an intervention and a low event rate to show lesser benefit because there is little room for improvement. However, even if such an interpretation is suggested by a meta-analysis, one must hesitate to extrapolate such a finding to an individual patient because populations in trials may not be evenly distributed as to risk. Whereas benefit could appear to accrue to all individuals across a given average risk level, it could, in fact, apply only to the few with a very high risk. This is another example of ecological fallacy.

OTHER TYPES OF META-ANALYSIS

Specific meta-analysis techniques have been developed for the synthesis of different types of studies. This section briefly addresses a few of them.

Network Meta-analysis

Until now, the article has discussed comparisons between two treatments. However, for several clinical questions, isolated pairwise comparisons are less informative and perhaps out of the typical clinical context. This may be especially true in the infectious diseases field: in the case of acute sinusitis, there are many antibiotics that are routinely used.[41] Why is the comparison between azithromycin and amoxicillin, for example, more interesting than a comparison among different macrolides and penicillins, or among cephalosporins, or folate inhibitors? It is increasingly appreciated that systematic reviews and meta-analyses should examine the comparative effectiveness across several (contemporary and realistic) treatment options.

Network meta-analysis (or multiple treatment meta-analysis) is an extension of the meta-analysis methodology to more than two comparisons.[42] To compare any two among several alternative treatments, network meta-analysis can use information from studies that perform direct (head-to-head) comparisons together with information from indirect comparisons (ie, by contrasting the treatments of interest with a common reference and deducing their relative effects).

Diagnostic and Prognostic Test Meta-analysis

Meta-analysis can also be used to summarize the performance of diagnostic and prognostic tests. Test performance is typically captured by its sensitivity (its ability to maximize true-positives) and its specificity (its ability to minimize false-positives), quantities readily available from a cross tabulation of index test and reference standard responses.[43] There is a tradeoff between the sensitivity and specificity of any test, with each of them diminishing as the other increases. Among other things,[44] the choice of the threshold for a positive test response affects sensitivity and specificity.[45] Separate meta-analyses of sensitivities and specificities fail to consider these correlated quantities jointly and may not be the best way to summarize test performance across different studies.

Alternative methods capture the tradeoff between sensitivity and specificity by calculating a summary receiver operating characteristic curve (SROC) (**Fig. 5**).[46] Recent advances in the methodology of meta-analysis (eg, bivariate meta-analysis of sensitivity and specificity[47] and hierarchical SROC analyses[48,49]) address many of the limitations of the classical SROC-based analyses, but will not be discussed here.

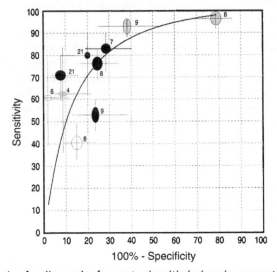

Fig. 5. SROC analysis of radiography for acute sinusitis (using sinus puncture as a reference standard). Studies are represented by ellipses whose horizontal and vertical axes are proportional to the weight of their specificity (more accurately its complement, 100% - specificity, or the false-positive rate) and sensitivity, respectively. The thin horizontal and vertical lines are the confidence intervals that accompany the (complement of) specificity and the sensitivity of each study. A perfect study would have a sensitivity and specificity of 100%, and would fall in the upper left corner of the graph. The solid curve is the SROC line that describes the tradeoff between the aforementioned quantities in the included studies. The color of the ellipses codes for the definition of a positive radiograph across studies (*black*, sinus fluid or opacity; *gray* sinus fluid or opacity or mucus membrane thickening; *white*, sinus opacity). Compared with puncture (considered more accurate), radiography offers moderate ability to diagnose acute sinusitis (area under the SROC curve approximately 0.83; an area of 1.00 would imply perfect diagnostic ability and an area of 0.50 absence of diagnostic ability). (*From* Engels EA, Terrin N, Barza M, et al. Meta-analysis of diagnostic tests for acute sinusitis. J Clin Epidemiol 2000;53:856; with permission.)

Other Types of Meta-analysis

Finally, there are many methodologies for advanced meta-analysis that have been developed to address specific concerns, including meta-analysis of individual participant data,[50,51] multivariate meta-analysis,[52-54] and special types of meta-analysis in genetics.[55]

FINAL REMARKS

Meta-analysis is no longer a novelty in medicine. Systematic reviews with quantitative syntheses are now routinely published and are used by practitioners and policy decision-makers. Meta-analysis offers the potential to address questions that individual studies lack the power to address. Most importantly, it provides a framework to explore and explain between-study heterogeneity, potentially affording insights into the mechanisms of effects, and a means to identify populations most likely to benefit from an intervention.

Meta-analysis has its acknowledged limitations and criticisms, many of which stem from weaknesses of the primary data. Numerous empiric studies have been conducted over the past decades to advance the understanding of how best to assess primary studies and interpret results of meta-analyses. Standards by which to conduct and report meta-analyses have been published to improve the quality of reporting.[56,57]

The best meta-analysis cannot compensate for limitations and defects in the primary studies. However, meta-analysts should always aim to present meaningful and clinically relevant analyses of the available data. For example, for several clinical questions (and perhaps more so for infectious diseases rather than other medical domains) the issue is the comparative effectiveness of several contemporary and routinely used treatment alternatives. In such instances, pairwise comparisons between any two interventions—isolated from the remaining options—are perhaps not as meaningful as network meta-analysis. Recent advances in meta-analysis methodology provide the statistical tools to perform such comparative effectiveness reviews.

This article has attempted to introduce the reader to the principles, practicalities, and pitfalls of meta-analysis in a readable manner. In an era in which meta-analyses in virtually every specialty are appearing almost daily, it is important for readers to be informed about the strengths and weaknesses of this fascinating analytical field.

REFERENCES

1. Glass GV. Primary, secondary and meta-analysis of research. Educational Researcher 1976;5:3–8.
2. Trikalinos TA, Churchill R, Ferri M, et al. Effect sizes in cumulative meta-analyses of mental health randomized trials evolved over time. J Clin Epidemiol 2004;57: 1124–30.
3. French SD, McDonald S, McKenzie JE, et al. Investing in updating: how do conclusions change when Cochrane systematic reviews are updated? BMC Med Res Methodol 2005;5:33.
4. Moher D, Tsertsvadze A, Tricco AC, et al. When and how to update systematic reviews. Cochrane Database Syst Rev 2008;MR000023.
5. Pearson K. Report on certain enteric fever inoculation statistics. BMJ 1904;3: 1243–6.

6. Chalmers TC, Matta RJ, Smith H Jr, et al. Evidence favoring the use of anticoagulants in the hospital phase of acute myocardial infarction. N Engl J Med 1977; 297:1091–6.

7. Lau J, Ioannidis JP, Schmid CH. Quantitative synthesis in systematic reviews. Ann Intern Med 1997;127:820–6.

8. Jordan H, Lau J. Linking pharmacoeconomic analyses to results of systematic review and meta-analysis. Expert Rev Pharmacoeconomics Outcomes Res 2003;3:89–96.

9. Balk EM, Lau J, Bonis PA. Reading and critically appraising systematic reviews and meta-analyses: a short primer with a focus on hepatology. J Hepatol 2005; 43:729–36.

10. Counsell C. Formulating questions and locating primary studies for inclusion in systematic reviews. Ann Intern Med 1997;127:380–7.

11. Schulz KF, Chalmers I, Grimes DA, et al. Assessing the quality of randomization from reports of controlled trials published in obstetrics and gynecology journals. JAMA 1994;272:125–8.

12. Juni P, Witschi A, Bloch R, et al. The hazards of scoring the quality of clinical trials for meta-analysis. JAMA 1999;282:1054–60.

13. Lau J, Ioannidis JP, Schmid CH. Summing up evidence: one answer is not always enough. Lancet 1998;351:123–7.

14. Hedges LV, Olkin I. Statistical methods for meta-analysis. San Diego (CA): Academic Press Inc.; 1985.

15. Normand SL. Meta-analysis: formulating, evaluating, combining, and reporting. Stat Med 1999;18:321–59.

16. Simpson E. The interpretation of interaction in contingency tables. J Roy Stat Soc Series B 1951;13:238–41.

17. Altman DG, Deeks JJ. Meta-analysis, Simpson's paradox, and the number needed to treat. BMC Med Res Methodol 2002;2:3.

18. Higgins JP, Thompson SG. Quantifying heterogeneity in a meta-analysis. Stat Med 2002;21:1539–58.

19. Mantel N, Haenszel W. Statistical aspects of the analysis of data from retrospective studies of disease. J Natl Cancer Inst 1959;22:719–48.

20. Yusuf S, Peto R, Lewis J, et al. Beta blockade during and after myocardial infarction: an overview of the randomized trials. Prog Cardiovasc Dis 1985;27:335–71.

21. Cochran W. The combination of estimates from different experiments. Biometrics 1954;10:101–29.

22. Hardy RJ, Thompson SG. Detecting and describing heterogeneity in meta-analysis. Stat Med 1998;17:841–56.

23. Sidik K, Jonkman JN. A comparison of heterogeneity variance estimators in combining results of studies. Stat Med 2007;26:1964–81.

24. DerSimonian R, Laird N. Meta-analysis in clinical trials. Control Clin Trials 1986;7: 177–88.

25. Huedo-Medina TB, Sanchez-Meca J, Marin-Martinez F, et al. Assessing heterogeneity in meta-analysis: Q statistic or I2 index? Psychol Methods 2006; 11:193–206.

26. Lau J, Schmid CH, Chalmers TC. Cumulative meta-analysis of clinical trials builds evidence for exemplary medical care. J Clin Epidemiol 1995;48:45–57.

27. Ioannidis JP, Lau J. State of the evidence: current status and prospects of meta-analysis in infectious diseases. Clin Infect Dis 1999;29:1178–85.

28. Engels EA, Schmid CH, Terrin N, et al. Heterogeneity and statistical significance in meta-analysis: an empirical study of 125 meta-analyses. Stat Med 2000;19: 1707–28.
29. Ioannidis JP, Trikalinos TA, Ntzani EE, et al. Genetic associations in large versus small studies: an empirical assessment. Lancet 2003;361:567–71.
30. Thompson SG, Sharp SJ. Explaining heterogeneity in meta-analysis: a comparison of methods. Stat Med 1999;18:2693–708.
31. Thompson SG, Higgins JP. How should meta-regression analyses be undertaken and interpreted? Stat Med 2002;21:1559–73.
32. Ioannidis JP, Cappelleri JC, Sacks HS, et al. The relationship between study design, results, and reporting of randomized clinical trials of HIV infection. Control Clin Trials 1997;18:431–44.
33. Schmid CH, Stark PC, Berlin JA, et al. Meta-regression detected associations between heterogeneous treatment effects and study-level, but not patient-level, factors. J Clin Epidemiol 2004;57:683–97.
34. Berlin JA, Santanna J, Schmid CH, et al. Individual patient- versus group-level data meta-regressions for the investigation of treatment effect modifiers: ecological bias rears its ugly head. Stat Med 2002;21:371–87.
35. Glasziou PP, Irwig LM. An evidence based approach to individualising treatment. BMJ 1995;311:1356–9.
36. Schmid CH, Lau J, McIntosh MW, et al. An empirical study of the effect of the control rate as a predictor of treatment efficacy in meta-analysis of clinical trials. Stat Med 1998;17:1923–42.
37. Dohoo I, Stryhn H, Sanchez J. Evaluation of underlying risk as a source of heterogeneity in meta-analyses: a simulation study of Bayesian and frequentist implementations of three models. Prev Vet Med 2007;81:38–55.
38. Sharp SJ, Thompson SG. Analysing the relationship between treatment effect and underlying risk in meta-analysis: comparison and development of approaches. Stat Med 2000;19:3251–74.
39. Obonyo CO, Juma EA, Ogutu BR, et al. Amodiaquine combined with sulfadoxine/pyrimethamine versus artemisinin-based combinations for the treatment of uncomplicated falciparum malaria in Africa: a meta-analysis. Trans R Soc Trop Med Hyg 2007;101:117–26.
40. Obonyo CO, Lau J. Efficacy of *Haemophilus influenzae* type b vaccination of children: a meta-analysis. Eur J Clin Microbiol Infect Dis 2006;25:90–7.
41. Lau J, Zucker D, Engels EA, et al. Diagnosis and treatment of acute bacterial rhinosinusitis. Evid Rep Technol Assess (Summ) 1999;9:1–5.
42. Lumley T. Network meta-analysis for indirect treatment comparisons. Stat Med 2002;21:2313–24.
43. Loong TW. Understanding sensitivity and specificity with the right side of the brain. BMJ 2003;327:716–9.
44. Leeflang MM, Bossuyt PM, Irwig L. Diagnostic test accuracy may vary with prevalence: implications for evidence-based diagnosis. J Clin Epidemiol 2008;62: 5–12.
45. Leeflang MM, Deeks JJ, Gatsonis C, et al. Systematic reviews of diagnostic test accuracy. Ann Intern Med 2008;149:889–97.
46. Littenberg B, Moses LE. Estimating diagnostic accuracy from multiple conflicting reports: a new meta-analytic method. Med Decis Making 1993;13:313–21.
47. Reitsma JB, Glas AS, Rutjes AW, et al. Bivariate analysis of sensitivity and specificity produces informative summary measures in diagnostic reviews. J Clin Epidemiol 2005;58:982–90.

48. Rutter CM, Gatsonis CA. A hierarchical regression approach to meta-analysis of diagnostic test accuracy evaluations. Stat Med 2001;20:2865–84.
49. Engels EA, Terrin N, Barza M, et al. Meta-analysis of diagnostic tests for acute sinusitis. J Clin Epidemiol 2000;53:852–62.
50. Olkin I, Sampson A. Comparison of meta-analysis versus analysis of variance of individual patient data. Biometrics 1998;54:317–22.
51. Steinberg KK, Smith SJ, Stroup DF, et al. Comparison of effect estimates from a meta-analysis of summary data from published studies and from a meta-analysis using individual patient data for ovarian cancer studies. Am J Epidemiol 1997;145: 917–25.
52. Arends LR. Multivariate meta-analysis: modelling the heterogeneity. Rotterdam: Erasmus University; 2006.
53. Riley RD, Abrams KR, Sutton AJ, et al. Bivariate random-effects meta-analysis and the estimation of between-study correlation. BMC Med Res Methodol 2007;7:3.
54. Trikalinos TA, Olkin I. A method for the meta-analysis of mutually exclusive binary outcomes. Stat Med 2008;27:4279–300.
55. Trikalinos TA, Salanti G, Zintzaras E, et al. Meta-analysis methods. Adv Genet 2008;60:311–34.
56. Moher D, Cook DJ, Eastwood S, et al. Improving the quality of reports of meta-analyses of randomised controlled trials: the QUOROM statement. Quality of Reporting of Meta-analyses. Lancet 1999;354:1896–900.
57. Stroup DF, Berlin JA, Morton SC, et al. Meta-analysis of observational studies in epidemiology: a proposal for reporting. Meta-analysis of Observational Studies in Epidemiology (MOOSE) group. JAMA 2000;283:2008–12.

Identifying Risk Factors for Infections: The Role of Meta-analyses

Evelina Tacconelli, MD, PhD*, Maria A. Cataldo, MD, PhD

KEYWORDS

• Meta-analysis • Risk factors • Infection • Longitudinal studies

RISK FACTORS FOR INFECTIONS: LIMITS OF ANALYSIS

Infections are a major cause of morbidity and mortality worldwide. Characterization of risk factors for infections allows prediction of the probability of developing infection among specific populations; this aids in understanding pathophysiologic mechanisms and is useful for defining prevention strategies. A variety of studies were performed to identify factors that predispose to microbiologic agent transmission and the development of disease.[1] Some risk factors, such as immunodeficiency status or presence of severe underlying diseases, old age, hospitalization, surgical procedures, use of invasive devices, and exposure to antimicrobial therapy, predispose to bacterial and viral infections whereas some factors are associated only with a specific infection. Any factor, such as intravascular devices, wounds, or large burns, that weakens the host defenses increases the likelihood of sepsis. Cigarette smoking, use of a nasogastric tube, mechanical ventilation, presence of tracheostomy, or reduced consciousness increases the risk for pneumonia. Urinary tract infections are more frequent among women, patients who have urinary catheters, and those who have abnormalities of the urinary tract. Presence of sinusitis or otitis, cerebrospinal fluid leak, and living in close quarters predispose to the occurrence of meningitis.[1]

The ability to detect meaningful statistical associations between infection and risk factors is dependent on the accuracy and reliability of variables definition. Some syndromes may be caused by more than one etiologic agent and, conversely, some agents may lead to a broad spectrum of infections. Statistical association may represent a true causal relationship or a confounding association with another risk factor. Biologic plausibility of the association also is demonstrated. To control for confounding and to determine whether or not any of the risk factors are associated independently with an infection, multivariate regression analysis usually is performed.[2]

Department of Infectious Diseases, UniversitÁ Cattolica Sacro Cuore, Largo F. Vito 8, 00168 Roma, Italy
* Corresponding author.
E-mail address: etacconelli@rm.unicatt.it (E. Tacconelli).

Infect Dis Clin N Am 23 (2009) 211–224
doi:10.1016/j.idc.2009.01.011
0891-5520/09/$ – see front matter © 2009 Elsevier Inc. All rights reserved.

id.theclinics.com

Randomized controlled trials (RCTs) are considered the gold standard of epidemiologic research. Analysis of infections' risk factors, however, generally cannot be tested in randomized experiments and relies mainly on nonexperimental observational studies. An exception might be considered the analysis of the efficacy of antibiotic prophylaxis of bacterial infections that usually are designed as a RCT. The majority of studies are cohort (retrospective or prospective), case control, cross sectional, or ecologic. For example, in an outbreak of *Salmonella enteritidis* that occurred in Minnesota, the results of a case-control study promptly identified the ice cream made by a national producer as the source of the infection.[3] A historical example of cohort study for defining risk factors for infections is represented by the cohort of homosexual men that helped to evaluate risk factors for transmission of HIV, hepatitis B virus, and hepatitis C virus (HCV).[4,5]

Although specific methodologic principles of case-control studies have been outlined in an effort to improve these types of study designs and their conclusions, case-control studies continue to have limitations: methodologic issues, including patient population under study; different definitions for selection of the control group; matching criteria; and grouping of antimicrobial classes.[6,7] In many cases, the magnitude of association, for example between antibiotic therapy and development of antibiotic-resistant infections, is still under evaluation. Risk factor studies of antibiotic-resistant bacteria usually try to control for the risk attributable to comorbidity using a numeric index. The index used most often is the Charlson comorbidity index, which generates a composite value of pre-existing medical conditions and was validated in a patient population with end-stage renal diseases.[8] The scoring system was never validated, however, in patients who had infections resulting from antibiotic-resistant bacteria. A new approach was proposed by McGregor and colleagues using new aggregate comorbidity measures based on the Chronic Disease Score for assessing the comorbidity attributable risk in patients who have infections caused by antibiotic-resistant bacteria, such as methicillin-resistant *Staphylococcus aureus* (MRSA) and vancomycin-resistant enterococci (VRE).[9] A major problem that affects the analysis of the relationship between risk factors and infections resulting from antibiotic-resistant bacteria is represented by the design of studies that mostly are retrospective case control. Other significant biases are related to the context where data are gathered (outbreaks or endemic situations) or to special patient populations (such as ICU patients). More important, the majority of studies did not differentiate between infection and colonization. Kaye and colleagues underlined that a major flaw in case-control studies analyzing risk factors for antibiotic-resistant infections is related to the selection of control groups not always selected independently of their exposure status.[10] The majority of published studies compared infections resulting from antibiotic-resistant bacteria to those caused by antibiotic-susceptible ones.[11,12] Controls must be selected, however, among patients who do not have infection by the target microorganism and should come from the source population.[4] A way to overcome this problem is a case-case control study where two groups of different cases (infected by antibiotic-resistant or antibiotic-susceptible bacteria) are compared with randomized patients who do not have the infection. This study design allows a comparison of two risk models.[7]

Of 47 studies published up to 2007 analyzing the impact of antibiotic therapy on the acquisition of MRSA infection or colonization, 22 (47%) were retrospective and 32 (68%) selected controls among patients who had infection resulting from methicillin-susceptible *S aureus* (MSSA).[13] Nine studies (19%) did not differentiate between infection and colonization. Definition of infection varied deeply among studies. Some of them focused on a specific infection (ie, bacteremia or skin infection or ventilator-associated pneumonia) whereas others included cases independent of the type of infections. Among 25 articles studying risk factors for infections resulting from extended-spectrum β-lactamases (ESBL)-producing *Escherichia coli* and *Klebsiella pneumoniae*, 22 were case-control studies (88%) and 7 (28%) did not differentiate between infection and colonization.[14]

Harris and colleagues[15] analyzed potential bias that might arise in studies of antimicrobial resistant organisms resulting from control group misclassification if control patients are required to have at least one clinical culture. Investigators performed two case-control studies. In the first group, control patients were randomly selected whereas in the second group they had to have at least one negative clinical culture. Statistical analysis showed that requiring control patients to have at least one clinical culture introduced a selection bias likely because it eliminated patients who had a less severe illness.

Other shortcomings of published studies for risk factors of infections is the definition of "time-at-risk period" for previous antibiotic exposure that ranged, in different studies, from a few days to 1 year.[13] Such a huge difference among studies analyzing the same risk factor (ie, antibiotic usage) introduces significant bias and heterogeneity.

Definition of risk factors also might vary among case-control and cohort studies. Prior antibiotic use may be defined as a categoric (eg, exposure or no exposure) or a continuous variable (eg, measured in days of exposure).[14] Identifying one individual antibiotic as the independent risk factor for emergence of resistance in patients receiving multiple antibiotics is difficult. In a systematic review on risk factors for infection with ESBL-producing *E coli* and *K pneumoniae*, investigators observed that methods used to describe prior antibiotic exposure significantly varied across studies.[14] Results from two multivariable models that used different methodologic approaches differed substantially. Specifically, use of third-generation cephalosporins was a risk factor for infection with ESBL-producing *E coli* and *K pneumoniae* when antibiotic use was described as a continuous variable but not when antibiotic use was described as a categoric variable. The use of different methods may alter the identified antimicrobial risk factors substantially, which has important implications for the resultant interventions regarding antimicrobial use.

In studies that investigated the association between risk factors and antibiotic-resistant infections, it often is assumed that the bacteria under investigation are resistant to a single antibiotic, when, in fact, a subset of these bacteria may be resistant to multiple antimicrobials.[16] The distinction between single drug versus multiple drug resistance is important to address because exposure to one antimicrobial may select for resistance to several unrelated antimicrobials among the multiple drug-resistant bacteria compared with the single drug–resistant bacteria. The assumption of single drug resistance among cases, therefore, may lead to erroneous conclusions about exposure to specific antibiotics. In a prospective study identifying risk factors for colonization with ceftazidime-resistant gram-negative bacilli, exposure to second- and third-generation cephalosporins and extended-spectrum penicillins were identified as independent risk factors.[17] It is likely that a subset of the ceftazidime-resistant gram-negative bacilli was co-resistant to extended-spectrum penicillins. The association between exposure to extended-spectrum penicillins and colonization with ceftazidime-resistant gram-negative bacilli may have differed if the selection of cases was restricted to gram-negative bacilli resistant only to ceftazidime.

Many studies have explored the risk factors associated with infection or colonization resulting from antimicrobial-resistant *Pseudomonas aeruginosa*.[18–25] The results of these studies differ substantially regarding the individual antimicrobials identified as independent risk factors. Because the selection pressure of one antimicrobial can lead to the selection for bacteria resistant not only to that antimicrobial but to other unrelated antimicrobials, through co- and cross-resistant mechanisms, the impact of individual antimicrobial exposure to the emergence of resistance cannot be assessed adequately without taking into consideration resistance to other antimicrobials. The authors sought to demonstrate that the identification of risk factors associated with antimicrobial-resistant pathogens requires analysis of the complete susceptibility profile of the pathogen under investigation.[26] The hypothesis was that because many single drug–resistant pathogens are resistant to other antimicrobials, an accurate assessment of the independent risk factors, in particular individual antimicrobial exposure, would require distinguishing between single drug and multiple drug resistance. Therefore, the authors compared the risk factors associated with harboring *P aeruginosa* isolates resistant only to ciprofloxacin to those associated with *P aeruginosa* isolates resistant to multiple antimicrobials. Substantial differences in the risk factors between the two groups were identified.

EXAMPLES OF META-ANALYSES OF RISK FACTORS FOR INFECTIONS

In recent years, systematic reviews and meta-analysis of observational studies increasingly have been used to address risk factors for infections (**Table 1**). Three major groups of interest might be defined: risk factors for HIV and HCV transmission; risk factors for bacterial infections; and risk factors for antibiotic-resistant infections.

Meta-analyses of Risk Factors for HIV and Hepatitis C Virus Transmission

HIV transmission and related risk factors have been studied extensively since the beginning of the epidemic. Such studies are important particularly for planning prevention campaigns in the community and to explore possible reasons for the rapid and largely unexplained growth of HIV in the general population in Eastern and Southern Africa. Among them, studies of HIV risk factors in sub-Saharan Africa presented evidence relevant to ongoing debates about the contributions of sexual transmission to the epidemic in Africa. Five meta-analysis reported on sexual risk factors for HIV infection.[27–31] Sex partners, history of paid sex, exposure to medical injections, and infection with herpes simplex virus type 2 (HSV-2) or other sexually transmitted infections each were showed significant in all reviews. The relevance of these meta-analyses was mainly for the definition of infection control measures to reduce HIV transmission, in particular among people who have high rates of partner change, such as female sex workers and their male clients. Even in high prevalence settings, prevention among people who have high rates of partner change is likely to reduce transmission overall. The principal limitations of these meta-analyses, however, are represented by the design of included studies as mostly cross sectional. This means that exposure and HIV status had been determined at the same time. The common route of transmission of HIV and HSV-2 might have had a confounding effect. Moreover, the choice of risk factors usually was limited. Heterogeneity of risk from each study and misclassification of exposure were present because they were self-reported. A meta-analysis by Baral and colleagues[27] showed that men who have sex with men (MSM) from low- and middle-income countries are in urgent need of prevention and care and seem understudied and underserved. The meta-analysis was able to show that significant differences in odd ratios (ORs) for HIV infection among MSM were seen when comparing low- and middle-income countries. Low-income countries had an OR of 7.8, whereas middle-income countries had an OR of 23.4. Stratifying the pooled ORs by whether or not a country had a substantial number of intravenous drug users (IDUs) resulted in an OR of 12.8 in countries where IDU transmission was prevalent and 24.4 where it was not. The investigators concluded that MSM have a markedly greater risk for being infected with HIV compared with general population samples from low- and middle-income countries in the Americas, Asia, and Africa. The majority of the studies, however, used convenience samples and were cross sectional, so may not be representative of MSM. There also was a lack of controls because the Joint United Nations Program on HIV/AIDS general population prevalence estimates for each country were used as the unexposed population. Finally, a portion of the difference in ORs seen between strata may be explained by a ceiling effect.

Another relevant meta-analysis for policy makers working on HIV transmission showed a significant association between oral contraceptive use and HIV-1 seroprevalence or seroincidence, suggesting that for women at risk for HIV-1 infection, oral contraceptive use for prevention of pregnancy should be accompanied by condom use for prevention of HIV-1 infection.[32]

Discordant results were observed from three meta-analyses reporting on circumcision as a risk factor for sexually transmitted diseases (STDs) and HIV transmission.[33–35] Van Howe[33] in 1999 observed that circumcision did not have any impact on HIV transmission. A few years later Weiss and colleagues,[34,35] through two different meta-analyses, proved that circumcised men are at lower risk for chancroid and syphilis with less association with HSV-2. A possible explanation of different results might be related to the significant heterogeneity between studies on syphilis and to misclassification bias. Design of included studies (mostly cross-sectional and case-control) did not allow determining the temporal sequence of circumcision and infection. This would tend to underestimate any protective effect of male circumcision.

Epidemiology of HCV transmission also represents an important topic for meta-analyses. A recent meta-analysis of Xia and colleagues[36] demonstrated that, in China, there was no significant difference in the risk for HCV infection among needle-sharing IDUs and non–needle-sharing IDUs. A longer duration of IDU was associated with increased HCV prevalence. High-risk sexual practices were strongly associated with drug injection behaviors. Co-infection with HIV greatly increased the probability of HCV infection among IDUs, whereas the probability of hepatitis B virus infection remained similar for HCV-positive and HCV-negative IDUs.

Meta-analyses of Risk Factors for Bacterial Infections

Risk factors for bacterial infections have been analyzed extensively because of the high morbidity and mortality associated with these infections.[15] Li and colleagues[37] demonstrated, in 13 studies, that the child of a parent who smokes has approximately twice the risk of a parent who does not smoke for having a serious respiratory tract infection requiring hospitalization in early life. This association was pronounced in children younger than age 2 and diminished after age 2. The investigators stressed the need for new public health campaigns to discourage smoking in the presence of young children. Of particular interest are meta-analyses of risk factors for bacterial infections in immunocompromised patients. Vamvakas[38] demonstrated that allogeneic blood transfusion increases the risk for postoperative bacterial infection. Their results provided overwhelming evidence that allogeneic blood transfusion was associated with a significantly increased risk for postoperative bacterial infection in surgical patients.

Two systematic reviews of the literature were performed to identify risk factors associated with *Clostridium difficile* infection.[39,40] In a meta-analysis by Bignardi, two main outcomes were considered: *C difficile* diarrhea and *C difficile* carriage. A qualitative assessment, based on a set of defined and consistently applied criteria,

Table 1
Examples of meta-analyses on risk factors for infections

First Author, Year of Publication [ref.]	Risk Factor(s)/ Infection (Setting)	Included Studies, n	Study Design	Main Results	Major Limits
Safdar 2008[42]	MRSA colonization/ MRSA infection	10	Clinical trial, case-control, cohort	MRSA colonization increases the risk for MRSA infection	Significant between studies heterogeneity; differences in severity of illness, frequency of sampling to detect colonization, choice of patients population
Tacconelli 2008[13]	Antimicrobial therapy/ MRSA acquisition	76	Case-control, cohort, cross-sectional	Antimicrobial exposure increases the risk for MRSA acquisition	Significant between studies heterogeneity; case definition bias; control selection bias
Baral 2007[27]	MSM/HIV infection (low- and middle-income countries)	83	Convenience samples, cross-sectional	MSM have a greater risk for being infected with HIV	Study design; control selection bias
Chen 2007[28]	Sexual behaviors/HIV infection (Africa)	68	Cross-sectional, case-control, longitudinal	Number of partners, paid sex, HSV-2 infection increase the risk for HIV transmission	Significant heterogeneity of risks; misclassification of exposures; limited choice of risk factors
Weiss 2006[34]	Male circumcision/genital herpes, syphilis, and chancroid	26	Cross-sectional, case-control, cohort	Circumcision decreases the risk for chancroid and syphilis; less association with genital herpes	Significant heterogeneity between studies; misclassification of serologic status and of circumcision status

Vamvakas 2002[38]	Allogeneic and autologous blood transfusion/ postoperative infections	5	RCTs	No difference in risk for infection	Case definition bias
Thomas 2003[40]	Antimicrobial therapy/ C difficile acquisition	48	Cross-sectional, case-control, cohort	Antibiotic exposure increases the risk for C difficile acquisition	Control group selection bias; lack of precision in the effect estimates
Bignardi 1998[39]	Risk factors/ C difficile acquisition	30	Clinical trial, case-control, cohort	Increasing age, underlying diseases, nonsurgical gastrointestinal procedures, nasogastric tube, antiulcer medications, stay on ICU, duration of hospital stay and antibiotic course, administration of multiple antibiotics increases the risk for C difficile acquisition	Control group selection bias; study design; inadequate sample size; inadequate control of confounders; diagnostic bias
Carmeli 1999[43]	Vancomycin use/VRE acquisition	20	Case-control	Vancomycin use increases the risk for VRE acquisition	Significant between studies heterogeneity; control group selection bias

seemed the best approach for risk factors other than antibiotic use, as an approach based on meta-analysis would have used only the information provided by a minority of the studies. Risk factors for which there was evidence suggestive or consistent with an association with *C difficile* diarrhea were increasing age, severity of underlying diseases, nonsurgical gastrointestinal procedures, presence of a nasogastric tube, antiulcer medications, stay on ICU, duration of hospital stay and of antibiotic course, and administration of multiple antibiotics. Exposure to an antibiotic was shown to be statistically significantly associated with *C difficile* diarrhea and *C difficile* carriage. The meta-analysis approach enabled the ranking of individual antibiotics in relation to the risk for *C difficile* infection, although the 95% CIs often were wide and overlapping. Major limits of this meta-analysis were use of incorrect control groups, study design, inadequate sample sizes, and inadequate control of confounders in the included studies. Diagnostic bias also might be present in studies that identified cases through the clinical management of patients.[39] A few years later, in their meta-analysis, Thomas and colleagues[40] confirmed that although the majority of studies of *C difficile* found an association with various antibiotics, antibiotic classes, or components of antibiotic administration, most were limited in their ability to establish a causal relationship by the use of incorrect control groups, the presence of bias, inadequate control of confounding, and small sample sizes. The limitations identified in their review prevented the pooling of results in a meta-analysis.

An interesting approach to studying risk factors for infections was used by Lin and colleagues,[41] documenting the effects of smoking and solid-fuel use on tuberculosis in China. The investigators used a time-based, multiple risk factor, modelling study. They modeled future tuberculosis incidence, taking into account the accumulation of hazardous effects of risk factors on chronic obstructive pulmonary disease and lung cancer over time and dependency of the risk for tuberculosis infection on the prevalence of disease. The investigators demonstrated that complete cessation of smoking and solid-fuel use by 2033 would reduce projected annual tuberculosis incidence in 2033 by 14% to 52% if 80% directly observed therapies coverage is sustained.

Meta-analyses of Risk Factors for Antibiotic-Resistant Infections

Published evidence suggests that previous colonization is a prerequisite for subsequent infection for many bacteria, such as MRSA and VRE. Studies have found that colonization with MRSA poses a greater risk for clinical infection than colonization with MSSA. A systematic review by Safdar and Bradley[42] provided an overall estimate of the risk for infection after colonization with MRSA compared with colonization by MSSA. Ten observational studies, with a total of 1170 patients, were identified that provided data on MSSA and MRSA colonization and infection. Investigators demonstrated that colonization by MRSA was associated with a fourfold increase in risk for infection. Main limits were that studies differed particularly in the choice of patient population, severity of illness, and frequency of sampling to detect colonization. The authors' group performed a meta-analysis on the association between antibiotic therapy and the development of MRSA colonization or infection, including 67 studies for a total of 24,230 patients. Antibiotic exposure was determined in the 126 ± 184 (mean $\pm$ SD) days preceding MRSA isolation. The risk for acquiring MRSA was increased by 1.8-fold in patients who had taken antibiotics.[13] Carmeli and colleagues[43] studied the association between antecedent vancomycin treatment and hospital-acquired VRE. A total of 20 studies described in 15 published reports was included in the analysis. When results from all 20 studies were combined, the pooled OR was 4.5 but the test for heterogeneity was highly significant. The five studies that used patients who had vancomycin-susceptible enterococci as controls found a stronger association than the 15 studies that used controls who had no VRE isolated. After restricting the analysis to the latter studies only, no heterogeneity was evident in the unadjusted study results. Patients who had VRE had stayed in the hospital much longer than control patients. Studies that adjusted for this difference found only a small and nonsignificant association between vancomycin treatment and VRE (pooled OR 1.4; 95% CI, 0.74–2.60). Investigators also detected publication bias, favoring report of studies that found a large measure of association. They reported strong association between vancomycin treatment and hospital-acquired VRE results from the selection of the reference group, confounding by duration of hospitalization, and publication bias.

IS META-ANALYSIS OF RISK FACTORS FOR BACTERIAL INFECTIONS JUSTIFIED?

The limitations of meta-analysis of RCTs have been discussed extensively.[44] Some of the criticisms include publication and citations bias, misclassification bias, selection and inclusion bias, and combination of heterogeneous data. Bias in location of studies interest RCT and observational studies.[45] Meta-analyses published in English language received more attention. Egger and colleagues[46] examined this issue for literature published in German. Their findings showed that for publications of RCTs from German-speaking Europe, an English language bias exists and that ignoring trials published in German is problematic. The same situation is likely in relation to other languages, in particular European languages. Strikingly different results in meta-analysis can be obtained depending on which studies are selected. Meta-analysis reduces random error but does not necessarily reduce systematic error and may even increase it. Meta-analysis involves the same issues as in a report on a single study, and quantitative and narrative elements are required. An advantage of meta-analyses is that possible biases can be addressed using actual data rather than hypothetical examples. Therefore, it is evident that meta-analysis of observational studies poses additional challenges compared with meta-analysis of RCTs. Results of observational studies should be presented with a description of the unit, and OR risk or hazard ratio should be given with CIs. Analysis of the quality of studies should be performed. Cohort studies should be analyzed with particular regard toward selection of cohorts and comparability of the same. Assessment of the definition of infection should be clear.

Results of these meta-analyses can be difficult to interpret because of the many limits related to longitudinal studies. Without randomization, study quality usually is lower. Heterogeneity is common and might be related to exposure (nature, level, and measure), populations studied, outcomes measured, and lack of control of confounding factors.

Confounding

Confounding factors are factors that are associated with the outcome of interest and the exposure of interest (such as length of hospitalization and nosocomial infections). Carmeli and colleagues,[43] in their meta-analysis on association between antibiotic exposure and VRE, showed that only studies not accounting for confounders (length of hospitalization) showed an association between VRE and previous antibiotic therapy. Even after the adjustment for confounding factors, however, residual confounding remains a potentially serious problem. In observational studies that seek information on infection risk factors, the use of the overall risk ratio may be contentious. The evidence available from observational studies on the causal relation between a risk factor and infection can be interpreted only if there is enough information about confounding and measurement bias. That is the reason why summary estimates from the meta-analysis of observational studies should be considered cautiously. Moreover, when looking at risk factors for infections, controlling for confounders might not be as straightforward. For sexually transmitted infections, for example, adjustment for potential confounding factors might not be possible, given the various causal pathways. Wald and Link[31] reviewed the contribution of HSV-2 infection to the risk for HIV acquisition. Nine cohort and nested case-control studies documented that HSV-2 infection before HIV acquisition was associated with a risk estimate of 2.1 (95% CI, 1.4–3.2); for 22 case-control and cross-sectional studies, the risk estimate was 3.9 (95% CI, 3.1–5.1). Investigators concluded that control strategies for HSV-2 need to be incorporated into control of STDs to prevent HIV transmission. Because HIV and HSV-2 infections are STDs, however, concerns about confounding of the effect of HSV-2 on HIV acquisition by sexual behaviors should be taken into account. The studies that indicate the increased risk for HSV-2 in HIV-infected persons underscores the potential for confounding by sexual behaviors in cross-sectional surveys.

Heterogeneity

The investigation of heterogeneity between studies is a main task in each meta-analysis and is present in observational studies. Presence of heterogeneity of risks from single studies reduces the confidence in the validity of summary estimate for the risks. Heterogeneity should be analyzed with appropriate tests and graphically visualized using plots with single studies grouped according to specific covariates.[47] An important method to investigate heterogeneity is sensitivity analysis (eg, calculating a pooled estimate only for subgroups of studies to investigate variations of the OR). In a meta-analysis on the role of previous antibiotic therapy in the development of MRSA colonization or infection, the authors explored potential sources of heterogeneity through subgroup and sensitivity analysis. The subgroup analysis was performed through metaregression that tests whether or not trial attributes are associated with the study results. Subgroup analysis was performed stratifying for sampling frame for inclusion, definition of case subjects and controls, study design, geographic area of the study, presence of adjustment of covariates, and length of antibiotic exposure period.[13] The forest plots stratified for community and nosocomial/health care–associated MRSA isolation showed a significant disadvantage of patients previously treated with antibiotic therapy. The risk was higher among community-acquired versus nosocomial/health care–associated cases and among infected patients versus colonized ones. Heterogeneity was reduced among prevalence surveys. Using regression analysis the presence of heterogeneity was associated with the length of potential exposure period (more or less than 180 days) for antibiotics.

Misclassification Bias

In meta-analyses analyzing risk factors for infections, misclassification bias might be common. In their meta-analysis, Safdar and Bradley[42] observed that there were differences among studies regarding the frequency of sampling to detect MRSA colonization. It is possible that differential frequency of sampling may have resulted in detection of more patients with colonization in one group than the other. This differential misclassification of exposure would be expected to have an impact on results. Chen and colleagues, in their meta-analysis on sexual risk factors for HIV infection in sub-Saharan Africa, used self-report of exposure to sex partner, paid sex, and STD introducing a significant misclassification bias.[28]

Analysis of Quality

Assessment of quality of observational studies is more difficult than for RCTs and other experimental studies. Quality assessment methods for observational studies have not been well worked out and, although several scales have been elaborated, none of them have been fully validated. The Newcastle-Ottawa Scale has been developed to assess the quality of nonrandomized studies in meta-analysis and has been partly validated.[48] This scale is recommended by the Cochrane Non-Randomized Studies Methods Working Group. A star system has been developed in which a study is judged on three broad perspectives. For cohort studies, the scale takes into account selection of cohorts (representativeness of the exposed cohort, selection of the nonexposed cohort, ascertainment of exposure, and demonstration that outcome of interest was not present at start of study), comparability of cohorts (on the basis of the design or analysis), and outcome (assessment of outcome and adequacy of follow up of cohorts). For case-control studies, the scale looks at selection of case and controls (adequacy of case definition, representativeness of the cases, selection of controls, definition of controls), comparability of cases and controls (on the basis of the design or analysis), and exposure (ascertainment of exposure and non-response rate). Thomas and colleagues,[40] in their systematic review on antibiotic and *C difficile* diarrhea, analyzed study quality. Among 45 studies (23 case-control and 22 cross-sectional), only 33 studies were judged to have used appropriate control groups.

Publication Bias

Publication bias always is a concern in meta-analysis. Research projects with statistically significant results are more likely to be published than works with nonsignificant results. In a retrospective survey, 487 research projects approved by the Central Oxford Research Ethics Committee between 1984 and 1987 were studied for evidence of publication bias.[49] Studies with statistically significant results were more likely to be published than those finding no difference between the study groups. The impact of publication bias was greater with observational and laboratory-based experimental studies than with RCTs. Publication bias might be responsible of an overestimate of risk-factor associations in published work and may compromise the validity of meta-analyses, which often include only published data. Thus, a prerequisite in the analysis and interpretation of results of systematic review is to take into account publication bias.

SUMMARY

Systematic review and meta-analysis are assuming greater importance in influencing policy makers and clinical opinion worldwide. Many discussions and publications have considered the merits of meta-analysis of epidemiologic data.[50] Some observers suggest that meta-analysis of observational studies should be abandoned altogether.[51] In the authors' opinion, statistical combination of observational studies should not be a primary goal of a review. Analysis of heterogeneity between longitudinal studies, however, would provide more insights than mathematical calculation of the summary risk. Meta-analyses of risk factors for infections should strictly follow guidelines for meta-analyses of observational studies. A study protocol should be written in advance, completed literature searches performed, and studies selected in a reproducible and objective fashion. Biologic plausibility must be addressed. The reported findings should be interpreted with caution, taking into account the limitations of various methodologic aspects of risk factors studies. An important role for meta-analyses in this field would be to clarify hypotheses to be formulated for future studies and stress limitations strictly related to studies on risk factors for bacterial and viral infections.

REFERENCES

1. Mandell GL, Bennett JE, Dolin R. Principles and practice of infectious diseases. 6th edition. New York: Churchill Livingstone; 2005.
2. Study design and conduct. In: Rothman KJ, Greenland S, editors. Modern epidemiology. Philadelphia: Lippincott–Raven; 1998. p. 67–180.
3. Hennessy TW, Hedberg CW, Slutsker L, et al. A national outbreak of Salmonella enteritidis infections from ice cream. The Investigation Team. N Engl J Med 1996;334(20):1281–6.
4. Osmond DH, Charlebois E, Sheppard HW, et al. Comparison of risk factors for hepatitis C and hepatitis B virus infection in homosexual men. J Infect Dis 1993;167(1):66–71.
5. Moss AR, Osmond D, Bacchetti P, et al. Risk factors for AIDS and HIV seropositivity in homosexual men. Am J Epidemiol 1987;125(6):1035–47.
6. Harris AD, Karchmer TB, Carmeli Y, et al. Methodological principles of case-control studies that analysed risk factors for antibiotic resistance: a systematic review. Clin Infect Dis 2001;32:1055–61.
7. Harris AD, Samore MH, Lipsitch M, et al. Control-group selection importance in studies of antimicrobial resistance: examples applied to Pseudomonas aeruginosa, Enterococci, and Escherichia coli. Clin Infect Dis 2002;34:1558–63.
8. Charlson ME, Pompei P, Ales KL, et al. A new method of classifying prognostic comorbidity in longitudinal studies: development and validation. J Chronic Dis 1987;40(5):373–83.
9. McGregor JC, Perencevich EN, Furuno JP, et al. Comorbidity risk-adjustment measures were developed and validated for studies of antibiotic-resistant infections. J Clin Epidemiol 2006;59(12):1266–73.
10. Kaye KS, Harris AD, Samore M, et al. The case-case-control study design: addressing the limitations of risk factor studies for antimicrobial resistance. Infect Control Hosp Epidemiol 2005;26(4):346–51.
11. Lee SO, Kim NJ, Choi SH, et al. Risk factors for acquisition of imipenem-resistant Acinetobacter baumannii: a case-control study. Antimicrob Agents Chemother 2004;48(1):224–8.
12. Manzur A, Vidal M, Pujol M, et al. Predictive factors of meticillin resistance among patients with Staphylococcus aureus bloodstream infections at hospital admission. J Hosp Infect 2007;66(2):135–41.
13. Tacconelli E, De Angelis G, Cataldo MA, et al. Does antibiotic exposure increase the risk of methicillin-resistant Staphylococcus aureus (MRSA) isolation? A systematic review and meta-analysis. J Antimicrob Chemother 2008;61(1):26–38.
14. Hyle EP, Bilker WB, Gasink LB, et al. Impact of different methods for describing the extent of prior antibiotic exposure on the association between antibiotic use and antibiotic-resistant infection. Infect Control Hosp Epidemiol 2007;28(6):647–54.
15. Harris AD, Carmeli Y, Samore MH, et al. Impact of severity of illness bias and control group misclassification bias in case-control studies of antimicrobial-resistant organisms. Infect Control Hosp Epidemiol 2005;26:342–5.
16. D'Agata EMC. Rapidly rising prevalence of nosocomial multidrug-resistant gram-negative bacilli: a 9-year surveillance study. Infect Control Hosp Epidemiol 2004;25:842–6.

17. D'Agata E, Venkataraman L, DeGirolami P, et al. The molecular epidemiology of acquisition of ceftazidime-resistant gram-negative strains in a non-outbreak setting. J Clin Microbiol 1997;35:2602–5.
18. Trouillet JL, Vuagnat A, Combes A, et al. Pseudomonas aeruginosa ventilator-associated pneumonia: comparison of episodes due to piperacillin-resistant versus piperacillin-susceptible organisms. Clin Infect Dis 2002;34:1047–54.
19. Muder RR, Brennen C, Drenning SD, et al. Multiply antibiotic-resistant gram-negative bacilli in a long-term care facility: a case-control study of patient risk factors and prior antibiotic use. Infect Control Hosp Epidemiol 1997;18:809–13.
20. Paramythiotou E, Lucet J, Timsit J, et al. Acquisition of multidrug-resistant Pseudomonas aeruginosa in patients in intensive care units: role of antibiotics with antipseudomonal activity. Clin Infect Dis 2004;38:670–7.
21. Defez C, Fabbro-Peray P, Bouziges N, et al. Risk factors for multidrug-resistant Pseudomonas aeruginosa nosocomial infection. J Hosp Infect 2004;57:209–16.
22. Cao B, Wang H, Sun H, et al. Risk factors and clinical outcomes of nosocomial multidrug resistant Pseudomonas aeruginosa infections. J Hosp Infect 2004;57:112–8.
23. Harris AD, Perencevich E, Roghmann MC, et al. Risk factors for piperacillin-tazobactam-resistant Pseudomonas aeruginosa among hospitalized patients. Antimicrob Agents Chemother 2002;46:854–8.
24. Harris AD, Smith D, Johnson JA, et al. Risk factors for imipenem-resistant Pseudomonas aeruginosa among hospitalized patients. Clin Infect Dis 2002;34:340–5.
25. Tacconelli E, Tumbarello M, Bertagnolio S, et al. Multidrug-resistant Pseudomonas aeruginosa bloodstream infections: analysis of trends in prevalence and epidemiology. Emerg Infect Dis 2002;8:220–1.
26. D'Agata EM, Cataldo MA, Cauda R, et al. The importance of addressing multidrug resistance and not assuming single-drug resistance in case-control studies. Infect Control Hosp Epidemiol 2006;27(7):670–4.
27. Baral S, Sifakis F, Cleghorn F, et al. Elevated risk for HIV infection among men who have sex with men in low- and middle-income countries 2000–2006: a systematic review. PLoS Med 2007;4(12):e339.
28. Chen L, Jha P, Stirling B, et al. Sexual risk factors for HIV infection in early and advanced HIV epidemics in sub-Saharan Africa: systematic overview of 68 epidemiological studies. PLoS ONE 2007;2(10):e1001.
29. Freeman EE, Weiss HA, Glynn JR, et al. Herpes simplex virus 2 infection increases HIV acquisition in men and women: systematic review and meta-analysis of longitudinal studies. AIDS 2006;20(1):73–83.
30. Gisselquist D, Potterat JJ. Review of evidence from risk factor analyses associating HIV infection in African adults with medical injections and multiple sexual partners. Int J STD AIDS 2004;15(4):222–33.
31. Wald A, Link K. Risk of human immunodeficiency virus infection in herpes simplex virus type 2-seropositive persons: a meta-analysis. J Infect Dis 2002;185(1):45–52.
32. Wang CC, Reilly M, Kreiss JK. Risk of HIV infection in oral contraceptive pill users: a meta-analysis. J Acquir Immune Defic Syndr 1999;21(1):51–8.
33. Van Howe RS. Circumcision and HIV infection: review of the literature and meta-analysis. Int J STD AIDS 1999;10(1):8–16.
34. Weiss HA, Thomas SL, Munabi SK, et al. Male circumcision and risk of syphilis, chancroid, and genital herpes: a systematic review and meta-analysis. Sex Transm Infect 2006;82(2):101–10.
35. Weiss HA, Quigley MA, Hayes RJ. Male circumcision and risk of HIV infection in sub-Saharan Africa: a systematic review and meta-analysis. AIDS 2000;14(15):2361–70.

36. Xia X, Luo J, Bai J, et al. Epidemiology of hepatitis C virus infection among injection drug users in China: systematic review and meta-analysis. Public Health 2008;122(10):990–1003.
37. Li JS, Peat JK, Xuan W, et al. Meta-analysis on the association between environmental tobacco smoke (ETS) exposure and the prevalence of lower respiratory tract infection in early childhood. Pediatr Pulmonol 1999;27(1):5–13.
38. Vamvakas EC. Meta-analysis of randomized controlled trials comparing the risk of postoperative infection between recipients of allogeneic and autologous blood transfusion. Vox Sang 2002;83(4):339–46.
39. Bignardi GE. Risk factors for Clostridium difficile infection. J Hosp Infect 1998; 40(1):1–15.
40. Thomas C, Stevenson M, Riley TV. Antibiotics and hospital-acquired Clostridium difficile-associated diarrhoea: a systematic review. J Antimicrob Chemother 2003;51(6):1339–50.
41. Lin HH, Murray M, Cohen T, et al. Effects of smoking and solid-fuel use on COPD, lung cancer, and tuberculosis in China: a time-based, multiple risk factor, modelling study. Lancet 2008;372(9648):1473–83.
42. Safdar N, Bradley EA. The risk of infection after nasal colonization with Staphylococcus aureus. Am J Med 2008;121(4):310–5.
43. Carmeli Y, Samore MH, Huskins C. The association between antecedent vancomycin treatment and hospital-acquired vancomycin-resistant enterococci: a meta-analysis. Arch Intern Med 1999;159(20):2461–8.
44. Egger M, Smith GD. Meta-analysis. Potentials and promise. BMJ 1997;315(7119): 1371–4.
45. Egger M, Smith GD. Bias in location and selection of studies. BMJ 1998; 316(7124):61–6.
46. Egger M, Zellweger-Zähner T, Schneider M, et al. Language bias in randomised controlled trials published in English and German. Lancet 1997;350(9074):326–9.
47. Egger M, Davey Smith G, Schneider M, et al. Bias in meta-analysis detected by a simple, graphical test. BMJ 1997;315(7109):629–34.
48. Wells GA, Shea B, O'Connell D, et al. The Newcastle-Ottawa Scale (NOS) for assessing the quality of nonrandomized studies in meta-analyses. Department of Epidemiology and Community Medicine, University of Ottawa, Canada. Available at: http://ohri.ca/programs/clinical_epidemiology/oxford.htm. Accessed February 28, 2009.
49. Easterbrook PJ, Berlin JA, Gopalan R, et al. Publication bias in clinical research. Lancet 1991;337(8746):867–72.
50. Einarson TR, Leeder JS, Koren G. A method for meta-analysis of epidemiological studies. Drug Intell Clin Pharm 1988;22(10):813–24.
51. Shapiro S. Meta-analysis/Shmeta-analysis. Am J Epidemiol 1994;140:771–8.

An Overview of Meta-analyses of Diagnostic Tests in Infectious Diseases

Mario Cruciani, MD[a,b,c,*], Carlo Mengoli, MD[d]

KEYWORDS

- Review • Meta-analyses • Diagnostic test
- Infectious diseases • Tuberculosis

Meta-analytic techniques for combining diagnostic studies in order to improve estimation of test accuracy are being developed and improved.[1–8] Systematic reviews of diagnostic studies involve additional challenges to those of intervention research.

Studies are observational in nature and prone to various biases. In addition, there is more variation between studies in methods, manufacturers, procedures, and outcome measurement scales used to assess test accuracy than in randomized controlled trials, which generally causes marked heterogeneity in results. The use of statistical methods to combine test accuracy studies is particularly challenging, not the least because test accuracy is conventionally represented by a pair of statistics (most often sensitivity and specificity) and not by a single effect measure, such as odds ratio or relative risk.

Previous research on systematic reviews of diagnostic tests noted poor methods and reporting. Irwig and colleagues[9] reviewed 11 meta-analyses published from 1990 to 1991 and drew up guidelines to address key areas where reviews were deficient. Schmid and colleagues[10] reported preliminary results on methods used for searching strategies and meta-analyses in 189 systematic reviews, and Whiting and colleagues[11] reported on the extent of quality assessment within diagnostic reviews. Mallett and colleagues[12] evaluated systematic reviews of diagnostic tests in cancer, with an emphasis on methods and reporting. Dinnes and colleagues[13] evaluated how heterogeneity had been examined in systematic reviews of diagnostic test accuracy.

[a] Center of Preventive Medicine & HIV Outpatient Clinic, V. Germania 20, 37135 Verona, Italy
[b] Consultant in Infectious Diseases, G. Fracastoro Hospital, San Bonifacio, Verona, Italy
[c] Infectious Diseases Specialty School, University of Padua, Italy
[d] Department of Histology, Microbiology and Medical Biotechnology, University of Padua, via Gabelli 63, 35100 Padua, Italy
* Corresponding author. Center of Preventive Medicine & HIV Outpatient Clinic, V. Germania 20, 37135 Verona, Italy.
E-mail address: crucianimario@virgilio.it (M. Cruciani).

Infect Dis Clin N Am 23 (2009) 225–267
doi:10.1016/j.idc.2009.01.010
0891-5520/09/$ – see front matter © 2009 Elsevier Inc. All rights reserved.

id.theclinics.com

Literature evaluating systematic reviews on accuracy of diagnostic tests, including those in the field of infectious diseases, is growing year after year, and these studies can be difficult and time consuming to identify and appraise. This overview was designed to summarize the main findings of systematic reviews of diagnostic tests in patients who have infectious diseases, appraising their quality and highlighting their relative strengths and weaknesses.

MATERIAL AND METHODS

Criteria for Considering Studies Included in this Overview

The authors searched the following electronic databases to find reports of relevant meta-analyses published between inception and September 2008: MEDLINE, EMBASE, and Database of Abstracts of Reviews of Effectiveness (DARE). Electronic searching was done independently by one of the authors. For the search, language restriction was not applied. The following search terms were used: diagnostic test(s)/diagnostic studies AND meta-analyses; diagnostic test(s)/diagnostic studies AND infectious diseases; and infectious diseases AND meta-analyses. Titles and abstracts of references identified by the search for potential relevance were screened. Complete copies were obtained of the publications judged potentially relevant for the review.

Reviews were included if they assessed a diagnostic test for presence or absence of an infection or for detecting the presence of an infectious agent; reported accuracy of the test assessed by comparison to concurrent reference tests; assessed whether or not there was an attempt to combine data from primary studies in a quantitative way; and listed references for included studies. Reviews addressing test development and diagnostic effectiveness or cost effectiveness were excluded.

Validity Assessment

The authors assessed the quality of each identified review according to Mallett and colleagues[12] The assessment produced is based on previous publications related to studies of diagnostic tests and on guidelines for meta-analyses evaluating diagnostic test.[4,6–9,11] The review evaluated methods and reporting of systematic reviews of diagnostic tests for cancer across nine domains: (1) review objectives and search strategy, (2) participants and clinical setting, (3) index test, (4) reference test, (5) study design, (6) study results, (7) graphs and meta-analyses, (8) quality and bias, and (9) procedures used in the review. For evaluation, the authors used the same framework, with few modifications. The authors introduced three items to evaluate heterogeneity in the reported meta-analyses.

The authors evaluated items examining questions at review, study, and individual test level. Results evaluated the methods and reporting of the review. Primary diagnostic studies often are poorly reported and, therefore, when meta-analyses reported information as sought but not found in the included studies, this information was counted as reported.

RESULTS

The search generated 503 references of possible relevance to this review, of which 432 were excluded on the basis of title or abstract. Seventy-one potentially eligible meta-analyses were assessed further, and 55 of those studies were included in the review.[14–68] There were 54 reviews in English and one in Spanish.[49] Sixteen articles were excluded from the assessment for various reasons, including two written in Korean for which a translation was not available,[69,70] three duplicates of previous publications,[71-73] five reviews,[74-78] two articles reporting guidelines,[79,80] one prevalence study,[81] two studies reporting sensitivity data only,[82,83] and a survey for diagnostic laboratories.[84] The mean number of primary studies included in the review was 29 ± 20 (median 23, range 5–96); overall, the 55 meta-analyses reported data from 1596 primary studies. The number of manuscripts published in the medical literature increased over the years. Two articles were published in 1992, four in 1996, two in 1997, two in 1998, one in 1999, five in 2000, two in 2001, two in 2002, two in 2003, four in 2004, six in 2005, nine in 2006, eleven in 2007, and three in 2008.

Table 1 shows the findings across the nine assessment domains. Items are classified according to whether or not they relate to the review, to a single test within the review, or to a single study within the review.

Objectives, Inclusion Criteria, and Search

A systematic review of diagnostic accuracy begins by defining the clinical context and developing a precise description of the diagnostic question for which test accuracy is to be assessed. This part of the process is similar to the development of the protocol for a primary study. It includes specification of the clinical question determining potential use of the test under investigation, technical characteristics of the tests, conditions under which the tests are interpreted, and reference information used in the assessment of test accuracy.[85]

In all 55 of the selected reviews the primary purpose was to assess test accuracy; few did so as part of a clinical guideline or as a general overview of diagnostic tests and none had economic evaluation as objective (see Table 1). Sixty-seven percent of the 55 reviews stated inclusion criteria. An electronic search was reported in all but one of the reviews. Literature retrieval methods were described in 54 of the 55 meta-analyses, and 52 used MEDLINE searching. Sixty percent (33/55) of the reviews searched two or more electronic databases; EMBASE was searched in 28 (50%) reviews; and 45 articles (81.8%) gave their search terms.

Description of Target Condition, Patients, and Clinical Setting

The reviews covered different types of diagnostic tests and infections. Types of diagnostic tests varied, but in the large majority they were laboratory tests and to a lesser extent imaging tests, pathology/cytology tests, and clinical examinations. There were 25 meta-analyses investigating diagnostic tests for bacterial infections,[14-38] four for fungal infections (including *Pneumocystis carinii*),[39-42] six for viral infections,[43-48] six for protozoan infections,[49-54] and 14 investigating diagnostic tests applied to different clinical syndromes and conditions,[55-68] including osteomyelitis,[55,67,68] meningitis,[58] acute sinusitis,[60,61] catheter-related blood stream infection and bacteremia,[57,63-66] urinary tract infections,[59,62] and diarrhea.[56] One third of the articles evaluated tests for the diagnosis of tuberculosis.[21-38] Some of these studies reported the yield of diagnostic tests in patients who had specific clinical conditions, including pulmonary tuberculosis,[21,34] extrapulmonary tuberculosis (peritonitis, pleuritis, pericarditis, meningitis, and lymphadenitis),[22,24,29,32,33,35,37] and latent infection.[36,38] Other studies investigated the diagnostic yield for the detection of *Mycobacterium tuberculosis* in clinical specimens,[23,25,28,30,31] or for the detection of resistance to antiimycobacterial agents.[26,27]

Clinical relevance and reliability require reporting of information on the target condition, patients, and clinical setting.[86] The clinical setting was stated clearly in 38 of 55 (69.1%) of the evaluated reviews. Details of patient characteristics for individual studies were extracted in 18 studies (32%), but they were reported in only 14 (25.5%) of the reviews. Less than half of the reviews reported country where the

Table 1
Assessment of reviews of diagnostic test accuracy in infectious diseases according to objectives and search, participants and clinical setting, study design, index test, reference test, graphic display of data, study results, quality evaluation, and methods of meta-analyses

Assessments Items	No. of Reviews	%
1. Objectives and search	55	100
Objective:		
• To review accuracy of diagnostic test	55	100
Other objectives:		
• Clinical guidelines	3	5.5
• General overview of disease	2	3.6
• Health economic study	0	0
Inclusion criteria of review stated[a]	37	67.3
Table of study characteristics included[a]	48	87.3
Search		
• Electronic search	54	98.1
• Use of MEDLINE	52	94.5
• ≥ 2 database	33	60
• Search terms specified	45	81.8
2. Participants and clinical setting		
Clinical setting stated[a]	38	69.1
Details of pts characteristics for individual studies[b]		
• Reported	14	25.5
• Information extracted but not reported	4	7.3
Patients demographics reported[b]		
• Age	13	23.6
• Sex	6	10.9
• Sex not applicable	3	5.5
• Country	25	45.5
3. Study design	55	100
Details of individual design assessed for individual studies[b]		
• Reported at least one aspect per study[d]	36	65.5
• Extracted but not reported at least one aspect per study[b]	12	21.8
Reporting of consecutive/non-consecutive study design[c]		
• All study design are not reported or unclear	30	54.5
• Consecutive study and/or randomized only	8	14.5
• Mix of consecutive, non-consecutive and randomized studies	17	30.9
Reporting of prospective/retrospective study design[c]		
• Prospective studies only	6	10.9
• Retrospective studies only	1	1.8
• Report study designs include prospective and/or retrospective	32	58.2
• Some study design are not reported or unclear	10	18.2
• All study design are not reported or unclear	20	36.4
Test Masking[a]		
• Test masking discussed in review	38	69.1
Type of test masking discussed:		
• Masking both ways between reference and index test	18	32.7
• Index test masked to reference test	7	12.7
• Reference test masked to index test	3	5.5
• Other (between two index tests or unspecified)	10	18.2

(continued on next page)

Table 1
(continued)

Assessments Items	No. of Reviews	%
4. Index test		
Index test[a]	55	100
• Single index test reported in review	20	36.4
• Multiple index test reported in review	35	63.6
• Index test not reported or unclear	0	
• Definition of positive test results given[c]	28	50.9
• Index test reported for each study[b]	46	83.6
• Time period between index test and reference test reported[c]	5	9.1
• Uninterpretable test results reported[c]	2	3.6
5. Reference test		
Reference test[a]		
• Single reference test reported in review	11	20
• multiple reference test reported in review	36	65.5
• Reference test not reported or unclear	8	14.5
Reference test for each study[b]		
• Reported	41	74.5
• Extracted but not reported	8	14.5
• Not reported or unclear	8	14.5
6. Graphical display of data[a]	55	100
• No graph	7	12.7
• Any graph	48	87.3
Type of graph[a]		
• Summary ROC graph	42	76.4
• Forest plots of sensitivity/specificity	26	47.3
• Other plots	18	32.7
7. Study results		
Study results reported for all studies[b]		
• Sensitivity	44	80
• Specificity	44	80
• Two measures of test accuracy	36	65.5
• Sample size	45	81.8
• Prevalence	35	63.6
2x2 tables results for each study[b]		
• Reported or can be calculated from review	30	54.5
• Extracted but not reported	20	36.4
• Not extracted or unclear	5	9.1
Confidence interval for individual studies	32	58.2
8. Quality	55	100
Quality of included studies assessed[a]		
• Formal assessment	35	63.6
• Discussion only	7	12.7
Bias assessment		
• Formal assessment	14	25.5
• Statistical test	11	20
• Funnel plots	12	21.8
• Discussion only	22	40
Heterogeneity assessment		
• Formal assessment (statistical heterogeneity)	33	60
• Clinical assessment	22	40
• Source of heterogeneity investigated	31	56.4

(continued on next page)

Table 1 (continued)		
Assessments Items	**No. of Reviews**	**%**
9. Method of meta-analyses:		
• Pool accuracy measures separately	sensitivity/ specificity	
• Likelihood ratio	52	94.5
• Summary ROC	19	34.5
• Other	40	72.7
	16	29.1
Confidence interval for meta-analyses	43	78.2
	42	76.4

[a] Related to review.
[b] Related to individual studies.
[c] Related to single test within review.
[d] Any of prospective/retrospective, consecutive/case-control, masking.

studies were carried out; age was reported in one quarter of the reviews; and gender of patients rarely was reported.

Study Design

Consecutive prospective recruitment from a clinically relevant population of patients with masked assessment of index and reference tests is the recommended design to minimize bias and ensure clinical applicability of study results. Cohort studies assemble patients at risk for a disease in whom the new test and the reference test are performed. By contrast, case-control studies assemble patients who have the disease and controls who do not have the disease (on the basis of the reference test results) and compare the index test results in the two groups. Therefore, case-control studies tend to be at higher risk from bias: the prevalence of the target disorder tends to be higher than in cohort studies (or than in practice); and cases and controls often are selected from opposite ends of the disease spectrum (eg, severe cases and healthy controls).

Whether or not consecutive recruitment was used in primary studies was not reported or was unclear in 30 of the 55 reviews examined (see **Table 1**). Few reviews limited inclusion to study designs less prone to bias, namely consecutive (14.5%) or prospective (10.9%) studies.

Sixty-nine percent of the articles (38/55) discussed test masking. Reviews sometimes omitted information that had been collected: for example, 21.8% (12/55) of reviews extracted information on study design for individual studies but did not report it.

Description of Index and Reference Tests

Index and reference tests need to be described clearly for a review to be clinically relevant and transparent and to allow readers to judge the potential for incorporation and verification biases (see also bias assessment). In this review, 63.6% of the meta-analyses reported a multiple index test and 36.4% reported a single reference test. Half of the reviews (28/55) reported the definition of a positive result for the index test (**Table 4**).

Ninety-five percent (47/55) reported the reference tests used in the review, and 74.5% (41/55) reported reference tests for each included study. The reference test was not reported or was unclear in eight reviews (14.5%). The reference test more commonly was multiple (36/55; 76.9%).

Reporting of Individual Study Results and Graphic Presentation

The two measures of diagnostic accuracy reported most commonly are sensitivity (that is, the probability that a test result is positive in patients who have the disease of interest) and specificity (the probability that a test result is negative in patients who do not have the disease of interest). The diagnostic odds ratio (DOR), defined as the product (true positive × true negative)/(false positive × false negative), represents another overall index of test accuracy.

If there is evidence that the diagnostic threshold varies between studies, the best summary of the diagnostic test results is provided by the summary receiver operating characteristic method (ROC).[87] ROC curve is a graph of the sensitivity on the vertical axis against the false-positive rate (1–specificity) on the horizontal axis.[3,87] The position of the ROC curve depicts the diagnostic performance of the test. A poor test is close to the rising diagonal, whereas an (almost) perfect test produces a line close to the point where specificity = sensitivity = 1. If the curve is reasonably symmetric, the overall test accuracy (DOR) is independent from the threshold point chosen. Alternatively, if the curve is asymmetric, a threshold effect is present.

Another measure of test performance is the positive likelihood ratio, (LR+) defined as the positive ratio (LR+) of the probability of a particular test result in people who have disease (sensitivity) to the probability of the same test result in people who do not have the disease (1-specificity). Moreover, the negative likelihood ratio (LR-) is defined as the ratio (1-sensitivity)/specificity. If the sampling method provides an implicit evaluation of the disease prevalence (as happens with cohort-type or cross-sectional design) positive predictive values and negative predictive values also can be derived immediately. Because this information is not available with the case-control design, in order to estimate the predictive values, the prevalence information must be obtained in an independent way, often from previous statistical data (Bayesian approach). If the prevalence of the disease (which is a proportion, i.e. a probability) is converted to pre-test odds = prevalence/(1 - prevalence), the product of the latter by the positive likelihood ratio is the post-test odds. This in turn can be converted to post-test probability (positive predictive value) = post-test odds/(1 + post-test odds). Similarly, the negative predictive value can be obtained from the disease non-prevalence and the negative likelihood ratio.

The simplest way to combine studies of diagnostic accuracy is to estimate weighted averages of sensitivity, specificity, or likelihood ratio. Moreover, the same approach can be used for DOR. These procedures can be coupled with forest plots. The homogeneity of the results provided by the studies can be tested using standard χ^2 test.[88]

The authors assessed the detail level used to report the results of individual studies. Eighty percent of the articles reported sensitivities and specificities data for individual studies; other reported measures of test accuracy were likelihoods ratios, DOR, and predictive values (**Table 5**). More than half (30/55) of the reviews provided adequate information to derive 2 × 2 tables for all included studies.

Of the 55 reviews, 48 (87.3%) contained graphs of study findings. Summary ROC curves were presented in 76% of the reviews and forest plots of sensitivity and specificity in 47%; other graphs presented were funnel plots to visually inspect for publication bias.[89]

Quality and Methods of Meta-analyses

Quality assessment is as important in systematic reviews of diagnostic accuracy studies as it is in any other review. If the results of individual studies are biased and

Table 2
Key features of meta-analyses evaluating diagnostic accuracy of tests for bacterial infections (excluding mycobacteria)

First Author, Year (Ref)	Object, Clinical Setting, and Condition	No. Studies; Inclusion Criteria[a]	Index Test	Standard Reference Test	Study Design and Relevance of Population Studied	Main Findings of the Review
Reed, 1996[14]	Evaluation of sputum Gram's stain in patients who had community-acquired pneumococcal pneumonia	12; criteria partially stated	Sputum Gram's stain	Multiple: culture of sputum, transtracheal aspirate, bronchial aspirate, or combinations	Prospective studies and retrospective chart review	Test sensitivity and specificity varied markedly among studies
Loy, 1996[15]	Evaluation of serologic kits for Helicobacter pylori	21; not stated	Different kits of ELISA, one kit of latex agglutination	Culture, culture and histology, culture + histology + urease testing on biopsy	Study design and participants not specified	Accuracy of serologic tests might not be adequate for clinical decision making
Mol, 1997[16]	Evaluation of chlamydial antibodies in women who had subfertility and tubal pathology	23; stated	Different antibody assays: ELISA, immunofluorescence (IF), micro-IF, immunoperoxidase	Laparoscopy	Consecutive and nonconsecutive patients included	The discriminative capacity of chlamydial antibodies in the diagnosis of tubal pathology is comparable to hysterosalpingography
Koumans, 1998[17]	Evaluation of nonculture tests for Neisseria gonorrhoeae in endocervical or male urethral specimens	21; partially stated	Nucleic acid hybridization (Pace 2 or 2c) or amplification (ligase chain reaction [LCR] or polymerase chain reaction [PCR]) tests	Culture	Study design and participants not specified	In settings were optimization of culture is difficult, NAA more reliable than nucleic acid probe or culture

Study	Aim	Number of studies included[a]	Tests evaluated	Reference standard	Study design and patient characteristics	Conclusions
Roberts, 2000[18]	Evaluation of serologic and urea breath test (UBT) for H pylori infection	30; not stated	UBT and serology enzyme immunoassay [EIA], ELISA, latex agglutination)	Different combinations of histology, culture, urease, campylobacter-like organisms test, UBT, microscopy, UBT	Study design and patient characteristics not stated/reported	The choice of H pylori diagnostic test should be influenced by prevalence of infection in the population
Watson, 2002[19]	Evaluation of diagnostic tests for Chlamydia trachomatis in asymptomatic, sexually active populations	30; broad inclusion criteria used	PCR and LCR, gene probes, EIA, IF, leukocyte esterase test	Culture, or an expanded reference standards of two nonculture tests	Various study designs included; inclusion of consecutive patients reported	NAA tests in noninvasive samples (urine) are more effective at detecting asymptomatic chlamydial infection than conventional tests
Gisbert, 2006[20]	Evaluation of different tests for H pylori in patients who had gastrointestinal bleeding	23; not stated	Rapide urease test, histology, culture, UBT, stool antigen test, serology	Not reported (at least one independent diagnostic method)	Study design not specified	UBT shows high accuracy in patients who had gastrointestinal bleeding. The investigators' conclusions should be interpreted with some degree of caution given the limitationsin primary studies and in review reporting

[a] Inclusion criteria related to study design, participants, and outcomes measures.

Table 3
Key features of meta-analyses evaluating diagnostic accuracy of tests for mycobacterial infections

First Author, Year (Ref)	Object, Clinical Setting, and Condition	No. Studies; Inclusion Criteria*	Index Test	Standard Reference Test	Study Design and Relevance of Population Studied	Main Findings of the Review
Sarmiento, 2003[21]	Evaluation of PCR for diagnosis of smear-negative pulmonary tuberculous (TB)	50; not stated	Various PCR procedures	Culture, smear, or combined (culture + clinical, or biopsy	Study design and patient characteristics not stated/reported.	PCR not consistently accurate to be routinely recommended in this setting.
Pai M, 2003[22]	NAA tests for the diagnosis of TB meningitis	45; inclusion criteria related to study design not stated	Various in-house (PCR or nested PCR) or commercial tests (Amplicor, Cobas Amplicor, Amplified M. tuberculosis Drect Test (MTD), LCx)	Culture ± microscopy, microbiology + clinical diagnosis; clinical diagnosis + response to therapy + other laboratory tests	Mostly consecutive and prospective	NAA commercial tests show potential role in the diagnosis of TB meningitis. Case-control studies produced DOR twice as large as DOR from cross-sectional studies.
Cruciani, 2004[23]	Evaluation of nonradiometric BACTEC system for detection of mycobacteria in clinical specimens (mostly from respiratory tract)	10; not stated	BACTEC 960/MGIT	BACTEC 460 ± solid media	Consecutive and random sampling methods in patients who had suspected pulmonary or extrapulmonary TB	BACTEC 960/MGIT shows elevated diagnostic accuracy, although BACTEC 460 + solid media remains the reference standard.

Study	Test/Condition	Number of studies; inclusion criteria	Test	Reference standard	Study design	Conclusions
Pai, 2004[24]	NAA tests for the diagnosis of TB pleuritis	40; inclusion criteria related to study design not stated	Various in-house PCR technique or commercial tests (Amplicor, MTD, LCx)	Culture; culture + clinical; culture + biopsy	Mostly consecutive and prospective	NAA commercial tests show potential role in confirming TB pleuritis. Case-control studies produced DOR greater than those from cross-sectional studies.
Flores, 2005[25]	In-house NAA tests for the detection of M tuberculosis in sputum specimens	84; inclusion criteria related to study design not stated	Various in-house PCR techniques (nested or seminested, regular or multiplex)	Not clearly defined	60 cross-sectional and 24 case-control studies; patient characteristics not stated/reported.	In-house NAA tests provide highly heterogeneous estimates of accuracy.
Morgan, 2005[26]	Line probe assay (LiPA) for detection of rifampicin resistance in M tuberculosis in culture isolates and clinical specimens	15; inclusion criteria related to study participants not stated	INNO-LiPA Rif. TB kit	Proportion method, BACTEC 460, minimum inhibitory concentration method	No study prospectively enrolled consecutive patients; patient characteristics not stated/reported.	LiPA may have a potential role in ruling in and ruling out rifampicin resistance.
Pai, 2005[27]	Bacteriophage-based assay for detection of rifampicin resistance in M tuberculosis in culture isolates and clinical specimens	21; inclusion criteria related to study participants not stated	Commercial (FastPlaque-TB) and in-house assay	Proportion method, BACTEC 460, minimum inhibitory concentration method	Few studies included consecutive or randomly selected patients or specimens; patient characteristics not stated/reported.	Phage assay has variable specificity on culture isolates; additional studies are required to evaluate its role directly on sputum specimens.

(continued on next page)

Table 3
(continued)

First Author, Year (Ref)	Object, Clinical Setting, and Condition	No. Studies; Inclusion Criteria*	Index Test	Standard Reference Test	Study Design and Relevance of Population Studied	Main Findings of the Review
Kalantri, 2005[28]	Bacteriophage-based assay for detection of *M tuberculosis* in clinical specimens (sputum and others)	13; inclusion criteria related to study participants and study design not stated	Commercial (FastPlaque-TB and PhageTek) and in-house assay	BACTEC 460 ± Lowenstein-Jensen (LJ), LJ, LJ + MTD	Diagnostic cohort studies and case-control studies. Most included patients who had suspected pulmonary TB.	Phage assay has high specificity, variable sensitivity; diagnostic accuracy is slightly higher than that of microscopy.
Tuon, 2006[29]	Adenosine deaminase (ADA) adjunctive test for TB pericarditis in patients who had pericardial effusion	5; not stated	ADA activity in pericardial effusion	Culture from effusion or tissue, histopathology, granulomas in pericardial tissue associated with active TB in another site; clinical improvement after empiric TB therapy	Prospective studies, consecutive or random samples; case-control studies (control groups with other pericardial diseases)	ADA is a valuable adjunctive test in the diagnosis of TB pericarditis. These conclusion are hampered, however, by study design of primary studies.

Steingart, 2006[30]	Comparison of sputum processing methods with standard methods to improve the sensitivity of smear microscopy	46; all study design included; criteria related to study participants not stated	Various chemical processing methods, centrifugation force/speed, and time	Culture; studies without reference standard included.	Few studies recruited samples in consecutive/random manner; limited data on clinical status of patients and disease severity; and few studies defined criteria for pulmonary TB suspects.	The results suggest that processing sputum increased sensitivity compared to standard methods, but these conclusions are hampered by biases in primary studies.
Steingart, 2006[31]	Comparison of fluorescence microscopy with conventional microscopy for the diagnosis of TB	45; all study design included; criteria related to study participants not stated	Fluorescence microscopy	Culture; studies without reference standard included	One third of studies recruited samples in consecutive/random manner; limited data on clinical status of patients and disease severity, and few studies defined criteria for pulmonary TB suspects.	Within the limits in the review methods and in primary studies, the investigators conclude that fluorescence microscopy increased sensitivity compared to conventional microscopy but specificity was similar.

(continued on next page)

Table 3
(continued)

First Author, Year (Ref)	Object, Clinical Setting, and Condition	No. Studies; Inclusion Criteria*	Index Test	Standard Reference Test	Study Design and Relevance of Population Studied	Main Findings of the Review
Riquelme, 2006[32]	ADA in ascitic fluid as adjunctive test for the diagnosis of TB peritonitis	20; inclusion criteria related to study participants not stated	ADA levels in peritoneal by Giusti method	Culture or positive acid-fast stain from ascitic fluid or (biopsy showing granulomatous or caseous lesion); clinical improvement after empiric TB therapy	Prospective studies including consecutive patients; patient characteristics not reported.	Measurement of ADA level in ascetic fluid is a fast and accurate test for TB peritonitis. These conclusion are hampered, however, by limitations in review methods and in primary studies.
Steingart, 2007[33]	Commercial serologic antibody testing for the diagnosis of extrapulmonary TB	21; inclusion criteria related to study participants and study design not stated	Seven different commercial tests (Anda-Tb IgG in 48%)	Culture or positive acid-fast stain, or histolopathology (biopsy showing granulomatous or caseous lesion)	None of the studies reported the method of subject selection. Mostly retrospective data collection and differential verification. Clinical setting not reported.	Antibody testing has no role in the diagnosis of extrapulmonary TB. The quality of the articles evaluated was poor, and the results of the analyses extremely heterogeneous.

Steingart, 2007[34]	Commercial serologic antibody testing for the diagnosis of pulmonary TB	68 studies (27 articles); all study design included; only studies with bacteriologic confirmed TB included	Nine different commercial tests	Culture or acid-fast bacilli from sputum smear	Half of the studies collected data prospectively; one third used random/ consecutive recruitment. Clinical setting was not reported.	Antibody testing has little or no role in the diagnosis of pulmonary TB. Many of the primary studies were of poor quality.
Daley, 2007[35]	NAA tests for the diagnosis of TB lymphadenitis	49 (36 articles); inclusion criteria related to study design not stated; studies testing lymph node samples from patients who had suspected TB lymphadenitis included	In-house or commercial (Abbott LCx, Gen-Probe MTDT, BD ProbeTec, Roche Amplicor) NAA tests	Culture; smear microscopy; histology; response to empiric treatment	80% of studies cross-sectional, with consecutive/ random sampling; patients clinical characteristics in individual studies not reported.	The results were highly variable and inconsistent, precluding the determination of clinically meaningful estimates of accuracy.
Menzies, 2007[36]	Comparison of interferon-gamma (IFN-γ) release assays (IGRAs) with tuberculin skin tests for diagnosing latent T B infection	58; inclusion criteria related to study design and reference standard not stated	Various in-house or commercial versions of QuantiFeron or Elispot tests. Studies compared 1 or more tests with tuberculin skin test.	Most of the included studies did not use a reference standard for latent TB; they use active TB as a surrogate measure of latent TB.	50 cross-sectional studies, and 8 cohort studies with serial testing. Sensitivity assessed in patients who had active TB and contact of person who had active TB; specificity in studies that included healthy subjects.	IGRAs are promising and have excellent specificity, but further studies are required to better define their diagnostic performance.

(continued on next page)

Table 3
(continued)

First Author, Year (Ref)	Object, Clinical Setting, and Condition	No. Studies; Inclusion Criteria*	Index Test	Standard Reference Test	Study Design and Relevance of Population Studied	Main Findings of the Review
Jiang, 2007[37]	Evaluation of IFN-γ in pleural effusion for the diagnosis of TB pleurisy	22; inclusion criteria related to patient characteristics and reference standard not stated	IFN-γ assay methods include radioimmunoassay or ELISA,	Bacteriology, histology, clinical course	Included studies were prospective and retrospective; some used a cross-sectional design; patients clinical characteristics in individual studies not reported.	The investigators conclude that the test is sensitive and specific. These conclusions are hampered, however, by several limitations in review methods and in primary studies.
Pai, 2008[38]	An update of a previous meta-analyses[36] comparing IGRAs with tuberculin skin tests for diagnosing latent TB infection	38; inclusion criteria related to study design and reference standard not stated	Analyses limited to QuantiFERON-TB Gold, QuantiFERON-TB Gold In-Tube, T-SPOT.TB	Most of the included studies did not use a reference standard for latent TB.	All were cross-sectional studies.	Within the limits of the original studies, the review concludes that the specificity of IGRAs in detecting latent TB is good and unaffected by BCG vaccination status. Sensitivity is not consistent across tests and populations studied.

analyzed without any consideration of quality, then the results of the review also will be biased. Bias limits the validity of the study results, whereas variability may affect the generalizability of study results. A formal assessment of the quality of primary studies included in a review allows investigation of the effect of different biases and sources of variation on study results.

Several checklists for the assessment of the quality of studies about diagnostic accuracy exist; among them, QUADAS (quality assessment for diagnostic accuracy studies) is a valuable tool for the quality assessment of studies of diagnostic accuracy included in systematic reviews;[86] it includes items that cover bias, variability, and, to a certain extent, the quality of reporting. Sixty-three percent (35/55) of reviews in this overview presented a formal assessment of quality of included studies (see **Table 1**). For this purpose, various checklist were used, including QUADAS[86] and STARD (standards for reporting of diagnostic accuracy),[4] or criteria specified in previous publications.[3,6]

Bias Assessment

The most important potential sources of bias in assessing diagnostic accuracy are the use of inappropriate reference standard, the lack of independence of observations, and the presence of specific types of bias, including publication, spectrum, and verification bias.[2,89] Publication bias may arise because articles with more interesting or statistically significant results are more likely to be published than studies with less extreme results.[3]

Methods for dealing with publication bias have been developed,[3,90] but their applicability to diagnostic test assessment has not been explored. A formal assessment of bias (publication bias) was presented in a quarter of the analyzed reviews (14/55) by means of statistical tests or funnel plots. In 40% of the reviews (22/55), different types of bias were discussed, namely spectrum and verification bias. Overall, in 29 of the 55 reviews (52.7%) the spectrum of patients was representative of those patients who receive the test in clinical practice.

Heterogeneity Assessment

A formal assessment of heterogeneity by means of statistical tests was reported in 60% (33/55) of the reviews. More than half of the meta-analyses attempted to investigate statistically possible sources of variation, using subgroup analyses or regression analyses. The impact of clinical or sociodemographic variables was investigated in 22 (40%) of these reviews.

Methods of Meta-analyses

The majority of meta-analyses (52/55) was based on estimates of sensitivity and specificity from the primary studies. Forty studies (72.7%) estimated summary ROC curves, and 19 (34.5%) assessed likelihood ratio.

Main Findings from Individual Meta-analyses

In addition to a general assessment of meta-analyses, the main findings of individual meta-analyses included in the reviews are summarized. For this purpose, focus was on the following issues: objective and inclusion criteria of the review, clinical setting where the test was used and the disease prevalence, the index test and the reference standard evaluated, details of individual study design (eg, consecutive/randomized/nonconsecutive, prospective/retrospective, or case-control/cross-sectional), clinical relevance of patients included in the studies, and main conclusions of the review. These data are shown on separate tables related to studies evaluating

Table 4
Key features of meta-analyses evaluating diagnostic accuracy of tests for fungal infections

First Author, Year (Ref)	Object, Clinical Setting, and Condition	No. Studies; Inclusion Criteria*	Index Test	Standard Reference Test	Study Design and Relevance of Population Studied	Main Findings of the Review
Cruciani, 2002[39]	Comparison of sputum induction procedure with bronchoalveolar lavage (BAL) in the diagnosis of P carinii pneumonia (PCP) in HIV infected patients	7; inclusion criteria related to participants, reference standard and study design stated	Microscopic examination of sputum after induction procedure using conventional cytochemical staining methods and IF methods	BAL using conventional cytochemical staining methods and IF methods	All studies included consecutive HIV infected patients requiring fiberoptic bronchoscopy for suspected PCP or other pulmonary diseases.	In a setting of low prevalence of PCP, sputum induction, particularly with immunostaining, seems adequate for clinical decision making.
Pfeiffer, 2006[40]	Galactomannan assay for the diagnosis of invasive aspergillosis (IA) in patients who had immunodeficiency	27; inclusion criteria related to patient characteristics not stated; case-control studies excluded	Galactomannan assay with different cutoff to defining positivity (0.5–1.5)	Criteria of the European Organisation for Research and Treatment of Cancer (EORTC) or other criteria	Patients at risk for IA, including pateints who had hematologic malignancy, solid-organ and bone marrow transplant recipients. Subgroup analyses performed according to clinical characteristics of patient cutoff of GM, reference standard.	The galactomannan assay has moderate accuracy for diagnosis of IA in immunocompromised patients.

| Tuon, 2007[41] | PCR from BAL in patients at risk for IA | 15; inclusion criteria related to patients characteristics and study design not stated | Various in-house and commercial kits for NAA in BAL specimens | EORTC criteria in some studies; in other studies criteria not specified | Various study designs included; patient characteristic not reported. | The investigators support the clinical value of PCR on BAL specimens. The conclusions, however, are potentially vulnerable to biases introduced by methodologic flaws in the primary studies. |
| Mengoli, 2009[42] | Evaluation of PCR in patients at high risk for IA | 16; criteria of inclusion stated | Various in-house PCR procedures on serum/blood samples | EORTC criteria | Case-control study excluded. | PCR promising in the diagnosis of IA. The results also show that not all PCR tests are the same because some yielded much higher DORs than others. |

Table 5
Key features of meta-analyses evaluating diagnostic accuracy of tests for viral infections

First Author, Year (Ref)	Object, Clinical Setting, and Condition	No. Studies; Inclusion Criteria*	Index Test	Standard Reference Test	Study Design and Relevance of Population Studied	Main Findings of the Review
Owens, 1996[43]	To evaluate the sensitivity and specificity of PCR assay for the diagnosis of HIV infection in adults	96; no inclusion criteria related to study design and reference standard specified	DNA amplification by PCR on peripheral mononuclear blood cells	Details of the reference standards not fully reported. The investigators suggested EIA + confirmatory Western blot analyses or viral culture as examples of reference standards used.	The reporting of the characteristics of the included studies was poor.	The use of PCR for the diagnosis of HIV in adults should be limited to situations in which antibody tests are known to be insufficient.
Colin, 2001[44]	To evaluate sensitivity/specificity of third-generation serologic hepatitis C virus (HCV) diagnostic tests	6; criteria of inclusion stated	Eight types of ELISA (Ortho HCV 3.0, Abbott HCV EIA 3.0, Murex anti-HCV III, Inno-EIA, Cobas Core Anti-HCV EIA, Monolisa anti-HCV new antigen, Sorin ETI-AB-HCV, and Ubi 4.0) and two types of recombinant immunoblot assay (RIBA) (Chiron RIBA HCV 3.0 and Matrix HCV)	HCV RNA detection. Two studies, however, used ELISA as gold standard.	Screened population included blood donors, hemodialysis patients, consecutive patients who had documented non-A, non-B hepatitis.	Good sensitivity and specificity of ELISA 3, particularly in high risk patients.

Kowalsky, 2001[45]	Comparative evaluation of test performance among Food and Drug Administration–licensed EIA for HIV in population with different risk for acquiring the infection	49; no inclusion criteria related to study design and participants specified	Several EIAs for HIV antibody testing	Western blot, PCR, p24 antigen testing	High or low risk population screened. Quality of studies defined as low, moderate, or high, according to predefined criteria.	Differences in test performance among HIV EIA manufacturers were found.
Blacksell, 2006[46]	To evaluate the accuracy of rapid dengue virus diagnostic assays	11; no inclusion criteria relating to the study design were specified.	Studies that evaluated rapid point of care immunochromatographic tests (ICTs) for the detection of dengue virus immunoglobulin M (IgM) antibodies were eligible for inclusion. Assays limited to the detection of IgG and assays taking longer than 60 minutes to perform were excluded. All included studies evaluated the PanBio ICT.	The reference standards used were Panbio Duo ELISA, Panbio IgM ELISA, MRL IgM ELISA, AFRIMS MAC-ELISA, and hemagglutination inhibition test.	Both cohort (five studies) and case-control (six) design included. Disease severity and infectious status in individual studies often not reported	Rapid ICTs can be used to rule in and out infection with dengue virus but are more accurate when samples are collected later in the acute phase of infection.

(continued on next page)

Table 5
(continued)

First Author, Year (Ref)	Object, Clinical Setting, and Condition	No. Studies; Inclusion Criteria*	Index Test	Standard Reference Test	Study Design and Relevance of Population Studied	Main Findings of the Review
Pai NP, 2007[47]	To assess the diagnostic accuracy of rapid HIV tests in pregnancy and the feasibility, acceptability, and impact of testing in practice	17; no inclusion criteria were specified for reference standard and study design	Studies of rapid HIV test kits were eligible for the review. Limited details of the kits used in the included studies were reported, but the majority involved a blood test or an oral fluid test.	Various reference standard used, including EIA, performed once or twice with or without Western blot; one study used a single Western blot test.	The included studies were described as cross-sectional or surveys.	Rapid tests for HIV have high diagnostic accuracy and are feasible to perform in antenatal and delivery room settings. Issues about the generally poor quality and limited reporting of the included studies, however, make it difficult to be sure of the reliability of the conclusions.
Shaheen, 2007[48]	FibroTest and FibroScan for the prediction of HCV-related fibrosis	12; no inclusion criteria were specified for study design	FibroTest or FibroScan	Liver biopsy	Both retrospective and prospective studies included. Patient characteristics not reported.	FibroTest and FibroScan have excellent usefulness for identification of HCV-related cirrhosis but lesser accuracy for earlier stages.

diagnostic test of bacterial infections (other than tuberculosis) (**Table 2**), tuberculosis (**Table 3**), fungal infections (**Table 4**), viral infections (**Table 5**), protozoan infections (**Table 6**), and various clinical conditions and syndromes (**Table 7**).

In general, several reviews were identified that coupled good overall methods and reporting to a relevant clinical performance (eg, study performed in a group of subjects covering the spectrum of diseases likely encountered in the current or future use of a diagnostic test). Examples of such reviews can be found in references.[16,19,22–24,29,32–34,39,40,42,48,51,53,55,58–63,65–68] Overall, study quality was not related to publication year.

DISCUSSION

Although the current research relates to reviews on the diagnosis of infectious diseases, the authors believe that the results likely also are representative of other specialties. The assessment checklist mostly was based on a previous overview of systematic reviews in oncology,[12] and it probably could be applied to any medical topic. Some peculiarity of infectious diseases compared to other medical fields, however, may explain differences in characteristics of primary studies and systematic reviews of diagnostic test. For instance, the types of diagnostic tests used in infectious diseases are different from those in other medical specialties. Overviews of meta-analyses of diagnostic tests in all specialties and in cancer showed that approximately half of diagnostic tests were imaging tests, one third were laboratory tests, and the remaining were clinical tests.[9,12] In contrast, the majority of diagnostic tests evaluated in meta-analyses of infectious diseases were laboratory tests and a few were imaging or clinical tests.

Other overviews of reviews of diagnostic tests have highlighted the poor quality of the literature, in primary studies and in systematic reviews. The authors have found that an electronic search was reported in all but one of the reviews, and 60% of the reviews searched two or more electronic databases. Other surveys of systematic reviews have found a higher prevalence of reporting problems. In a review of meta-analyses of diagnostic tests across all specialties, Lijmer and colleagues[6] found that a systematic search was not reported in 7 of 26 reviews (26.9%), whereas the overview in oncology by Mallett and colleagues[12] showed that 37% of otherwise eligible reviews did not report an electronic search.

The authors found that only 20% of reviews reported that only one reference test was used, compared to 14% of the reviews in cancer. Multiple reference tests was reported in 65% of the reviews in infectious diseases compared to 53% of the reviews in cancer and 51% in the review by Mallett and colleagues.[12,13] The reference test was not reported or was unclear in 14.5% of reviews in infectious diseases compared to 32% in cancer. Altogether, these findings indicate the potential for heterogeneity as a result of difference reference tests in a large proportion of reviews.

Arroll and colleagues[91] found that 87% of primary diagnostic studies clearly defined positive and negative test results. Only 50% of reviews in the authors' study, and 40% of reviews in cancer, reported a definition of positive test results or reported that it was not available in the primary studies. It seems likely that key information available in primary studies often is omitted from systematic reviews.

Differences in demographic and clinical features between populations may produce measures of diagnostic accuracy that vary considerably, known as spectrum bias. Reported estimates of diagnostic accuracy may have limited clinical applicability (generalizability) if the spectrum of tested patients is not similar to the patients in whom the test will be used in practice. It is, therefore, of utmost importance that diagnostic test evaluation includes an appropriate spectrum of patients for the test under

Table 6
Key features of meta-analyses evaluating diagnostic accuracy of tests for protozoan infections

First Author, Year (Ref)	Object, Clinical Setting, and Condition	No. Studies; Inclusion Criteria*	Index Test	Standard Reference Test	Study Design and Relevance of Population Studied	Main Findings of the Review
Garduno-Espinosa, 1992[49]	Evaluation of the diagnostic performance of immunologic tests in amebic liver abscess using receiver operating characteristic curves	24; inclusion criteria related to study design and reference standard not stated	Indirect hemoagglutination, ELISA, IF, latex agglutination test, complement fixation, flocculation, radioimmunoassay, EIA	Identification of the parasite in pus, or a positivity of a test other than the index test, or combination of ≥3: clinical findings (liver enlargment, fever, pain in the right upper abdomen), ultrasounds, macroscopic characteristics of pus, gamagraphy.	Patients from original articles stratified according to the following conditions: amebic liver abscess, intestinal amebiasis, asymptomatic carriers, healthy controls, and controls with other clinical conditions.	A greater variation in the diagnostic efficiency of the test analyzed was identified.
Patel, 2000[50]	Review of diagnostic tests for vaginal trichomoniasis	35; inclusion criteria related to Patient characteristics and study design not stated	PCR techniques (six studies); ELISA (five); direct fluorescent-antibody assay (three); other techniques (six); various culture media (20)	Trichomonads culture ± wet mount. The investigators stated that it seems prudent to use only the culture media with the highest sensitivity (Diamond, Hollander, or CPM)	One third of studies were prospective evaluation of consecutive patients. The articles were graded according to whether or not they met validity criteria.	High variability of the diagnostic yield of different test evaluated. The methodologic quality of studies included was not always reported clearly, and several studies were of poor quality.

Wiese, 2000[51]	Cervical Papanicolaou's smear and wet mount for the diagnosis of vaginal trichomoniasis	31; inclusion criteria related to patient characteristics and study design not stated	Papanicolaou's smear and wet mount	Thricomonads culture, including Diamond, Hollander, CPLM, Oxoid, InPouch TV, AC medium, multiple culture, agar, Feiner Whittington	Women suspected of having trichomoniasis, in different setting (specialty sexually transmitted disease clinics, general clinics). 40% of studies were prospective evaluation of consecutive pateints. The articles were graded according to whether or not they met validity criteria.	A positive Papanicolaou's smear for trichomonads in settings with high prevalence (>20%) requires treatment. When the prevalence is low (1%), a culture should be performed. Specificity of wet mount is high but not sensitivity.
Cruciani, 2004[52]	Rapid test (Parasight-F) in the diagnosis of Plasmodium falciparum malaria	32; inclusion criteria related to patient characteristics not stated	Parasight-F test	Tick or thin blood smear	Sampling methods include consecutive patients and case-control. Diagnostic performance evaluated in people living in endemic areas and in travelers returning from endemic areas.	Parasight-F test could be of particular value in the diagnosis of P falciparum malaria in travelers returning from endemic areas.

(continued on next page)

Table 6
(continued)

First Author, Year (Ref)	Object, Clinical Setting, and Condition	No. Studies; Inclusion Criteria*	Index Test	Standard Reference Test	Study Design and Relevance of Population Studied	Main Findings of the Review
Marx, 2005[53]	Rapid test for malaria in travelers returning from endemic areas	21; inclusion criteria related to study design not stated	Various commercial rapid test (eg, Parasight-F, Path IC strip, ICT Pf/Pv, OptiMal) targeting HRP-2 (*P falciparum* only) or HRP-2 + aldolase, or LDH (targeting *P vivax*, *P malariae*, and *P ovale*)	Combination of microscopic examination (tick or thin blood smear) and PCR	Various study design included (six studies prospective, 10 enrolled consecutive patients). Subjects were nonimmune individuals who had suspected malaria returning from endemic areas. Studies with more than 10% of participants were immune excluded.	HRP-2 based tests were a useful adjunct to microscopy in ruling out *P falciparum* malaria in centers without major expertise in tropical medicine. More research is required for other species.
Chappuis, 2006[54]	Comparison of the performance of direct agglutination test and rK 39 dipstick for the diagnosis of visceral leishmaniosis	43; inclusion criteria for study design or reference standard not stated	Freeze-dried and aqueous antigen types of agglutination tests, and Kalazar Detect and other types of rK39 dipsticks. Studies of the rapid version of the direct agglutination test were excluded.	Microscopic examination of lymph node, bone marrow, or spleen aspirate; detection of parasites in culture or by PCR; or clinical response to antileishmanial drugs in patients who had clinically suspected disease who had positive serology results.	Various study designs included. Studies quality reported by QUADAS tool The primary studies included patients who had current clinical visceral leishmaniasis (not HIV infected) and various types of controls: (healthy and not healthy).	The diagnostic performance of the direct agglutination test and the rK39 dipstick for visceral leishmaniasis is good to excellent and seem comparable.

investigation. It also is important to provide a clear description of the population actually included in the study. Incorporation bias occurs when the experimental test is used as part of the reference strategy, leading to a lack of independence between the experimental test and the reference tests and to overestimation of sensitivity and specificity. Verification bias occurs where the decision to undertake or apply the reference test is influenced by the result of the experimental test (also called ascertainment bias or work-up bias).

Many studies the authors analyzed in this overview discussed different types of bias, but they did not always provide information to enable readers to assess the risk for bias. For instance, reporting of consecutive/nonconsecutive study design was not reported or was unclear in more than half of the reviews; 30% of the reviews included studies with a mix of consecutive and nonconsecutive recruitment of patients or specimens. Likewise, reporting of prospective/retrospective study design was not reported or was unclear in 36% of the reviews, and 18% of the reviews included subsets of studies that were unclear about this item or not reported it. Therefore, few reviews limited inclusion to study designs less prone to bias, namely consecutive (14.5%) or prospective (10.9%) studies; these findings are similar to those in the overview of cancer reviews, where only 8% and 12% of reviews, respectively, included consecutive or prospective studies only.[12]

Previous research in diagnostic studies has shown that case-control designs and nonconsecutive recruitment of patients can lead to bias and to overestimation of diagnostic accuracy.[5,6] Two of the reviews included in this overview provide a good example of this phenomenon.[22,24] In a systematic review of the diagnostic accuracy of nucleic acid amplification (NAA) for tuberculous meningitis, Pai and colleagues[22] provided estimates of test accuracy according to study design. As expected, case-control studies produced DOR twice as large as DOR from cross-sectional studies (86.5 and 43.3, respectively). Findings were much the same in another review by the same investigators of the diagnostic accuracy of NAA for tuberculous pleuritis: subgroup analyses of case-control studies produced a DOR of 68.3 compared to a DOR of 28.7 in cross-sectional studies.[24]

Interpretation of the results of the index test may be influenced by knowledge of the results of the reference standard and vice versa. This is known as review bias and may lead to an overestimation of diagnostic accuracy. The extent that this may affect test results is related to the degree of subjectiveness in the interpretation of the test result. In the authors' review, test masking was discussed in 69% of the meta-analyses, but a more detailed assessment of type of masking (eg, index test masked to reference test or reference test masked to index test) was reported less commonly.

Clinical setting was stated in 69% of reviews, but details of patient characteristics for individual studies were reported in only 25%. Detailed information about the clinical setting and patient characteristics are of utmost importance in diagnostic studies, because measures of diagnostic accuracy are generalizable only to settings that have a similar spectrum of patients, defined by the type and extent of disease in patients who have the disease of interest and the type and extent of differential diagnoses in the controls. This spectrum likely varies in different practice settings.[9]

Studies of diagnostic accuracy are reported with growing abundance. In order to be useful, a diagnostic test must be accurate, reproducible, feasible, and capable of assisting clinical decision, thus producing favorable outcomes. Although the reliability of the diagnostic prediction can be assessed in a relatively simple way, the other tasks are more difficult to achieve. Reproducibility can be addressed by studies of intra- and interobserver and laboratory variability. The capability of having an impact on clinical decisions depends on diagnostic yield evaluations, based on studies of pre- and

Table 7
Key features of meta-analyses evaluating diagnostic accuracy of tests for infectious diseases syndromes or conditions

First Author, Year (Ref)	Object, Clinical Setting, and Condition	No. Studies; Inclusion Criteria*	Index Test	Standard Reference Test	Study Design and Relevance of Population Studied	Main Findings of the Review
Littenberg, 1992[55]	Technetium (Tc) bone scanning in patients who had suspected osteomyelitis of the foot	10; no inclusion criteria were specified for study design and reference standard	Radionuclide scanning with Tc-isotopes, especially Tc-99m methylene diphosphonate	Combination of pathologic findings after surgery or biopsy and clinical follow-up after treatment	Patients who had diabetes or other vasculopathy and suspected osteomyelitis of the foot. Both retrospective and prospective studies included. Subgroups analyses according to study design, prevalence of the disease, clinical findings	Tc bone scanning in patients who had suspected osteomyelitis of the foot has poor diagnostic performance.
Huicho, 1996[56]	Evaluation of fecal screening tests in the workup of patients who had inflammatory diarrhea	25; no inclusion criteria were specified for study design	Fecal leukocytes, occult blood, fecal lactoferrin, and combination of fecal leukocytes with clinical data	Stool culture	Various study designs included (prospective/ retrospective), consecutive/ nonconsecutive). Patient characteristics not reported in all studies.	Fecal ferritin was the most accurate index test. Although the test is not specific for a particular pathogen, it seems highly sensitive for inflammatory bowel process.

| Siegman-Igra, 1997[57] | To evaluate the accuracy and cost-effectiveness of methods of diagnosing vascular catheter-related bloodstream infection | 22; no inclusion criteria relating to the reference standard and patient characteristics were specified | Three categories: catheter segment culture (qualitative, semiquantitative, and quantitative), culture of blood drawn through the catheter (unpaired qualitative, unpaired quantitative, and paired quantitative), and a group of miscellaneous methods (including direct staining methods, catheter site skin culture and hub culture). | In most studies, catheter-related bloodstream infection defined as the presence of clinical features of bloodstream infection, growth of the same organisms from peripheral blood and catheter segment or a blood culture aspirated from the catheter, and the absence of another possible source of infection. Studies that did not clearly state their reference standard were excluded. | No restrictions were placed on the study designs included | Quantitative catheter segment culture demonstrated the greatest accuracy for documenting catheter-related bloodstream infection. The conclusions of the review, however, are potentially vulnerable to biases introduced by methodologic flaws in the primary studies. |

(continued on next page)

Table 7
(continued)

First Author, Year (Ref)	Object, Clinical Setting, and Condition	No. Studies; Inclusion Criteria*	Index Test	Standard Reference Test	Study Design and Relevance of Population Studied	Main Findings of the Review
Gerdes, 1998[58]	To evaluate the potential benefits of using C-reactive protein (CRP) to discriminate between patients who had bacterial meningitis and patients who had other diseases, in particular aseptic meningitis	35; no inclusion criteria relating to the reference standard were specified	CRP in serum or cerebrospinal fluid	The investigators state that the final diagnosis of meningitis was based on generally accepted methods and principles.	Basing on study design (eg, cross-sectional versus case-control, prospective and consecutive enrollment), studies were characterized as being of "clinical performance" of a CRP test or not.	The post-test probability of not having bacterial meningitis, given a negative CRP test, is very high in the range of pretest probability (prevalence of bacterial meningitis) of 10%–30%. The conclusions, however, are potentially vulnerable to biases introduced by methodologic flaws in the primary studies.

| Gorelick, 1999[59] | To evaluate the performance of rapid diagnostic tests for urinary tract infection (UTI) in children | 26; the inclusion criteria were explicit and details of the included studies were presented | Urine dipstick for leukocyte esterase (LE) or nitrite; microscopic analyses of centrifuged or uncentrifuged urine sample for white blood cells; Gram's stain of uncentrifuged urine; or enhanced urinalysis (cell count and Gram's stain on uncentrifuged urine) | Quantitative or semiquantitative urine culture | In the eligible study, the screening test and the urine culture were performed on all participants, and the results of the screening test were not included in the definition of UTI. The validity of the included studies was not formally assessed. The settings included a laboratory, referral clinic, home, outpatient department, in patient ward, pediatric clinic, and emergency and acute care clinics. | Gram's stain and dipstick analyses for nitrite and LE perform similarly in detecting UTI in children, and are superior to microscopic analyses for pyuria. |

(continued on next page)

Table 7
(continued)

First Author, Year (Ref)	Object, Clinical Setting, and Condition	No. Studies; Inclusion Criteria*	Index Test	Standard Reference Test	Study Design and Relevance of Population Studied	Main Findings of the Review
Engels, 2000[60]	To evaluate diagnostic tests for acute sinusitis	13; only studies that evaluated each test on all subjects included. No inclusion criteria relating to the reference standard and patient characteristics were specified.	Clinical examination, radiography, ultrasonography, and sinus puncture/aspiration	No inclusion criteria were specified for the reference standard. The reference standard in each comparative study was based on a hierarchy of test accuracy, with the most accurate treated as the reference standard: sinus puncture, followed by radiography, ultrasonography, and then clinical criteria.	Patients had to present symptoms of acute sinusitis. The settings included hospital, ED, office practice (primary care or otolaryngologist. Verification bias was avoided by excluding studies where some patients did not undergo all of the tests being compared.	Radiography and clinical evaluation (especially risk scores) seem to provide useful information for diagnosis of acute sinusitis. Many studies were of poor quality.

| Varonen, 2000[61] | Evaluation of clinical examination, ultrasound and radiography as diagnostic measures for acute maxillary sinusitis (AMS) in unselected populations | 9; any prospective study comparing one of the diagnostic techniques being evaluated with an eligible reference test. No inclusion criteria relating to study design were specified. | Clinical examination, ultrasound, and radiography | Reference standard tests were sinus puncture (the gold standard) and CT. Some studies also used radiographs as part of their reference standard. | The participants had to be adults who had suspected AMS (symptoms for less than 3 months) in primary care or a comparable setting. The studies were set in general practice; ear, nose, and throat clinics; military clinics; and an emergency ward. Study design and patient characteristics often not reported in individual studies | Ultrasounds were slightly less accurate than radiography compared to sinus puncture; clinical examination seems unreliable in diagnosing AMS. |

(continued on next page)

Table 7
(continued)

First Author, Year (Ref)	Object, Clinical Setting, and Condition	No. Studies; Inclusion Criteria*	Index Test	Standard Reference Test	Study Design and Relevance of Population Studied	Main Findings of the Review
Deville, 2004[62]	Evaluation of the diagnostic accuracy of urine dipstick tests for detecting bacteriuria or UTI	72; no inclusion criteria for the study design were specified	Dipstick tests to detect the presence of nitrites or leukocyte esterase, in order to diagnose bacteriuria or UTI	Semiquantitative or quantitative urine culture. The urine sampling methods included suprapubic aspiration, catheterization, midstream collection, and bag collection.	All included studies seemed to be diagnostic cohorts.	Negative results for leukocyte esterase and nitrite seem rule out disease in all populations, but that positive results require confirmation.
Safdar, 2005[63]	Evaluation of the most accurate methods for the diagnosis of intravascular device (IVD)-related bloodstream infection	51; no inclusion criteria for the study design and participants were specified	Qualitative, semiquantitative, or quantitative culture of catheter segment, IVD-drawn quantitative or qualitative blood culture, paired quantitative blood cultures, and acridine orange leukocyte cytospin test	Various reference standards used, including qualitative and quantitative microbiologic methods (on catheter segment, blood culture) and clinical symptoms and signs of infection	Mostly diagnostic cohort studies. The study populations varied widely, from infants to adults and from general in patients to patients who had end-stage renal disease and patients in ICU.	Paired quantitative blood culture is the most accurate test for the diagnosis of IVD-related bloodstream infection.

| Uzzan, 2006[64] | Comparison of procalcitonin (PCT) and C-reactive protein (CRP) as diagnostic marker of sepsis, severe sepsis, or septic shock, in ICU, and after surgery and trauma | 33; no inclusion criteria for the study design, reference standard and participants were specified | PCT (LUMItest PCT test only, not assay on Kryptor) and CRP (various methods) | Investigators state that diagnosis of sepsis was not gold standard in critically ill patients | All studies but one had prospective design; 23 studies recluded consecutive patients. Most studies used the term, sepsis, as a mixture of sepsis, severe sepsis, and septic shock, compared with nonseptic systemic inflammatory response syndrome (SIRS). | The investigators conclude that PCT represents a good biologic marker for sepsis, severe sepsis, or septic shock in ICU. These conclusions should be interpreted with caution, given the problems with reference standard for the clinical conditions under investigation. |
| Jones, 2007[65] | PCT as diagnostic marker of bacteremia in the emergency department (ED) population | 17; studies were graded according to sampling methods and clinical characteristics of patients | PCT | Blood culture | Outpatient populations (adult and pediatric) studied in the ED or at admission to the hospital. Studies with consecutive or random sampling in patients who had signs and symptoms of infection analyzed separately from case-control studies or other studies. | The performance of PCT test for identifying bacteremia in ED patients was found moderate. |

(continued on next page)

Table 7
(continued)

First Author, Year (Ref)	Object, Clinical Setting, and Condition	No. Studies; Inclusion Criteria*	Index Test	Standard Reference Test	Study Design and Relevance of Population Studied	Main Findings of the Review
Tang, 2007[66]	Accuracy of PCT for diagnosis of sepsis in critically ill patients. Most studies were in ICU, some in ED	18; inclusion criteria for the study design not specified	PCT	Sepsis definition of the American College of Chest Physicians/Society of Critical Care Medicine Consensus Conference, and infection confirmed by culture	A subgroup of studies evaluated the test's real-life performance in patients suspected as having the disorder; another subgroup evaluated the performance in patients who had and did not have the disease of interest.	PCT cannot reliably differentiate sepsis from other noninfectious causes of SIRS in critically ill adult patients.
Kapoor, 2007[67]	To evaluate the accuracy of MRI for osteomyelitis of the foot and to compare its performance with Tc-99m bone scanning, plain radiography and white blood cell studies	16; no inclusion criteria for the study design and reference standard were specified. Patients suspected of having osteomyelitis of the foot or ankle, or who had foot infection, were eligible for inclusion	Studies of MRI were eligible for inclusion. The review also compared MRI with Tc-99m bone scanning, plain radiography, and white blood cell studies in studies that directly compared the modalities	The reference standards used in the primary studies included biopsy; some studies did not specify a reference standard.	Nine studies were prospective and six of these included consecutive patients.	MRI can be used to rule in or rule out foot osteomyelitis and is superior to Tc-99m bone scanning, plane radiography and white blood cell studies.

| Dinh, 2008[68] | Evaluation of the physical examination and imaging test for osteomyelitis in diabetic patients who had foot ulcers | 9; no inclusion criteria for the study design were specified | Several diagnostic methods evaluated: clinical examination features (ulcer appearance, ulcer size, presence of exposed, or palpable bone), plain radiography, MRI, nuclear medicine bone scan, and indium-labeled leukocyte scan | Histopathologic examination or microbiologic culture of bone specimens | All but one of the included studies was prospective; recruitment consecutive in four, not reported in five. All studies avoided the workup bias, 44% the review bias. | MRI is the most accurate imaging test for diagnosis of osteomyelitis. |

post-test clinical decision making. The feasibility issue implies the evaluation of the costs, risks, and acceptability of a test. The aptitude to improve clinical outcome is accomplished best by means of randomized trials, cohort or case-control studies in which the predictor variable is receiving the test, and an outcome that includes morbidity, mortality, or costs related to the disease or to its treatment. This information still is sparse in studies of diagnostic test performance, and improvement is awaited along this line of research.

The first meta-analyses of diagnostic testing of infectious diseases the authors found is dated 1992. Since then, the number of published articles has increased, and those published in the past 3 years (2006–2008) equal the number of articles published in the previous 13 years (1992–2005). Therefore, it is conceivable that the number will increase significantly in the near future. The execution and reporting of systematic reviews of diagnostic tests need to be improved. The authors' assessment of meta-analyses of diagnostic tests in infectious diseases has underlined problems in several of the key steps of reviews, namely reporting detailed information about the study design, reference and index tests characteristics, and patient characteristics of the included primary studies, and to a lesser extent, in review methods.

ACKNOWLEDGMENTS

The authors thank Claudia Rimondo for helpful advice in preparing the manuscript.

REFERENCES

1. Deeks JJ. Systematic reviews in health care: systematic reviews of evaluations of diagnostic and screening tests. BMJ 2001;323(7305):157–62.
2. Begg CB. Biases in the assessment of diagnostic tests. Stat Med 1987;6(4): 411–23.
3. Irwig L, Bossuyt PMM, Glasziou P, et al. Designing studies to ensure that estimates of test accuracy are transferable. BMJ 2002;324(7338):669–71.
4. Bossuyt PMM, Reitsma JB, Bruns DE, et al. The STARD statement for reporting studies of diagnostic accuracy: explanation and elaboration. Ann Intern Med 2003;138(1):W1–12.
5. Whiting P, Rutjes AWS, Reitsma JB, et al. Sources of variation and bias in studies of diagnostic accuracy: a systematic review. Ann Intern Med 2004;140(3): 189–202.
6. Lijmer JG, Mol BW, Heisterkamp S, et al. Empirical evidence of design-related bias in studies of diagnostic tests. JAMA 1999;282(11):1061–6.
7. Sheps SB, Schechter MT. The assessment of diagnostic tests. A survey of current medical research. JAMA 1984;252(17):2418–22.
8. Deville WL, Buntinx F, Bouter LM, et al. Conducting systematic reviews of diagnostic studies: didactic guidelines. BMC Med Res Methodol 2002;2:9.
9. Irwig L, Tosteson AN, Gatsonis C, et al. Guidelines for meta-analyses evaluating diagnostic tests. Ann Intern Med 1994;120(10):667–76.
10. Schmid C, Chung M, Chew P, et al. Survey of diagnostic test meta-analyses. In: 12th Cochrane Colloquium, Ottawa; October 2–6, 2004.
11. Whiting P, Rutjes AWS, Dinnes J, et al. A systematic review finds that diagnostic reviews fail to incorporate quality despite available tools. J Clin Epidemiol 2005; 58(3):1–12.
12. Mallett S, Deeks JJ, Halligan S, et al. Systematic reviews of diagnostic tests in cancer: review of methods and reporting. BMJ 2006;333(7565):413.

13. Dinnes J, Deeks J, Kirby J, et al. A methodological review of how heterogeneity has been examined in systematic reviews of diagnostic test accuracy. Health Technol Assess 2005;9:1–128.
14. Reed WW, Byrd GS, Gates RH, et al. Sputum gram's stain in community-acquired pneumococcal pneumonia: a meta-analyses. West J Med 1996; 165(4):197–204.
15. Loy CT, Irwig LM, Katelaris PH, et al. Do commercial serological kits for *Helicobacter pylori* infection differ in accuracy: a meta-analyses. Am J Gastroenterol 1996;91(6):1138–44.
16. Mol BW, Dijkman B, Wertheim P, et al. The accuracy of serum chlamydial antibodies in the diagnosis of tubal pathology: a meta-analyses. Fertil Steril 1997;67:1031–7.
17. Koumans EH, Johnson RE, Knapp JS, et al. Laboratory testing for *Neisseria gonorrhoeae* by recently introduced nonculture tests: a performance review with clinical and public health considerations. Clin Infect Dis 1998;27(5):1171–80.
18. Roberts AP, Childs SM, Rubin G, et al. Tests for *Helicobacter pylori* infection: a critical appraisal from primary care. Fam Pract 2000;17(Suppl 2):S12–20.
19. Watson EJ, Templeton A, Russell I, et al. The accuracy and efficacy of screening tests for *Chlamydia trachomatis*: a systematic review. J Med Microbiol 2002; 51(12):1021–31.
20. Gisbert JP, Abraira V. Accuracy of *Helicobacter pylori* diagnostic tests in patients with bleeding peptic ulcer: a systematic review and meta-analyses. Am J Gastroenterol 2006;101(4):848–63.
21. Sarmiento OL, Weigle KA, Alexander J, et al. Assessment by meta-analyses of PCR for diagnosis of smear-negative pulmonary tuberculosis. J Clin Microbiol 2003;41(7):3233–40.
22. Pai M, Flores LL, Pai N, et al. Diagnostic accuracy of nucleic acid amplification tests for tuberculous meningitis: a systematic review and meta-analyses. Lancet Infect Dis 2003;3(10):633–43.
23. Cruciani M, Scarparo C, Malena M, et al. Meta-analyses of BACTEC MGIT 960 and BACTEC 460 TB, with or without solid media, for detection of mycobacteria. J Clin Microbiol 2004;42(5):2321–5.
24. Pai M, Flores LL, Hubbard A, et al. Nucleic acid amplifiaction tests in the diagnosis of tuberculous pleuritis: a systematic review and meta-analyses. BMC Infect Dis 2004;4:6.
25. Flores LL, Pai M, Colford JM Jr, et al. In-house nucleic acid amplification tests for the detection of Mycobacterium tuberculosis in sputum specimens: meta-analyses and meta-regression. BMC Microbiol 2005;3(5):55.
26. Morgan M, Kalantri S, Flores L, et al. A commercial line probe assay for the rapid detection of rifampicin resistance in *Mycobacterium tuberculosis*: a systematic review and meta-analyses. BMC Infect Dis 2005;5:62.
27. Pai M, Kalantri S, Pascopella L, et al. Bacteriophage-based assays for the rapid detection of rifampicin resistance in *Mycobacterium tuberculosis*: a meta-analyses. J Infect 2005;51(3):175–87.
28. Kalantri S, Pai M, Pascopella L, et al. Bacteriophage-based tests for the detection of *Mycobacterium tuberculosis* in clinical specimens: a systematic review and meta-analyses. BMC Infect Dis 2005;5:59.
29. Tuon FF, Litvoc MN, Lopes MI. Adenosine deaminase and tuberculous pericarditis–a systematic review with meta-analyses. Acta Trop 2006;99(1):67–74.
30. Steingart KR, Ng V, Henry M, et al. Sputum processing methods to improve the sensitivity of smear microscopy for tuberculosis: a systematic review. Lancet Infect Dis 2006;6(10):664–74.

31. Steingart KR, Henry M, Ng V, et al. Fluorescence versus conventional sputum smear microscopy for tuberculosis: a systematic review. Lancet Infect Dis 2006;6(9):570–81.
32. Riquelme A, Calvo M, Salech F, et al. Value of adenosine deaminase (ADA) in ascitic fluid for the diagnosis of tuberculous peritonitis: a meta-analyses. J Clin Gastroenterol 2006;40(8):705–10.
33. Steingart KR, Henry M, Laal S, et al. A systematic review of commercial serological antibody detection tests for the diagnosis of extrapulmonary tuberculosis. Thorax 2007;62(10):911–8.
34. Steingart KR, Henry M, Laal S, et al. Commercial serological antibody detection tests for the diagnosis of pulmonary tuberculosis: a systematic review. PLoS Med 2007;4(6):e202.
35. Daley P, Thomas S, Pai M. Nucleic acid amplification tests for the diagnosis of tuberculous lymphadenitis: a systematic review. Int J Tuberc Lung Dis 2007; 11(11):1166–76.
36. Menzies D, Pai M, Comstock G. Meta-analyses: new tests for the diagnosis of latent tuberculosis infection. Areas of uncertainty and recommendations for research. Ann Intern Med 2007;146(5):340–54.
37. Jiang J, Shi HZ, Liang QL, et al. Diagnostic value of interferon-gamma in tuberculous pleurisy: a metaanalyses. Chest 2007;131(4):1133–41.
38. Pai M, Zwerling A, Menzies D. Systematic review: T-cell-based assays for the diagnosis of latent tuberculosis infection: an update. Ann Intern Med 2008; 149(3):177–84.
39. Cruciani M, Marcati P, Malena M, et al. Meta-analyses of diagnostic procedures for *Pneumocystis carinii* pneumonia in HIV-1-infected patients. Eur Respir J 2002; 20(4):982–9, Review.
40. Pfeiffer CD, Fine JP, Safdar N. Diagnoses of invasive aspergillosis using a galactomannan assay: a meta-analyses. Clin Infect Dis 2006;42(10):1417–27.
41. Tuon FF. A systematic literature review on the diagnosis of invasive aspergillosis using polymerase chain reaction (PCR) from bronchoalveolar lavage clinical samples. Rev Iberoam Micol 2007;24(2):89–94, Review.
42. Mengoli C, Cruciani M, Barnes RA, et al. Performance of polymerase chain reaction for diagnosing invasive aspergillosis: systematic review and meta-analyses. Lancet Infect Dis 2009;9(2):89–96.
43. Owens DK, Holodniy M, McDonald TW, et al. A meta-analytic evaluation of the polymerase chain reaction for the diagnosis of HIV infection in infants. JAMA 1996;275(17):1342–8.
44. Colin C, Lanoir D, Touzet S, et al. Sensitivity and specificity of third-generation hepatitis C virus antibody detection assays: an analyses of the literature. J Viral Hepat 2001;8(2):87–95.
45. Kowalski J, Tu XM, Jia G, et al. A comparative meta-analyses on the variability in test performance among FDA-licensed enzyme immunosorbent assays for HIV antibody testing. J Clin Epidemiol 2001;54(5):448–61.
46. Blacksell SD, Doust JA, Newton PN, et al. A systematic review and meta-analyses of the diagnostic accuracy of rapid immunochromatographic assays for the detection of dengue virus IgM antibodies during acute infection. Trans R Soc Trop Med Hyg 2006;100(8):775–84.
47. Pai NP, Tulsky JP, Cohan D, et al. Rapid point-of-care HIV testing in pregnant women: a systematic review and meta-analyses. Trop Med Int Health 2007; 12(2):162–73.

48. Shaheen AA, Wan AF, Myers RP. FibroTest and FibroScan for the prediction of hepatitis C-related fibrosis: a systematic review of diagnostic test accuracy. Am J Gastroenterol 2007;102(11):2589–600.
49. Garduño-Espinosa J, Martínez-García MC, Rendón-Macías E, et al. [Diagnostic performance of immunologic tests in amebic liver abscess using receiver operating characteristic curves]. Rev Invest Clin 1992;44(3):373–82 [in Spanish].
50. Patel SR, Wiese W, Patel SC, et al. Systematic review of diagnostic tests for vaginal trichomoniasis. Infect Dis Obstet Gynecol 2000;8(5–6):248–57.
51. Wiese W, Patel SR, Patel SC, et al. A meta-analyses of the Papanicolaou smear and wet mount for the diagnosis of vaginal trichomoniasis. Am J Med 2000; 108(4):301–8.
52. Cruciani M, Nardi S, Malena M, et al. Systematic review of the accuracy of the ParaSight-F test in the diagnosis of *Plasmodium falciparum* malaria. Med Sci Monit 2004;10(7):MT81–8.
53. Marx A, Pewsner D, Egger M, et al. Meta-analyses: accuracy of rapid tests for malaria in travelers returning from endemic areas. Ann Intern Med 2005; 142(10):836–46.
54. Chappuis F, Rijal S, Soto A, et al. A meta-analyses of the diagnostic performance of the direct agglutination test and rK39 dipstick for visceral leishmaniasis. BMJ 2006;333(7571):723.
55. Littenberg B, Mushlin AI. Technetium bone scanning in the diagnosis of osteomyelitis: a meta-analyses of test performance. Diagnostic Technology Assessment Consortium. J Gen Intern Med 1992;7(2):158–64.
56. Huicho L, Campos M, Rivera J, et al. Fecal screening tests in the approach to acute infectious diarrhea: a scientific overview. Pediatr Infect Dis J 1996;15(6): 486–94.
57. Siegman-Igra Y, Anglim AM, Shapiro DE, et al. Diagnosis of vascular catheter-related bloodstream infection: a metaanalyses. J Clin Microbiol 1997;35(4): 928–36.
58. Gerdes LU, Jørgensen PE, Nexø E, et al. C-reactive protein and bacterial meningitis: a meta-analyses. Scand J Clin Lab Invest 1998;58(5):383–93.
59. Gorelick MH, Shaw KN. Screening tests for urinary tract infection in children: a meta-analyses. Pediatrics 1999;104(5):e54.
60. Engels EA, Terrin N, Barza M, et al. Meta-analyses of diagnostic tests for acute sinusitis. J Clin Epidemiol 2000;53(8):852–62.
61. Varonen H, Makela M, Savolainen S, et al. Comparison of ultrasound, radiography, and clinical examination in the diagnosis of acute maxillary sinusitis: a systematic review. J Clin Epidemiol 2000;53(9):940–8.
62. Devillé WL, Yzermans JC, van Duijn NP, et al. The urine dipstick test useful to rule out infections. A meta-analyses of the accuracy. BMC Urol 2004;2(4):4.
63. Safdar N, Fine JP, Maki DG. Meta-analyses: methods for diagnosing intravascular device-related bloodstream infection. Ann Intern Med 2005;142(6):451–66.
64. Uzzan B, Cohen R, Nicolas P, et al. Procalcitonin as a diagnostic test for sepsis in critically ill adults and after surgery or trauma: a systematic review and meta-analyses. Crit Care Med 2006;34(7):1996–2003.
65. Jones AE, Fiechtl JF, Brown MD, et al. Procalcitonin test in the diagnosis of bacteremia: a meta-analyses. Ann Emerg Med 2007;50(1):34–41.
66. Tang BM, Eslick GD, Craig JC, et al. Accuracy of procalcitonin for sepsis diagnosis in critically ill patients: systematic review and meta-analyses. Lancet Infect Dis 2007;7(3):210–7.

67. Kapoor A, Page S, Lavalley M, et al. Magnetic resonance imaging for diagnosing foot osteomyelitis: a meta-analyses. Arch Intern Med 2007;167(2):125–32.
68. Dinh MT, Abad CL, Safdar N. Diagnostic accuracy of the physical examination and imaging tests for osteomyelitis underlying diabetic foot ulcers: meta-analyses. Clin Infect Dis 2008;47(4):519–27.
69. Hwang SH, Oh HB, Choi SE, et al. [Meta-analyses for the pooled sensitivity and specificity of hepatitis B surface antigen rapid tests]. Korean J Lab Med 2008; 28(2):160–8 [in Korean].
70. Kim S, Oh HB, Cha CH, et al. [Quality evaluation of the performance study of diagnostic tests using STARD checklist and meta-analyses for the pooled sensitivity and specificity of third generation anti-HCV EIA tests]. Korean J Lab Med 2006;26(4):307–15 [in Korean].
71. Lau J, Zucker D, Engels EA, et alIn: Diagnosis and treatment of acute bacterial rhinosinusitis, 9. Rockville (MD): Agency for Health Care Policy and Research. Evidence Report/Technology Assessment; 1999.
72. Benninger MS, Sedory Holzer SE, Lau J. Diagnosis and treatment of uncomplicated acute bacterial rhinosinusitis: summary of the Agency for Health Care Policy and Research evidence-based report. Otolaryngol Head Neck Surg 2000;122(1):1–7.
73. Shaheen AA, Myers RP. Systematic review and meta-analyses of the diagnostic accuracy of fibrosis marker panels in patients with HIV/hepatitis C coinfection. HIV Clin Trials 2008;9(1):43–51.
74. Scott JD, Gretch DR. Molecular diagnostics of hepatitis C virus infection: a systematic review. JAMA 2007;297(7):724–32.
75. Evans R, Ho-Yen DO. Evidence-based diagnosis of toxoplasma infection. Eur J Clin Microbiol Infect Dis 2000;19(11):829–33.
76. Pai M, Riley LW, Colford JM Jr. Interferon-gamma assays in the immunodiagnosis of tuberculosis: a systematic review. Lancet Infect Dis 2004;4(12):761–76.
77. Dumler JS. Molecular diagnosis of Lyme disease: review and meta-analyses. Mol Diagn 2001;6(1):1–11.
78. Prandini N, Lazzeri E, Rossi B, et al. Nuclear medicine imaging of bone infections. Nucl Med Commun 2006;27(8):633–44.
79. Guidelines for laboratory evaluation in the diagnoses of Lyme disease. American College of Physicians. Ann Intern Med 1997;127(12):1106–8.
80. Tugwell P, Dennis DT, Weinstein A, et al. Laboratory evaluation in the diagnosis of Lyme disease. Ann Intern Med 1997;127(12):1109–23.
81. Hörman A, Korpela H, Sutinen J, et al. Meta-analyses in assessment of the prevalence and annual incidence of Giardia spp. and Cryptosporidium spp. infections in humans in the Nordic countries. Int J Parasitol 2004;34(12):1337–46.
82. Mase SR, Ramsay A, Ng V, et al. Yield of serial sputum specimen examinations in the diagnosis of pulmonary tuberculosis: a systematic review. Int J Tuberc Lung Dis 2007;11(5):485–95.
83. Attia J, Hatala R, Cook DJ, et al. Does this adult patient have acute meningitis? JAMA 1999;282(2):175–81.
84. Müller I, Brade V, Hagedorn HJ, et al. Is serological testing a reliable tool in laboratory diagnosis of syphilis? Meta-analyses of eight external quality control surveys performed by the German infection serology proficiency testing program. J Clin Microbiol 2006;44(4):1335–41.
85. Gatsonis C, Paliwal P. Meta-analyses of diagnostic and screening test accuracy evaluations: methodologic primer. AJR Am J Roentgenol 2006;187(2):271–81.

86. Whiting P, Rutjes AW, Reitsma JB, et al. The development of QUADAS: a tool for the quality assessment of studies of diagnostic accuracy included in systematic reviews. BMC Med Res Methodol 2003;3:25.
87. Moses LE, Shapiro D, Littenberg B. Combining independent studies of a diagnostic test into a summary ROC curve: data-analystic approaches and some additional considerations. Stat Med 1993;12(14):1293–316.
88. Deeks JJ. Systematic reviews of evaluations of diagnostic and screening tests. In: Egger M, Davey Smith G, Altman DG, editors. Systematic reviews in health care. Meta-analyses in context. 2nd edition. London: BMJ Books; 2001. p. 248–83.
89. Egger M, Davey Smith G, Schneider M, et al. Bias in meta-analyses detected by a simple, graphical test. BMJ 1997;315(7109):629–34.
90. Begg CB, Berlin JA. Publication bias and dissemination of clinical research. J Natl Cancer Inst 1989;81(2):107–15.
91. Arroll B, Schechter MT, Sheps SB. The assessment of diagnostic tests: a comparison of medical literature in 1982 and 1985. J Gen Intern Med 1988;3(5):443–7.

Meta-analyses on the Optimization of the Duration of Antimicrobial Treatment for Various Infections

Petros I. Rafailidis, MD, MSc, MRCP[a], Anastasios I. Pitsounis, MD[a],
Matthew E. Falagas, MD, MSc, DSc[a,b,*]

KEYWORDS

- Meta-analyses • Duration • Antibiotics • Treatment • Short
- Long • Infections • Optimisation

Thirteen relevant meta-analyses (MAs) were identified. A variety of infections were the focus in these MAs: acute bacterial meningitis in one, acute otitis media in one, acute bacterial sinusitis in one, streptococcal tonsillopharyngitis in two, infectious exacerbations of chronic bronchitis in two, community-acquired pneumonia (CAP) in two, acute pyelonephritis in one, acute cystitis in two, and brucellosis in one. The herein reviewed MAs indicate that a short-duration treatment seems to be as effective as a longer course of antibiotic treatment in such infections as acute otitis media, acute bacterial sinusitis, CAP, infectious exacerbations of chronic bronchitis, and acute pyelonephritis. In the case of acute cystitis, clinical success is not different in the comparators, whereas a better bacteriologic cure rate is evident in the long-duration regimens. In the case of streptococcal tonsillopharyngitis and brucellosis, patients receiving longer courses of antibiotics have better clinical and bacteriologic cure rates. MAs can have a decisive role to estimate the optimal duration of treatment for various infections with far-reaching implications for clinical practice. The duration of antibiotic treatment

The authors have no conflicts of interest and have not received any sponsorship for writing this article.
[a] Alfa Institute of Biomedical Sciences, 9 Neapoleos Street and Kifisias Avenue, 151 23 Marousi, Athens, Greece
[b] Department of Medicine, Tufts University School of Medicine, 136 Harrison Avenue, Boston, MA 02110, USA
* Corresponding author. Alfa Institute of Biomedical Sciences, 9 Neapoleos Street and Kifisias Avenue, 151 23 Marousi, Athens, Greece.
E-mail address: m.falagas@aibs.gr (M.E. Falagas).

Infect Dis Clin N Am 23 (2009) 269–276
doi:10.1016/j.idc.2009.01.009
0891-5520/09/$ – see front matter © 2009 Elsevier Inc. All rights reserved.

id.theclinics.com

can be shortened in a variety of common bacterial infections without compromising patients' outcomes.

The duration of antibiotic treatment is often a dilemma for physicians as to whether a short or a lengthier regimen is more appropriate. A longer than necessary duration of treatment is unwanted for several reasons. The longer the drug is administered to a patient, the greater the risk for toxicity. Recent data suggest that a significant number of patients taking antibiotics present to the emergency departments of hospitals with a variety of adverse events.[1] Moreover, longer treatment is more expensive to the patient and to the health care system. In addition, resistance of the microorganisms responsible for the infection may be more likely to develop when patients are exposed to longer courses of antibiotics;[2] antimicrobial resistance can increase the days of hospitalization, morbidity, or mortality.[3] Finally, patient compliance is another potential benefit of short-duration antibiotic regimens. It is mandatory to evaluate whether a shorter-duration antibiotic regimen for the treatment of a disease is as effective as a longer one and therefore preferable.

It is not surprising that a significant number of randomized control trials (RCTs) have been conducted to examine the optimal duration of antibiotic treatment for various infections. Conflicting results of these RCTs may only further perpetuate the question regarding the ideal duration of antibiotic treatment. This problem may be solved by the panorama of these studies, with the use of MAs. Specifically, the results of all the RCTs on each specific field can be examined, analyzed, and evaluated by the use of MAs.

LITERATURE REVIEW

In this study the Medline, Scopus, and Cochrane online medical databases were searched for MAs investigating RCTs that examined the duration of treatment for the respected diseases. This study is restricted to humans and articles written in the English language. Only MAs that included a comparison of the same antibiotic in both treatment groups (short-duration arm and long-duration arm), either as the only focus of the MA or at least in a subset analysis, were further reviewed. This approach was used because significant differences in pharmacokinetic properties (ie, half-time) of one antibiotic in comparison with another antibiotic may introduce heterogeneity in the comparison of short- versus long-duration antibiotic regimens. A total of 13 relevant MAs were retrieved: one for acute bacterial meningitis, one for acute otitis media, one for acute bacterial sinusitis, two for streptococcal tonsillopharyngitis, two for infectious exacerbations of chronic bronchitis, two for CAP, one for acute pyelonephritis, two for cystitis in women, and one for brucellosis.

RELEVANT META-ANALYSES
Acute Bacterial Meningitis

Karageorgopoulos and colleagues[4] have performed a MA to study the clinical effectiveness and safety of short duration of antimicrobial treatment versus long duration in acute bacterial meningitis. Five RCTs with an open-label design involving children (age range, 3 weeks–16 years) were included. No difference could be shown in the comparison of short-duration (4–7 days) with long-duration (7–14 days) treatment with intravenous ceftriaxone regarding the clinical outcomes of this MA. Specifically, there was no difference in the end-of-therapy clinical success (five RCTs; 383 patients; fixed effect model [FEM]; odds ratio [OR], 1.24; 95% confidence interval [CI], 0.73–2.11) or in the long-term neurologic complications (five RCTs; 367 patients; FEM; OR, 0.60; 95% CI, 0.29–1.27). In addition, long-term hearing impairment (four RCTs;

241 patients; FEM; OR, 0.59; 95% CI, 0.28–1.23) was not different in the two treatment arms. Total adverse events did not differ between the short and long comparators (two RCTs; 122 patients; FEM; OR, 1.29; 95% CI, 0.57–2.91).

Acute Otitis Media

Kozyrskyj and colleagues[5] examined in a MA short-duration versus long-duration antibiotic treatment administered to children (age, 4 weeks–18 years) with acute otitis media. It was examined whether less than 7 days of antibiotic treatment versus 7 days or more of antibiotic treatment was a better choice. The primary outcome in this MA was treatment failure defined as lack of clinical resolution or relapse or recurrence of acute otitis media during a period of 31 days after treatment start. In the subset analysis of RCTs that examined the same antibiotic administered in both arms, no statistical difference was found regarding the primary outcome in the comparison of the short-duration (administered for 5 days) and the long-duration (administered for 8–10 days) antibiotic regimens (five RCTs; 1832 patients; OR, 1.54; 95% CI, 1.21–1.95) for the 8- to 30-day period and (four RCTs; 1629 patients; OR, 1.25; 95% CI, 0.90–1.74) for the 20- to 30-day period.

Acute Bacterial Sinusitis

In the only MA in this field,[6] 12 RCTs (10 double-blinded) involving adult patients with radiologically confirmed acute bacterial sinusitis were included. There was no difference in the comparison of short-duration (3–7 days) with long-duration treatment (6–10 days) regarding clinical outcomes. Specifically, clinical success (12 RCTs; 4430 patients; FEM; OR, 0.95; 95% CI, 0.81–1.12) and relapses of symptoms and signs (five RCTs; 1396 patients; FEM; OR, 0.95; 95% CI, 0.63–1.42) were not different in the comparators. No difference was evident regarding bacteriologic efficacy (three RCTs; 511 microbial strains; FEM; OR, 1.30; 95% CI, 0.62–2.74). Adverse events were not different in the comparators (10 RCTs; 4172 patients; random effects model; OR, 0.88; 95% CI, 0.71–1.09). In contrast, in the subset analysis comparing 5- with 10-day regimens, adverse events were fewer with short-course treatment (five RCTs; 2151 patients; FEM; OR, 0.79; 95% CI, 0.63–0.98).

Streptococcal Tonsillopharyngitis

Two MAs examining the duration of treatment for streptococcal tonsillopharyngitis were retrieved. Casey and Pichichero[7] examined in their MA the bacterial and clinical cure rates of short-duration and long-duration antibiotic regimens in both children and adult patients. Five of the included 22 RCTs compared the same antibiotic administered in the treatment arms. Specifically, three studies compared cephalosporins in both treatment arms, administered for 5 days in the short arm and 10 days in the long arm, and two RCTs compared 5-day with 10-day penicillin regimens. There was no difference regarding the bacterial cure rate of the 5-day course cephalosporin therapy versus that of the 10-day course (three RCTs; 773 patients; OR, 0.70; 95% CI, 0.42–1.14). In contrast, the bacterial cure rate was significantly lower for the short (5-day) penicillin duration regimen (two RCTs; 309 patients; OR, 0.29; 95% CI, 0.13–0.63) in comparison with the long (10-day) penicillin regimen. Similarly, the clinical cure rate was lower with the short-duration penicillin regimen (OR, 0.28; 95% CI, 0.08–0.91).

Falagas and colleagues[8] studied 11 RCTs in patients with streptococcal (GAS) tonsillopharyngitis comparing short-duration (penicillin V [3–7 days], oral cephalosporins [5–7 days], intramuscular ceftriaxone [1 day], clindamycin [5 days], in five, four, one, and one RCTs, respectively) with long-duration treatment (7–10 days for oral agents, 3 days for ceftriaxone). The primary outcome of this MA was microbiologic eradication of GAS in the treatment arms of 5 to 7 days versus 10 days; this was worse for the short-duration comparators in the total study population (eight RCTs; 1607 patients; FEM; OR, 0.49; 95% CI, 0.32–0.74) and was also inferior in the subset analysis of children and adolescents (six RCTs; 1258 patients; FEM; OR, 0.63; 95% CI, 0.40–0.98). In subset analyses of the primary outcome, however, microbiologic eradication was lower only in patients who received penicillin V (three RCTs; 500 patients; OR, 0.36; 95% CI, 0.13–0.99) and not in those who received cephalosporins.

In addition, bacteriologic relapse (with the same type of GAS) was not different in the comparators (five RCTs; 981 patients; OR, 1.74; 95% CI, 0.88–3.46), whereas bacteriologic recurrence (with a different type of GAS) was more likely in the short-duration arm (three RCTs; 698 patients; OR, 3.02; 95% CI, 1.06–8.56). Clinical success was less likely in patients treated for 5 to 7 days versus those who were treated for 10 days (five RCTs; 1217 patients; OR, 0.49; 95% CI, 0.25–0.96). Adverse events did not differ between the comparators.

Chronic Bronchitis

In the case of chronic bronchitis, two MAs were retrieved. In the first of them, Falagas and colleagues[9] examined short-duration versus long-duration antibiotic treatment in seven RCTs enrolling adult 3083 patients with acute exacerbations of chronic bronchitis. This study was aimed to evaluate the comparative effectiveness and safety of short (5 days) and long (7 or 10 days) duration of treatment. The drugs in the RCTs used in this MA were β-lactams (cefixime); macrolides (clarithromycin); and quinolones (oxifloxacin, levofloxacin, grepafloxacin, gatifloxacin). No difference was found between the short-duration and long-duration treatment arms with regard to treatment success in intention-to-treat (relative risk [RR], 0.99; 95% CI, 0.95–1.03), clinically evaluable (RR, 0.99; 95% CI, 0.96–1.02), or microbiologically evaluable (RR, 0.98; 95% CI, 0.93–1.02) patients. Short-duration treatment was associated with fewer adverse events than the long-duration arm (RR, 0.84; 95% CI, 0.72–0.97). El Moussaoui and colleagues[10] performed a MA examining the role of short-duration versus long-duration treatment in acute exacerbations of chronic bronchitis; in a subset analysis including six RCTs, comparing the same antibiotic in both comparator arms (5 versus 7–10 days), they found no difference in clinical cure at early follow-up (OR, 0.93; 95% CI, 0.78–1.11).

COMMUNITY-ACQUIRED PNEUMONIA

Dimopoulos and colleagues[11] studied a total of seven RCTs for CAP (five RCTs in adults and two in children). Adults were treated with amoxicillin, cefuroxime, ceftriaxone, telithromycin, and gemifloxacin; children received amoxicillin. The duration of treatment was 3 to 7 days in the short-treatment arm for adults (3 days in children), whereas it was 7 to 10 days in the long-treatment arm for adults (5 days in children). No difference was found regarding clinical success at end of therapy (six RCTs; 5115 patients [1103 adults, 4012 children]; FEM; OR, 0.90; 95% CI, 0.75–1.08), clinical success at late follow-up, microbiologic success (409 patients; FEM; OR, 1.03; 95% CI, 0.52–2.05); relapses (4187 patients; FEM; OR, 1.15; 95% CI, 0.81–1.63), mortality (seven RCTs; 5438 patients; FEM; OR, 0.57; 95% CI, 0.23–1.43), adverse events (five RCTs; 3214 patients; FEM; OR, 0.90; 95% CI, 0.72–1.13), or withdrawals as a result of adverse events. No differences were found in subset analyses of adults or children treated with no more than 5-day short-course regimens versus at least 7-day long-course regimens.

Haider and colleagues[12] examined three RCTs involving 5763 children (age, 2–59 months) treated for nonsevere CAP either with a short-duration regimen (3 days) or a long-duration regimen (5 days) of either amoxicillin (administered to 4012 patients) or trimethoprim-sulfomethoxazole (1751 patients). Different durations of treatment produced similar results in terms of clinical cure (RR, 0.99; 95% CI, 0.97–1.01); failure (RR, 1.07; 95 CI%, 0.92–1.25) of the treatment; and rate of relapse (RR, 1.09; 95% CI, 0.83–1.42).

ACUTE PYELONEPHRITIS

Kyriakidou and colleagues[13] examined four RCTs for patients diagnosed with acute pyelonephritis. Short-duration treatment was regarded as 7 to 14 days and long-duration treatment as 14 to 42 days. The antibiotics compared were pivampicillin plus pivmecillinam, trimethoprim-sulfamethoxazole, ampicillin, cephalexin, and fleroxacin. Differences were not found between the short- and long-duration treatment of acute pyelonephritis in terms of clinical success (four RCTs; 199 patients; OR, 1.27; 95% CI, 0.59–2.70); bacteriologic efficacy (four RCTs; 199 patients; OR, 0.80; 95% CI, 0.13–4.95); relapse (reappearance of the same strain in urine culture; four RCTs; 199 patients; OR, 0.65; 95% CI, 0.08–5.39); and recurrence (reappearance of a different strain in urine culture; OR, 1.39; 95% CI, 0.63–3.06). Adverse events (OR, 0.64; 95% CI, 0.33–1.25) and withdrawals caused by them (OR, 0.65; 95% CI, 0.28–1.55) did not vary significantly in the comparators.

CYSTITIS IN WOMEN

Katchman and colleagues[14] examined short-duration versus long-duration antibiotic treatment in women with cystitis. A short-duration treatment was regarded as 3 days and a long one as 5 to 10 days. The antibiotics used where quinolones, β-lactams, and combinations of sulfonamides and trimethoprim. There was no difference in short-term (within 2 weeks of follow-up) symptomatic failure in the comparison of short with long duration (14 RCTs examining 2678 patients; RR, 1.16; 95% CI, 0.96–1.41). Similarly, no difference was found in the comparison of short with long duration of antibiotic treatment in the long-term (within 8 weeks following treatment) symptomatic failure (eight RCTs examining 2121 patients; RR, 1.17; 95% CI, 0.99–1.38). In contrast, bacteriologic cure rates were better with the long-duration treatment. Specifically, short- term (within 2 weeks of follow-up) bacteriologic cure rate was better for the long-duration arm (18 RCTs examining 3146 patients; RR, 1.37; 95% CI, 1.07–1.74). Also, long-term bacteriologic cure rate was better for the long-duration (within 8 weeks of follow-up) arm (13 RCTs; 2502 patients; RR, 1.47; 95% CI, 1.22–1.77). Adverse effects were more common in the long-duration group (17 RCTs; 3852 patients; RR, 0.31; 95% CI, 0.19–0.53). Lutters and Vogt-Ferrier[15] in a recent MA found no difference regarding the persistence of urinary tract infection in 208 elderly women studied in two RCTs, which received the same antibiotic in the short-duration and long-duration comparator arms (RR, 1.0; 95% CI, 0.12–8.57).

BRUCELLOSIS

Skalsky and colleagues[16] examined RCTs that addressed the efficacy of different treatment regimens for the treatment of children and adults with brucellosis. Short versus long duration of the same or similar treatment was a subset analysis (four RCTs, 1442 patients) of this MA. A period of therapy for less than 30 days was regarded as short in contrast to more than 6 weeks, which was regarded as long.

Overall failure was significantly more common with short-treatment duration (RR, 3.08; 95% CI, 1.01–9.38). Both therapeutic failure (RR, 3.02; 95% CI, 1.03–8.80) and relapse (RR, 1.70; 95% CI, 1.19–2.44) was significantly more common with the shorter duration, without significant heterogeneity.

DISCUSSION

The findings of this review of MAs indicate that the duration of antibiotic treatment can be shortened, without compromising patients' outcomes, for such infections as acute otitis, acute bacterial sinusitis, CAP, infectious exacerbations of chronic bronchitis, and acute pyelonephritis. In the case of acute cystitis, clinical success was also not different in the comparators, whereas a better bacteriologic cure rate was evident in the long-course regimens. In contrast, patients with streptococcal tonsillopharyngitis and brucellosis had better clinical and bacteriologic cure rates with longer antibiotic regimens.

Specifically, the review of MAs shows that if antibiotic treatment is warranted, its duration can be reduced to 3 to 5 days for the treatment of acute otitis media; to 3 to 7 days for acute bacterial sinusitis; to 3 to 7 days for CAP in adults (and to 3 days in children); to 5 days for acute infectious exacerbation of chronic bronchitis; and to 7 to 14 days for acute pyelonephritis. These represent a net benefit of decreased antibiotic treatment duration of at least 3 to 5 days less for acute otitis media; 3 days less for acute bacterial sinusitis; 2 to 3 days less for acute infectious exacerbation of chronic bronchitis; 3 to 4 days for CAP (2 days for children); and 7 to 28 days for acute pyelonephritis.

The particular benefit that MAs confer in trying to estimate the ideal duration of anti-microbial treatment is that they provide a holistic view of a scientific theme with the use of analysis of aggregated data. For example, some RCTs may show a benefit depending on the particular duration of treatment, whereas others may not because their sample size is small and they are underpowered to show a benefit, even if one would exist. These conflicting results provide no help to the physician, because they do not convey any succinct and practical message. More so, isolated data may eventually give a distorted picture of how long an antibiotic treatment should last; this false perception has an impact on patients' clinical outcome. It is crucial, if not imperative, to provide a synthesis of the available data of the RCTs by MA. Even in the case that the findings of MAs are in congruence with the results of most of the RCTs they examine, they corroborate the findings of these RCTs and strengthen their conclusions by providing more accurate mathematical analysis.

A methodologic issue of the analysis that has to be emphasized is that included were only studies that compared the same antibiotic in both treatment arms. It is indisputable that newer antibiotics (once-daily administered macrolides and respiratory fluoroquinolones) have a pharmacodynamic advantage and are well-established therapeutic options. A comparison of one antibiotic in one arm (ie, erythromycin with a half-time of 2 hours[17]) with an antibiotic with a multifold half-time (azithromycin with a half-time of 40 hours[17]), however, may introduce difficulties in the interpretation of the results because the exact duration could only be approximated theoretically by post hoc analyses. Probably the most accurate information would be derived from RCTs examining the same antibiotic in both treatment arms.

MAs examining the issue of appropriate duration are not devoid of limitations. A small number of RCTs, especially if these have a small number of patients, in a specific field may be underpowered to show a potential statistical difference. The quality of the included RCTs is also an additional important factor for the quality of the MA results.

In addition, some of the RCTs are performed with an open label design, which intro-duces a degree of bias. Another potential source of bias is that in some of the RCTs no data regarding mortality are presented or there is no or minimal mortality in the patient population. This means that the degree of severity of the infection is mild to moderate in most of the RCTs included. For example, in the RCTs included in the MA regarding acute bacterial meningitis minimal mortality was reported. This may be caused by selection bias, because the most severe forms of acute bacterial menin-gitis may not be included in the studies examining short-duration versus long-duration antibiotic treatment. Another limitation is that a variety of antibiotics are administered to patients in each of the MA arms. Subset analyses of specific antibiotics may provide an answer, but may decrease even more the sample size needed to show a potential difference. The authors sought to minimize the effect of this heterogeneity by at least comparing the same antibiotic in the two arms of the included RCTs. Furthermore, one must acknowledge that the definition of a short-duration antibiotic regimen and a long-duration antibiotic regimen are partially arbitrarily chosen from researchers. In some instances, there is a minimal interception of the short and long antibiotic regimens (ie, the upper limit of days in the short-duration arm of one RCT may be close or even equal to the lower limit of days of another RCT). In any case this tangential approximation of limits does not interfere significantly with the deduction of logical conclusions. More so, by using a nihilistic approach to negate the significance of MAs one may deprive the conveyance of a clear message to practicing physicians.

By decreasing the duration of treatment for common infections there are many advantages: better patient compliance, less adverse effects, and lower financial burden both on a patient and societal level. In addition, less pressure for selection for resistant bacterial strains is also a potential benefit, although this outcome is not always examined in RCTs. Further research in bacterial infections that require pro-longed antibiotic therapy, such as osteomyelitis, septic arthritis, or endocarditis, is a true challenge for modern medicine.

MAs regarding the duration of antimicrobial treatment in various types of infections have shown that the reduction of the duration of antibiotic treatment is possible for a significant number of common bacterial infections. The potential gains of the specific MAs for patients and the community have to be capitalized through a shift in medical practice to prescribing antibiotics, when indicated, for shorter durations.

REFERENCES

1. Mitka M. Emergency departments see high rates of adverse events from antibi-otic use. JAMA 2008;30:1505–6.
2. Foxman B, Ki M, Brown P. Antibiotic resistance and pyelonephritis. Clin Infect Dis 2007;45:281–3.
3. Cosgrove SE, Carmeli Y. The impact of antimicrobial resistance on health and economic outcomes. Clin Infect Dis 2003;36:1433–7.
4. Karageorgopoulos DE, Valkimadi PE, Kapaskelis A, et al. Short versus long dura-tion antibiotic therapy for bacterial meningitis: a meta-analysis of randomized controlled trials. Arch Dis Child, in press.
5. Kozyrskyj AL, Hildes-Ripstein GE, Longstaffe SE, et al. Treatment of acute otitis media with a shortened course of antibiotics. JAMA 1998;279:1736–42.
6. Falagas ME, Karageorgopoulos DE, Grammatikos AP, et al. Effectiveness and safety of short versus long duration of antibiotic therapy for acute bacterial sinus-itis: a meta-analysis of randomized trials. Br J Clin Pharmacol 2009;67:161–71.

7. Casey JR, Pichichero ME. Meta-analysis of short course antibiotic treatment for group A streptococcal tonsillopharyngitis. Pediatr Infect Dis J 2005;24:909–17.

8. Falagas ME, Vouloumanou EK, Matthaiou DK, et al. Effectiveness and safety of short-course vs long-course antibiotic therapy for group A β-hemolytic streptococcal tonsillopharyngitis: a meta-analysis of randomized trials. Mayo Clin Proc 2008;83:880–9.

9. Falagas ME, Avgeri SG, Matthaiou DK, et al. Short- versus long-duration antimicrobial treatment for exacerbations of chronic bronchitis: a meta-analysis. J Antimicrob Chemother 2008;62:442–50.

10. El Moussaoui R, Roede BM, Speelman P, et al. Short-course antibiotic treatment in acute exacerbations of chronic bronchitis and COPD: a meta-analysis of double-blind studies. Thorax 2008;63:415–22.

11. Dimopoulos G, Matthaiou DK, Karageorgopoulos DE, et al. Short- versus long-course antibacterial therapy for community-acquired pneumonia: a meta-analysis. Drugs 2008;68:1841–54.

12. Haider BA, Saeed MA, Bhutta ZA. Short-course versus long-course antibiotic therapy for non-severe community-acquired pneumonia in children aged 2 months to 59 months. Cochrane Database Syst Rev 2008;2:CD005976.

13. Kyriakidou KG, Rafailidis P, Matthaiou DK, et al. Short versus long course antibiotic therapy for acute pyelonephritis in adults: a meta-analysis of randomized controlled trials. Clin Ther 2008;30:1859–68.

14. Katchman EA, Milo G, Paul M, et al. Three-day vs longer duration of antibiotic treatment for cystitis in women: systematic review and meta-analysis. Am J Med 2005;118:1196–207.

15. Lutters M, Vogt-Ferrier NB. Antibiotic duration for treating uncomplicated, symptomatic lower urinary tract infections in elderly women. Cochrane Database Syst Rev 2008;3:CD001535.

16. Skalsky K, Yahav D, Bishara J, et al. Treatment of human brucellosis: systematic review and meta-analysis of randomised controlled trials. BMJ 2008;336:701–4.

17. Mulazimoglou L, Tulkens PM, Van Bambeke F. Macrolides. In: Yu VL, Edwards G, McKinnon PS, et al. editors. Antimicrobial therapy and vaccines. Pittsburgh (PA): Esun Technologies, LLC; 2005. p. 243–79.

Combination Antimicrobial Treatment Versus Monotherapy: The Contribution of Meta-analyses

Mical Paul, MD[a,b,*], Leonard Leibovici, MD[b,c]

KEYWORDS

- Synergism • Combination antibiotic treatment • Beta-lactam
- Aminoglycoside • *Pseudomonas aeruginosa* • Meta-analysis
- Systematic review

WHY COMBINATION THERAPY?

The rationale for combination therapy is based on in vitro observations. The main effect cited in favor of combination therapy is synergism. A second effect, which assumes increasing importance nowadays, is the prevention of emergence of resistant bacteria following exposure to antibiotics. Synergy exists when the bacteriostatic or bacteriocidic effect of a combination is greater than the sum of the effects of each individual antibiotic.[1] Quantitatively, synergy has been defined as a $2 \log_{10}$ or greater reduction in bacterial count after an overnight incubation with the combination as compared with that of each antibiotic alone.[2,3] The development of resistance is related to this concept: it is assumed that improved bactericidal efficacy will suppress growth of partially resistant subpopulations and prevent the emergence of newly resistant isolates.

Regardless of the interaction between the antibiotics, combination therapy broadens the spectrum of coverage compared with that achieved with each drug alone (unless there is 100% cross-resistance between the antibiotics in the combination).

[a] Unit of Infectious Diseases, Rabin Medical Center, Beilinson Campus, Jabotinsky 39, Petah Tikva 49100, Israel
[b] Sackler Faculty of Medicine, Tel-Aviv University, Jabotinsky 39, Petah Tikva 49100, Israel
[c] Department of Medicine E, Rabin Medical Center, Beilinson Campus, Jabotinsky 39, Petah Tikva 49100, Israel
* Corresponding author.
E-mail address: pil1pel@zahav.net.il (M. Paul).

Infect Dis Clin N Am 23 (2009) 277–293
doi:10.1016/j.idc.2009.01.004
0891-5520/09/$ – see front matter © 2009 Elsevier Inc. All rights reserved.

Conversely, combination therapy may carry disadvantages. Antagonism has been observed in vitro with certain antibiotic combinations, adverse events certainly are expected to increase, and the effect on the development of resistance development actually might be detrimental. Exposure of the patient and the environment to more than one class of antibiotics might increase the risk of carriage and transmission of multidrug-resistant bacteria such as *Acinetobacter, Pseudomonas,* or the recently described carbapenem-resistant *Klebsiella pneumonia.*[4–6]

Synergism has been shown in vitro for many antibiotic combinations and bacterial species. Beta-lactam–aminoglycoside combinations have synergistic activity against gram-negative bacteria, including *Pseudomonas aeruginosa, Klebsiella, Enterobacter, Escherichia coli,* and other Enterobacteriaceae.[7] These observations have been applied to clinical practice as combination therapy for empiric treatment of severe infections in the hospital, treatment of *Pseuomononas aeruginosa* bacteremia, and the management of febrile neutropenia. Synergism between cell-wall active agents (beta-lactams and glycopeptides) and aminoglycosides against *Staphylococcus aureus* is assumed in the treatment of endocarditis.[1,8,9] The long-recognized double beta-lactam synergy (mainly ceftriaxone and ampicillin) against *Enterococcus* has been introduced recently into clinical practice for the management of enterococcal endocarditis.[10,11]

The concept of synergism has been proven for specific types of infection. Combination therapy is used in clinical practice to enhance cure and prevent the development of resistance. Antiretroviral combination therapy has revolutionized the treatment of HIV and AIDS, for the first time offering long-term viral suppression and prevention of resistant mutant development.[12–14] The fact that noncompliance with only less than 5% to 10% of the treatment regimen may result in treatment failure and development of resistance further reinforces the concept.[15–17] Combination treatment has proven advantages in and is used for the treatment of tuberculosis and brucellosis.[18,19] Based on similar concepts of synergistic antibiotic activity, sequential rather than combination therapy has been advocated recently for treatment of *Heliobacter pylori.*[20] The synergistic combination of sulfamethoxazole and trimethoprim and, more recently, quinupristin-dalfopristin is used commonly.

This article focuses on combination therapy for infections commonly encountered in the hospital and on the contribution of systematic reviews and meta-analysis to the understanding of the overall clinical benefit and detriments associated with combination therapy.

IS CLINICAL PROOF NECESSARY? FROM THE LABORATORY TO EVIDENCE-BASED MEDICINE

Phenomena observed in the laboratory may not be replicated in the host. Laboratory methods to evaluate synergism, including the checkerboard method, killing curves, and disc or strip diffusion, all have in common the use of measured antibiotic concentrations administered at precise time points and tested against a standard inoculum of bacteria.

Antibiotic concentrations in the host are determined by the dose, volume of distribution, and elimination rate of the antibiotic.[3] Initially, the patient's age, weight, volume status, renal or hepatic function, and other individual patient characteristics affect the concentration of antibiotic achieved in blood. Other pharmacokinetic characteristics of specific antibiotics, such as sequestration in specific tissues, further complicate this equation. Only unbound drug is active in vivo; thus hypoalbuminemia commonly present during infections affects the concentration of the antibiotic that actually is active.

Furthermore, antibiotic activity is required at the site of infection. This activity, in turn, is determined by the amount of drug that is filtered from the vascular compartment to the infected tissue and the activity of the antibiotic at the site of infections. Aminoglycosides, for example, are relatively inactive in anaerobic and acidic environments because the first phase of their penetration into bacterial cells, the slow energy-dependent phase, is inhibited at low pH and anaerobic conditions.[19,21] Bacterial concentrations in the host obviously are highly variable, depending on the severity, type, and location of infection. These factors lead to the conclusion that phenomena observed in vitro cannot be assumed to occur straightforwardly in vivo. Clinicians should base their practice on empiric evidence showing an overall benefit to the individual patient.[22] Antibiotic combinations may be associated with adverse events that mitigate the clinical benefit of synergism. In antibiotic pharmacodynamics, even the basic benefit observed in vitro cannot be assumed to exist in vivo without empiric evidence.

WHAT ARE THE CLINICAL QUESTIONS AND HOW SHOULD THEY BE ANSWERED?

The questions are seemingly trivial: will synergistic antibiotic combinations improve the patient's outcome following an infection, and will these combinations prevent the development of resistance? The answer actually is more complex.

Consider the benefit of beta-lactam–aminoglycoside combinations for *Pseudomonas aeruginosa*. A direct clinical assessment of in vitro synergy would compare treatment with a beta-lactam versus treatment with the same beta-lactam combined with an aminoglycoside in patients who have *Pseudomonas aeruginosa* infections. However, outcomes are affected by the time of initiation of antibiotic treatment: the sooner, the better.[23–26] Thus, the use of the antibiotics being tested must be commenced empirically, before documentation of *Pseudomonas aeruginosa*. To test for synergistic activity against *Pseudomonas aeruginosa*, a clinical trial must recruit empirically a huge cohort of patients to assess outcomes among patients who have *Pseudomonas aeruginosa* infections. No such trial has been performed. Rather, clinical trials recruited a sample of patients who had sepsis, or even a sample more likely to be infected by *Pseudomonas aeruginosa,* and assessed outcomes for all patients assuming that the difference with regard to *Pseudomonas aeruginosa* applies to the full cohort. Even if this assumption is true, some patients in the cohort will have other infections or polymicrobial infections. Combination therapy broadens the spectrum of coverage; thus, in the full cohort, the intervention tests synergism as well as broad- versus narrower-spectrum empiric therapy. Should a comparison actually be made between a broad-spectrum beta-lactam versus a narrower-spectrum beta-lactam combined with an aminoglycoside, so that the empiric coverage afforded by monotherapy will equal that afforded by the combination?

Consider the best trial design: a randomized, controlled trial recruiting a huge sample of patients likely to have an infection caused by *Pseudomonas aeruginosa* and empirically given beta-lactam monotherapy or beta-lactam–aminoglycoside combination therapy, subsequently analyzing the subset of patients who have predefined, clinically documented infections caused by *Pseumononas aeruginosa* susceptible to the beta-lactam; or a trial recruiting patients when *Pseudomonas aeruginosa* is identified and using a sample large enough to adjust for empiric treatment. What are the outcomes and how are they measured? In the laboratory, one measures the presence and concentration of bacteria. Clinical practice is much more complicated. A patient's outcome probably is related in some degree to the concentration of bacteria causing infection, but by no means is this relationship simple. Adverse events, superinfection, *Clostridium difficile*, and background diseases affect and mask the rate of cure. The signs and symptoms used to define cure are nonspecific and imprecise. Therapeutic interventions other than antibiotic treatment (eg, supportive care, drainage, and other surgical interventions) have a crucial effect on the outcome. In addition, different combinations of beta-lactams and aminoglycosides might have different efficacy. It is difficult to imagine a single randomized clinical trial that could take all these variables into account and provide a solid answer.

THE CONTRIBUTION OF META-ANALYSIS: GENERAL CONCEPTS

The general concepts underlying meta-analysis in infectious diseases are addressed in a separate article by Leibovici and Falagas in this issue. Combination therapy is one of the clinical questions to which meta-analyses have made a significant contribution. The primary randomized, controlled trials assessing combination therapy did not always address the clinical question of synergism or evaluate combination therapy versus monotherapy. Many trials compared a new beta-lactam antibiotic versus the standard of care at that time, that is, beta-lactam–aminoglycoside combination therapy. A composite outcome (eg, treatment success without modification) usually was chosen to permit a feasible sample size that would show non-inferiority of the new drug (although older trials in this area did not perform formal sample-size calculations). No trials, either those assessing a newly marketed beta-lactam tested as monotherapy or those directly assessing the addition of an antibiotic to the same comparator, were adequately powered to show differences in outcomes that matter to the individual patient (eg, survival). Systematic reviews and meta-analyses have used the evidence accumulated during many years to generate strong clinical conclusions regarding the clinical effects of combination therapy, as discussed later.

Systematic reviews and meta-analyses most frequently include only randomized, controlled trials, because this is the design on which evidence-based medicine relies. The effects of monotherapy versus combination therapy have been addressed by many observational studies.[27–36] Meta-analysis of observational studies can be performed, either using the unadjusted raw numbers (eg, crude deaths among patients who received combination therapy versus deaths among patients who received monotherapy) or adjusted effect estimates (eg, adjusted odds ratios for mortality with combination therapy). The advantages and disadvantages of random versus nonrandom comparisons for combination therapy are detailed in **Table 1**. Because only random assignment can ensure comparability of the study groups, the most appropriate design to assess combination therapy is a randomized, controlled trial. Observational studies, however, probably reflect real-life situations more accurately and can assess easily large populations of patients with rare conditions, such as *Pseudomonas aeruginosa* bacteremia. Systematic reviews including nonrandomized studies can assess whether the effects in these trials are biased.

The question of synergism typically involves a selected group of patients (eg, patients who have infections caused by *Pseudomonas aeruginosa* or *Staphylococcus aureus* or patients who have endocarditis). Subgroup analysis in meta-analyses refers to the meta-analysis of outcomes occurring in a defined subgroup of patients. The comparison is a valid random comparison if the subgroups can be well defined (eg, patients who have endocarditis or *Pseudomonas aeruginosa* bacteremia) and when all patients in the subgroup are evaluated. If the study assesses a subjective selection of patients in subgroups, these comparisons no longer are randomized. Subgroup

Table 1
Advantages and disadvantages of random versus nonrandom trial designs assessing combination therapy versus monotherapy

Variable	Randomized, Controlled Trials	Nonrandomized Comparisons
Selection of patients	Restrictions on inclusion criteria result in the selection of lower-risk patients.−	The study can address all patients observed in clinical practice.+
Comparability of patients receiving monotherapy versus combination therapy	Should be completely comparable if adequate sequence generation and concealment are maintained.+	Likely incomparable, the choice reflecting disease severity, likelihood of resistant bacteria, and underlying conditions such as renal function.− Adjusted analyses cannot correct for all differences.
Addressing specific patient subgroup (eg, infections caused by *Pseudomonas aeruginosa*)	Small sample sizes likely. When treatment is assigned empirically, analysis is based on nonrandomized patient subgroups.−	Larger sample sizes can be addressed.+
Treatment regimen	Well-defined by protocol. Treatment modifications controlled. Per-protocol analysis.+	Variable beta-lactam and aminoglycoside administration schedules used; frequent changes likely.−
Outcome assessment	As defined by protocol. Should include all patients if intention-to-treat analysis is performed.+	Adequate, as defined by protocol, if performed prospectively.+ Retrospective studies may not be able to perform adequate outcome assessment.−
Sample size	Small and probably insufficient to answer the study question among specific patient subgroups (eg, patients who have *Pseudomonas aeruginosa* infection).−	Large samples can be analyzed with some power to assess the intervention in the target group of patients.+

Abbreviations: + sign for advantage; − sign for disadvantage.

meta-analysis can be performed only if the study originally reported the outcomes for patients with the characteristic defining the subgroup. Although not always formally analyzed in the original studies because of the small number of patients and events, these data sometimes can be found in the narrative description of patients in whom the outcome occurred (eg, an individual description of each case of demise). A different technique for overcoming the need for data reported as outcome per patient with risk factor involves meta-regression. In this method, the characteristic of interest is regressed against the effect estimate of the study, taking into account the weight (or precision) of the study. Random-effects meta-regression also can include in the model residual heterogeneity that is not explained by the characteristic studied. For example, rather than a meta-analysis of deaths among patients who had *Pseudomonas aeruginosa* bacteremia, the effect estimates for death among all patients in each study can be regressed against the incidence of *Pseudomonas aeruginosa* bacteremia in that study. A significant result indicates that this variable affects the comparison, and this effect can be quantified. Subgroup analysis is easier to interpret clinically than meta-regression, because a measure of benefit or harm is given for patients who have a specific condition.

BETA-LACTAM–AMINOGLYCOSIDE COMBINATION THERAPY FOR *PSEUDOMONAS AERUGINOSA* AND OTHER GRAM-NEGATIVE INFECTIONS

The authors conducted a systematic review and meta-analysis including all randomized, controlled trials that compared beta-lactam monotherapy versus beta-lactam–aminoglycoside combination therapy, administered as empiric therapy, to hospitalized non-neutropenic patients who had sepsis (64 trials) and in the empiric treatment of febrile neutropenia (68 trials).[37–40] In the subset of studies that compared the same beta-lactam in both trial arms, mortality was similar with monotherapy and with combination therapy. Among non-neutropenic patients (nine trials) the relative risk for death was 1.03 (95% confidence interval [CI], 0.77–1.39), and among neutropenic patients (six trials) mortality was lower with monotherapy, but the results did not reach statistical significance (relative risk [RR] 0.77, 95% CI, 0.53–1.11).[41] In the subset of studies comparing different beta-lactams, mortality was lower with the broader-spectrum beta-lactam monotherapy, but results did not reach statistical significance: among non-neutropenic patients (31 trials) the RR was 0.85 (95% CI, 0.71–1.01), and among neutropenic patients (33 trials) the RR was 0.91 (95% CI, 0.77–1.09).[38] Overall, adverse events were significantly fewer with monotherapy. The RR for nephrotoxicity was 0.30 (95% CI, 0.23–0.39, 45) among non-neutropenic patients (45 trials) and was 0.45 (95% CI, 0.35–0.57) among patients who had neutropenia (37 trials). Length of hospital stay is a highly relevant outcome to the individual patient; comparative rates were reported only in 4 of 64 trials of non-neutropenic patients that could not be pooled; and in 3 of 68 trials of neutropenic patients, in which the duration of hospital stay was shorter with monotherapy than with combination therapy using a different beta-lactam.

All studies primarily reported an outcome of clinical failure, which was defined as persistence of clinical signs of infection or the need for antibiotic modification. This outcome favored combination therapy over monotherapy with the same beta-lactams and favored monotherapy in the comparison of different beta-lactams, clearly suggesting the likelihood of physicians' modifying antibiotic treatment in these mostly or wholly open trials. Therefore, the present authors did not attribute clinical significance to the results of this outcome.

The subgroups of patients who had gram-negative and *Pseudomonas aeruginosa* infections were very small. Among non-neutropenic patients, for trials comparing broad-spectrum beta-lactam monotherapy versus equivalent-spectrum combination therapy, the RR for mortality with documented gram-negative infections was 1.25 (95% CI, 0.85–1.95). In febrile neutropenia (14 trials), the relative risks for mortality in gram-negative infections (14 trials) and *Pseudomonas aeruginosa* infections (eight trials) were 0.62 (95% CI, 0.35–1.12) and 0.73 (95% CI, 0.26–2.02), respectively. Further analyses of bacteremic infections and *Pseudomonas aeruginosa* infections could not be performed because of the lack of data.

Hospital-acquired pneumonia, mainly ventilator-associated pneumonia, is a specific instance in which the question of combination therapy is highly pertinent. Patients in the ICU are sicker and are more likely to die without the most effective antibiotic treatment, frequently are colonized by resistant bacteria, but also are more susceptible to renal failure and the development of resistance and their consequences. Aarts and colleagues[42] compiled all randomized, controlled trials of empiric antibiotic treatment for ventilator-associated pneumonia. Eleven trials were identified that compared any monotherapy versus combination therapy consisting of a beta-lactam combined with an aminoglycoside or a quinolone. The pooled RR for all-cause mortality in the comparison of broad-spectrum monotherapy versus combination therapy (eight trials) was 0.94 (95% CI, 0.76–1.16). Although no statistically significant difference was demonstrated, based on the upper limit of the 95% confidence intervals (1,16), the authors concluded that combination therapy is unlikely to carry a benefit for patients who have ventilator-associated pneumonia. Moreover, in the subgroup of patients who had hospital-acquired pneumonia in the authors' review comparing beta-lactam monotherapy versus beta-lactam–aminoglycoside combination therapy among non-neutropenic patients, the RR for mortality was 0.75 (95% CI, 0.54–1.05) in favor of monotherapy, mostly broad spectrum (unpublished analysis from Ref. 38).

Elphick and Tan[43] assessed the effects of combination therapy for patients who had cystic fibrosis. *Pseudomonas aeruginosa* infections are nearly universal among these patients (100% in five and 98% in one of the eight trials included in this review). Only trials comparing beta-lactam versus the same beta-lactam combined with an amino-glycoside were included (eight trials overall), and the outcomes were appropriately different from those chosen for the assessment of sepsis. Very few data could be combined, but no advantage could be shown for combination therapy with regard to lung function and clinical scores. Adverse events were not significantly different (these trials assessed children). Eradication of *Pseudomonas aeruginosa* at end of therapy was significantly higher with combination therapy (three trials) (RR 5.63, 95% CI, 2.12–14.94), but baseline susceptibility to the beta-lactam was not reported. The number of readmissions (two trials) also favored combination therapy. Preventing the development of resistance in the individual is of major importance among patients who have cystic fibrosis; however the change in *Pseudomonas aeruginosa* suscepti-bility from baseline to end of follow-up was reported only in a single trial (where a trend favoring combination therapy was observed).

Bliziotis and colleagues performed a meta-analysis comparing beta-lactam combined with ciprofloxacin versus beta-lactam combined with an aminoglycoside for patients who had febrile neutropenia. Although synergy between ciprofloxacin and beta-lactams for gram-negative bacteria has been reported,[44–47] the interactions were variably additive or synergistic, and there was significant strain variability, with only 20% to 50% of *Pseudomonas aeruginosa* strains showing synergism.[48] Amino-glycoside–beta-lactam combinations are synergistic in vitro against more strains than quinolone–beta-lactam combinations.[49] Thus, this meta-analysis provides a good platform to assess the net clinical benefit of synergism, using regimens with comparable spectra of coverage. All-cause mortality was lower with ciprofloxacin combination therapy (but results did not reach statistical significance) in trials comparing the same beta-lactam (odds ratio [OR] 0.88, 95% CI, 0.50–1.51), and over-all (OR 0.85, 95% CI, 0.54–1.35). Nephrotoxicity was significantly less common with ciprofloxacin combination therapy (OR 0.30, 95% CI, 0.16–0.59).

The development of resistance following treatment with monotherapy versus combi-nation therapy was assessed in the previously described meta-analyses and in a meta-analysis considering this issue specifically.[50] The development of resistance can be assessed by comparing the overall rate of superinfections (assuming that breakthrough infections that develop during antibiotic treatment are resistant to the antibiotics used for treatment), by superinfections caused specifically by bacteria resistant to the adminis-tered antibiotic(s), by the development of resistance among originally infecting bacteria, and by colonization with bacteria resistant to the antibiotic(s). This assessment requires the performance of surveillance cultures. Data regarding these outcomes were lacking from most trials comparing monotherapy versus combination therapy. Surveillance cultures for assessing the acquisition of resistant strains were not performed or were not reported comparatively in most trials. Among non-neutropenic patients who had sepsis (27 trials), there were no differences between monotherapy and combination therapy with regard to rates of any superinfection (RR 0.76, 95% CI, 0.57–1.01), the development of resistance to the beta-lactam among pretreatment isolates (nine trials) (RR 0.88, 95% CI, 0.54–1.45), or colonization by resistant bacteria (14 trials) (RR 0.85, 95% CI, 0.65–1.10), but in all comparisons there was a trend favoring monotherapy rather than combination therapy.[38] Among patients who had neutropenia (28 trials), only overall bacterial superinfection rates could be compiled from the reported data, and there was no difference between monotherapy and combination therapy (RR 1.00, 95% CI, 0.86–1.18).[39] Even among patients who had cystic fibrosis the data were scarce, with only two trials reporting on the isolation of resistant isolates of *Pseudomonas aeruginosa* following treatment.[43] In two trials, strains resistant to the aminoglycoside or the beta-lactam at end of follow-up (2–8 weeks following treatment) were less frequent with monotherapy, but results did not reach statistical significance (RR 0.44, 95% CI, 0.17–1.14).

Proponents of combination therapy might claim that combination therapy is necessary nowadays to provide a broader spectrum of coverage empirically. In combination therapy, however, the added coverage is achieved through treatment with a single aminoglycoside. Observational data suggest that single-aminoglycoside therapy may be suboptimal for the treatment of severe gram-negative infections. In a meta-analysis including mostly observational studies, overall mortality among patients who had *Pseudomonas aeruginosa* bacteremia was lower with combination therapy than with beta-lactam or aminoglycoside monotherapy (OR 0.50, 95% CI, 0.30–0.79).[51] When the analysis was limited to beta-lactam monotherapy versus combination therapy, however, the OR was 1.31 (95% CI, 0.62–2.79).[52] In a large prospective study assessing patients who had gram-negative bacteremia, the adjusted OR for mortality in patients given empiric treatment with aminoglycoside monotherapy as compared with beta-lactam monotherapy was 1.3 (95% CI, 0.8–2.0) among all patients and 1.9 (95% CI, 0.9–4.0) among patients who had neutropenia. The present authors tried to assess the effects of single-aminoglycoside treatment on sepsis and gram-negative infections in randomized, controlled trials.[53] The notable finding was the lack of randomized, controlled trials assessing single-aminoglycoside therapy for sepsis; 31 of the 37 trials included in the review included only patients who had urinary tract infections, and the median rate of clinical sepsis in all included trials was 18%. Overall, microbiologic failure was significantly more frequent with aminoglycoside monotherapy (RR 1.44; 95% CI, 1.21–1.72).

In summary, all meta-analyses uniformly show that combination therapy does not improve clinical outcomes as compared with beta-lactam monotherapy. Combination therapy results in a significantly higher rate of adverse events, mainly nephrotoxicity, among adults. Microbiologic efficacy and the development of resistant strains were assessed imperfectly. Only among children who had cystic fibrosis could a favorable trend be observed for combination therapy, based on very few trials. Among all patients, if a microbiologic benefit exists, it was not translated into a clinical benefit. Using beta-lactam–aminoglycoside combination therapy to broaden the spectrum of coverage empirically might be unjustified, because outcomes for patients are better when a single broad-spectrum beta-lactam is used, and single-aminoglycoside therapy might be less effective than other antibiotics for severe gram-negative sepsis.

In an era of increasing multidrug-resistant bacteria in hospitals, trials assessing antibiotic combinations of second-line, last-resort, antibiotics for these infections (eg, colistin) might be warranted.[54] Further trials comparing beta-lactam–aminoglycoside combination therapy versus monotherapy with the same beta-lactam are warranted only among patient subgroups in which the question is still applicable (eg, patients who have *Pseudomonas aeruginosa* bacteremia).

COMBINATION THERAPY FOR ENDOCARDITIS AND OTHER GRAM-POSITIVE INFECTIONS

Falagas and colleagues searched systematically for prospective comparative studies that compared beta-lactam monotherapy versus combination therapy using the same beta-lactam combined with an aminoglycoside.[55] The main finding of this review was the lack of clinical studies. Only three randomized, controlled trials and one prospective clinical study assessed combination therapy for *Staphylococcus aureus* endocarditis, and a single randomized, controlled trial examined the question among patients who had penicillin-susceptible streptococci. No randomized trial or prospective clinical study on the treatment of enterococcal endocarditis was identified.

The OR for all-cause mortality with monotherapy versus combination therapy was 0.59 (95% CI, 0.21–1.66) for all studies combined and was 0.69 (95% CI, 0.26–1.86) for the four studies that included patients who had *Staphylococcus aureus* endocarditis (with an OR less than 1 favoring monotherapy). Excluding the one nonrandomized trial resulted in lower ORs. The wide CIs for these comparisons reflect the small number of patients and outcomes: 257 patients overall with an unadjusted pooled mortality rate of 7.4%. A successful outcome without the need for surgery was achieved more frequently with monotherapy in the trial assessing patients who had streptococcal endocarditis and in two trials assessing patients who had *Staphylococcus aureus* endocarditis, but the numbers were too small for a meaningful analysis. There was no difference in the rate of relapse after treatment completion (OR 0.79, 95% CI, 0.15–4.29). Nephrotoxicity was significantly less frequent with monotherapy (OR 0.38, 95% CI, 0.16–0.88), with a number of patients needed to harm of seven (95% CI, 5–37).

The present authors searched for all randomized trials comparing beta-lactam monotherapy versus beta-lactam–aminoglycoside combination therapy for treatment of sepsis caused by gram-positive bacteria and found only one additional trial that recruited patients who had *Staphylococcus aureus* infections (mostly nonbacteremic).[38] The pooled RRs were in agreement with those reported by Falagas and colleagues.[55] In five trials, microbiologic failure, usually defined as the persistence of positive cultures, was similar for combination and monotherapy (RR 0.89, 95% CI, 0.47–1.69).

In summary, no prospective studies to date support the widespread use of combination therapy for gram-positive infections in general and for endocarditis in particular. Rather, where examined (endocarditis caused by penicillin-susceptible streptococci and methicillin-susceptible *Staphylococcus aureus*), monotherapy resulted in similar or better outcomes than combination therapy and in significantly lower rates of adverse events. The evidence is limited by the paucity of trials and small number of patients evaluated. Increasingly, infections of prosthetic devices caused by gram-positive bacteria are being treated, and these infections were not assessed at all.

Pending further evidence, clinicians are advised to follow the current guidelines for the treatment of endocarditis, bearing in mind that most recommendations are based on nonrandomized studies or expert opinion.[56–59] High-level evidence is limited to the recommendation for beta-lactam monotherapy for penicillin-susceptible streptococci (minimum inhibitory concentration, 0.12 mg/L) and methicillin-susceptible *Staphylococcus aureus*. Further randomized, controlled trials are needed to clarify whether patients are best served by combination therapy.

COMBINATION THERAPY FOR ABDOMINAL INFECTIONS

Abdominal infections are among the common reasons for the administration of antibiotic combinations in the hospital. Combination therapy for this indication is used mainly to provide a broader spectrum of coverage for polymicrobial infections. A frequent question in practice is which single or combination drug regimen should be preferred. Pertinent issues include the importance of covering enterococci empirically, the benefit, detriments and costs associated with aminoglycoside use for anti–gram-negative coverage, and the importance of including anti-anaerobe coverage. With these infections, the success of therapy without surgical complications requiring re-intervention might be an important outcome in addition to the assessment of mortality. Patients who died from causes unrelated to the abdominal infection or who experienced severe adverse events but resolved their primary infection were considered as treatment success in some of these trials,[60] undermining the relevance of this outcome to the individual patient (who does not care about the reason for an adverse outcome).

Matthaiou and colleagues[61] compiled four randomized, controlled trials and one prospective comparative study comparing ciprofloxacin–metronidazole versus beta-lactam–based regimens Mortality was not significantly different (OR 1.10, 95% CI, 0.71–1.69). Successful treatment, defined as resolution of infection without the need for additional surgical or medical treatment, was significantly higher with ciprofloxacin–metronidazole (OR 1.69, 95% CI, 1.20–2.39) overall and also in the analysis limited to randomized, controlled trials. Comparative length of hospital stay was reported in only two studies and was similar in the two arms in one study and was shorter with ciprofloxacin in the other study.

The same authors performed a meta-analysis of randomized, controlled trials comparing clindamycin–aminoglycoside combination therapy versus beta-lactam monotherapy for intra-abdominal infections.[62] In 19 trials, all-cause mortality was higher with combination therapy, but results did not reach statistical significance (OR 1.25, 95% CI, 0.74–2.11). In 28 trials, treatment success, as previously defined, was achieved less frequently with combination therapy, with a large and highly significant effect estimate (OR 0.67, 95% CI, 0.55–0.81). Interestingly, the overall rate of adverse events was similar for the two groups (OR 1.05, 95% CI, 0.80–1.37), but antibiotic-associated diarrhea was less common with clindamycin–aminoglycoside than with beta-lactams (OR 0.68, 95% CI, 0.46–1.00), whereas nephrotoxicity was more frequent with the combination therapy (OR 3.7, 95% CI, 2.09–6.57).

The broader question regarding the use of an aminoglycoside as the anti–gram-negative agent in antibiotic combinations for intra-abdominal infections was addressed in a Cochrane review.[63] Aminoglycosides were assessed in combination with anti-anaerobe antibiotics (clindamycin or metronidazole) and compared with beta-lactam–based (18 trials) or quinolone-based (one trial) regimens. All-cause mortality was reported in only five trials and favored the non-aminoglycoside arm (RR 2.03, 95% CI, 0.88–4.71); results did not reach statistical significance. Treatment success was significantly less common with aminoglycosides (19 trials) (RR 0.65. 95% CI, 0.46–0.92), as was microbiologic success (six trials) (RR 0.49, 95% CI, 0.31–0.76). Length of hospital stay also favored the comparator, with a significant half-day reduction in hospital stay (five trials) (weighted mean difference 0.57, 95% CI, 0.06–1.07). In this review aminoglycosides also were assessed in combination with penicillin–beta-lactamase inhibitor, penicillin plus an anti-anaerobe, and broad-spectrum penicillin plus an anti-anaerobe, each comparison consisting of only a single trial. All showed the same trend of lower mortality and treatment failure with non-aminoglycoside comparator regimens. The respective RRs of mortality for these comparisons were 0.85 (95% CI, 0.37–1.97), 0.23 (95% CI, 0.01–4.24), and 0.10 (95% CI, 0–1.99), respectively, with an RR of less than 1 in favor of the comparator.

In the present authors' review comparing beta-lactam monotherapy and beta-lactam–aminoglycoside combination therapy, the analysis limited to patients who had intra-abdominal infections favored beta-lactam monotherapy for all-cause mortality: RR = 0.52 (95% CI, 0.26–1.05) for broad-spectrum beta-lactam (eight trials) and RR = 0.91 (95% CI, 0.54–1.55) for the comparison of same beta-lactams (one trial) (unpublished analysis from Ref. 38).

In summary, meta-analyses assessing combination therapy for intra-abdominal infections show that aminoglycoside-based combination regimens may be inferior to those in which beta-lactams are used to cover gram-negative bacteria. Although the outcome of treatment success strongly disfavors aminoglycoside combination therapy, the authors of the Cochrane review correctly pointed out a possible bias in the assessment of this rather subjective outcome in trials comparing a new antibiotic against the traditional aminoglycoside-based regimen. The objective outcome of all-cause mortality supports this overall conclusion, however. The importance of coverage against enterococci and anaerobes has not been assessed expressly in meta-analyses.

ANTIFUNGAL THERAPY

Combination therapy for fungal infections, mainly invasive candidiasis and aspergillosis, currently is attracting much attention. These severe infections are associated with high mortality, current treatment options are limited, and single drugs frequently are fungistatic. In vitro studies have identified many interactions that are dependent on the specific antifungal agent and the fungal species.[64,65] Amphotericin B–azole combinations, both acting on the fungal cell membrane, have generally antagonistic effects, although synergism has been shown for amphotericin B and voriconazole or posaconazole against Aspergillus. The recently introduced echinocandins might be better candidates for combination therapy, because they have a different mechanism of action (inhibition of 1,3-b-glucan synthase required for cell wall formation). Synergism in vitro between caspofungin and amphotericin B or voriconazole has been shown against Aspergillus. Flucytosine, acting through a different mechanism (inhibition of fungal protein synthesis) has been shown to interact synergistically with amphotericin B against many fungal species and with azoles against Candida. The clinical implications of these findings are unclear. Adverse events may be increased with drug combinations or decreased if combination therapy allows lower dosing of the individual drugs. To complicate matters further, interactions may be concentration dependent, even in in vitro models.[66,67]

The present authors compiled the evidence from randomized, controlled trials on treatment regimens for invasive candidal infections.[68] Two trials were found comparing fluconazole versus amphotericin B–flucytosine combination therapy, and a single trial compared fluconazole versus amphotericin B–fluconazole combination therapy. For the three trials combined there was no difference in all-cause mortality (RR 0.98, 95% CI, 0.75–1.30). Clinical and microbiologic failure favored combination therapy (RR 1.33, 95% CI, 1.01–1.76 and RR 2.21, 95% CI, 1.45–3.35, respectively) (three trials for all comparisons; unpublished analysis from Ref. 66). The results of the single trial assessing amphotericin B–fluconazole combination therapy were

---

Box 1
Key points

1. In patients who have sepsis, beta-lactam-aminoglycoside combination therapy does not improve patient-related outcomes, including mortality, when compared with beta-lactam monotherapy.

2. In patients who have sepsis, broad-spectrum beta-lactam monotherapy is associated with improved outcomes when compared with similar-spectrum beta-lactam–aminoglycoside combination therapy.

3. Clinical evidence is lacking for patients who have serious gram-negative and *Pseudomonas aeruginosa* infections; currently there is no evidence to show that combination therapy improves patient-related outcomes in these infections.

4. Beta-lactam aminoglycoside combination therapy has not been shown to prevent the development of resistance that will have clinical implications for the individual patient.

5. Among patients who have cystic fibrosis, combination therapy might have some microbiological benefit that has not been shown to translate to improved patient-related outcomes.

6. Combination therapy for gram-positive infections and endocarditis is unsupported currently by evidence from randomized trials or prospective studies. The few existing data do not point at an advantage for combination therapy.

7. The few antifungal combinations tested in randomized, controlled trials were found to improve clinical and microbiologic outcomes but not survival. Primary and salvage combination therapy for invasive fungal infections currently rests on experience from observational studies.

8. Recent systematic reviews and meta-analyses have allowed the examination of these broad clinical questions. No answer was available before the conduct of these systematic reviews, despite the existence of many randomized, controlled trials. Both the answers given here and the ability identify areas where evidence is lacking are the result of systematic reviews and meta-analyses.

---

similar to those assessing amphotericin B–flucytosine, although most in vitro studies predicted antagonism of this combination against *Candida*.

Two small, open-label, randomized, controlled trials have been published comparing liposomal amphotericin B monotherapy versus liposomal amphotericin B combined with caspofungin. One trial compared high-dose liposomal amphotericin B monotherapy (10 mg/kg) versus low-dose liposomal amphotericin B (3 mg/kg) combination therapy for proven or probable invasive aspergillosis.[69] The other used low-dose liposomal amphotericin B (3 mg/kg) in both arms and assessed persistently febrile neutropenic allogeneic hematopoietic stem cell recipients.[70] Favorable response was observed more commonly with amphotericin B –caspofungin combination therapy in the two trials combined (RR 1.53, 95% CI, 1.11–2.13; unpublished analysis by the present authors). Mortality was reported in one trial that was not powered to detect differences in survival.[69] No systematic review has tried to compile the clinical evidence on invasive aspergillosis. Guidance for clinical practice will have to await further trials and their systematic reviews on combination therapy for fungal infections.

SUMMARY

Systematic reviews and meta-analyses have put into perspective the clinical implications of in vitro synergy (**Box 1**). Randomized, controlled trials are the cornerstone of evidence-based medicine. The trials included in the meta-analyses described in this article are the building blocks of evidence. Individual trials, however, were individually underpowered to address the broader clinical question and relevant patient-related outcomes. On the question of combination therapy, meta-analyses have shaped the complete picture. The interactions observed in vitro have not been shown to improve patient-related outcomes.

Authors of systematic reviews have the privilege of considering and selecting the clinical outcomes most relevant for the individual patient. Thus, all-cause mortality, rather than treatment failure with antibiotic modifications or infection-related mortality, has been selected for the assessment of patients who had severe gram-negative infections and febrile neutropenia. Mortality and relapse were assessed for patients who had endocarditis, and clinical and lung function scores were assessed for patients who had cystic fibrosis. The authors hope that the dissemination of these reviews will lead clinicians and researchers to consider primarily these outcomes when appraising or designing clinical research. These are the outcomes that clinicians target when treating the patient.

Systematic reviews have the virtue of a broad, systematic, and explicit search. In some areas, such as the use of combination therapy to treat gram-positive infections in general, and specifically to treat endocarditis and *Pseudomonas aeruginosa* bacteremia, the main contribution of the reviews was to show that current practice is based on very limited clinical evidence. This finding does not refute current practice but should serve to guide future trials and opens the possibility for a different choice of therapy when standard guidelines are difficult to implement. The fact that to date no evidence has been accrued for these infections is not surprising. The clinical question of combination therapy is of no major interest to pharmaceutical companies sponsoring most trials; the infections are rare; and the study design is complex. This gap in knowledge calls for a new trial paradigm: collaborative investigator-initiated, multi-center trials. When randomized, controlled trials are unfeasible, the use of novel methods for adjustments in observational studies, such as propensity analyses using large databases, might approximate the true effect of combination therapy in a wider patient population.

REFERENCES

1. Acar JF. Antibiotic synergy and antagonism. Med Clin North Am 2000;84(6): 1391–406.
2. Levison ME. Pharmacodynamics of antibacterial drugs. Infect Dis Clin North Am 2000;14(2):281–91.
3. Hessen MT, Kaye D. Principles of selection and use of antibacterial agents. In vitro activity and pharmacology. Infect Dis Clin North Am 2000;14(2):265–79.
4. Schwaber MJ, Klarfeld-Lidji S, Navon-Venezia S, et al. Predictors of carbapenem-resistant *Klebsiella pneumoniae* acquisition among hospitalized adults and effect of acquisition on mortality. Antimicrobial Agents Chemother 2008;52(3):1028–33.
5. Tacconelli E, Cataldo MA, De Pascale G, et al. Prediction models to identify hospitalized patients at risk of being colonized or infected with multidrug-resistant *Acinetobacter baumannii* calcoaceticus complex. J Antimicrob Chemother 2008;62(5):1130–7.
6. Falagas ME, Kopterides P. Risk factors for the isolation of multi-drug-resistant *Acinetobacter baumannii* and *Pseudomonas aeruginosa*: a systematic review of the literature. J Hosp Infect 2006;64(1):7–15.

7. Giamarellou H. Aminoglycosides plus beta-lactams against gram-negative organisms. Evaluation of in vitro synergy and chemical interactions. Am J Med 1986;80(6B):126–37.
8. Bouza E, Munoz P. Monotherapy versus combination therapy for bacterial infections. Med Clin North Am 2000;84(6):1357–89.
9. Le T, Bayer AS. Combination antibiotic therapy for infective endocarditis. Clin Infect Dis 2003;36(5):615–21.
10. Gavalda J, Len O, Miro JM, et al. Brief communication: treatment of Enterococcus faecalis endocarditis with ampicillin plus ceftriaxone. Ann Intern Med 2007; 146(8):574–9.
11. Gavarlda J, Len O, Miro J, et al. Efficacy of ampicillin plus ceftriaxone in the treatment of enterococcal endocarditis. Presented at the 48th Annual ICAAC/IDSA 46th Annual Meeting. Washington, DC, October 25–28, 2008.
12. Jordan R, Gold L, Cummins C, et al. Systematic review and meta-analysis of evidence for increasing numbers of drugs in antiretroviral combination therapy. BMJ 2002;324(7340):757–60.
13. Bartlett JA, DeMasi R, Quinn J, et al. Overview of the effectiveness of triple combination therapy in antiretroviral-naive HIV-1 infected adults. AIDS 2001; 15(11):1369–77.
14. Holtzer CD, Roland M. The use of combination antiretroviral therapy in HIV-infected patients. Ann Pharmacother 1999;33(2):198–209.
15. Paterson DL, Swindells S, Mohr J, et al. Adherence to protease inhibitor therapy and outcomes in patients with HIV infection. Ann Intern Med 2000;133(1):21–30.
16. Bangsberg DR, Perry S, Charlebois ED, et al. Non-adherence to highly active antiretroviral therapy predicts progression to AIDS. AIDS 2001;15(9):1181–3.
17. Bangsberg DR, Acosta EP, Gupta R, et al. Adherence-resistance relationships for protease and non-nucleoside reverse transcriptase inhibitors explained by virological fitness. AIDS 2006;20(2):223–31.
18. Skalsky K, Yahav D, Bishara J, et al. Treatment of human brucellosis: systematic review and meta-analysis of randomised controlled trials. BMJ 2008;336(7646):701–4.
19. Mandell G, Bennett J, Dolin R. Principles and practice of infectious diseases. 6th edition. Philadelphia: Elsevier; 2005.
20. Jafri NS, Hornung CA, Howden CW. Meta-analysis: sequential therapy appears superior to standard therapy for Helicobacter pylori infection in patients naive to treatment. Ann Intern Med 2008;148(12):923–31.
21. Bryan LE, Kwan S. Roles of ribosomal binding, membrane potential, and electron transport in bacterial uptake of streptomycin and gentamicin. Antimicrobial Agents Chemother 1983;23(6):835–45.
22. Sackett DL, Rosenberg WM, Gray JA, et al. Evidence based medicine: what it is and what it isn't. BMJ 1996;312(7023):71–2.
23. McGregor JC, Rich SE, Harris AD, et al. A systematic review of the methods used to assess the association between appropriate antibiotic therapy and mortality in bacteremic patients. Clin Infect Dis 2007;45(3):329–37.
24. Kuti EL, Patel AA, Coleman CI. Impact of inappropriate antibiotic therapy on mortality in patients with ventilator-associated pneumonia and blood stream infection: a meta-analysis. J Crit Care 2008;23(1):91–100.
25. Leibovici L, Shraga I, Drucker M, et al. The benefit of appropriate empirical antibiotic treatment in patients with bloodstream infection. J Intern Med 1998;244(5):379–86.
26. Fraser A, Paul M, Almanasreh N, et al. Benefit of appropriate empirical antibiotic treatment: thirty-day mortality and duration of hospital stay. Am J Med 2006; 119(11):970–6.

27. Arich C, Gouby A, Bengler C, et al. [Comparison of the efficacy of cefotaxime alone and the combination cefazolin-tobramycin in the treatment of enterobacterial septicemia]. Pathol Biol (Paris) 1987;35(5):613–5 [in French].
28. Carbon C, Auboyer C, Becq-Giraudon B, et al. Cefotaxime (C) vs cefotaxime + amikacin (C + A) in the treatment of septicemia due to enterobacteria: a multicenter study. Chemioterapia 1987;6(2 Suppl):367–8.
29. Chow JW, Yu VL. Combination antibiotic therapy versus monotherapy for gram-negative bacteraemia: a commentary. Int J Antimicrob Agents 1999;11(1):7–12.
30. Furno P, Bucaneve G, Del Favero A. Monotherapy or aminoglycoside-containing combinations for empirical antibiotic treatment of febrile neutropenic patients: a meta-analysis. Lancet Infect Dis 2002;2(4):231–42.
31. Hilf M, Yu VL, Sharp J, et al. Antibiotic therapy for Pseudomonas aeruginosa bacteremia: outcome correlations in a prospective study of 200 patients. Am J Med 1989;87(5):540–6.
32. Kuikka A, Valtonen VV. Factors associated with improved outcome of Pseudomonas aeruginosa bacteremia in a Finnish university hospital. Eur J Clin Microbiol Infect Dis 1998;17(10):701–8.
33. Leibovici L, Paul M, Poznanski O, et al. Monotherapy versus beta-lactam-aminoglycoside combination treatment for gram-negative bacteremia: a prospective, observational study. Antimicrobial Agents Chemother 1997;41(5):1127–33.
34. Mendelson MH, Gurtman A, Szabo S, et al. Pseudomonas aeruginosa bacteremia in patients with AIDS. Clin Infect Dis 1994;18(6):886–95.
35. Siegman-Igra Y, Ravona R, Primerman H, et al. Pseudomonas aeruginosa bacteremia: an analysis of 123 episodes, with particular emphasis on the effect of antibiotic therapy. Int J Infect Dis 1998;2(4):211–5.
36. Tapper ML, Armstrong D. Bacteremia due to Pseudomonas aeruginosa complicating neoplastic disease: a progress report. J Infect Dis 1974;130(Suppl 0):S14–23.
37. Paul M, Benuri-Silbiger I, Soares-Weiser K, et al. Beta lactam monotherapy versus beta lactam-aminoglycoside combination therapy for sepsis in immunocompetent patients: systematic review and meta-analysis of randomised trials. BMJ 2004;328(7441):668–72.
38. Paul M, Silbiger I, Grozinsky S, et al. Beta lactam antibiotic monotherapy versus beta lactam-aminoglycoside antibiotic combination therapy for sepsis. Cochrane Database Syst Rev 2006;(1):CD003344.
39. Paul M, Soares-Weiser K, Grozinsky S, et al. Beta-lactam versus beta-lactam-aminoglycoside combination therapy in cancer patients with neutropaenia. Cochrane Database Syst Rev 2003;(3):CD003038.
40. Paul M, Soares-Weiser K, Leibovici L. Beta lactam monotherapy versus beta lactam-aminoglycoside combination therapy for fever with neutropenia: systematic review and meta-analysis. BMJ 2003;326(7399):1111–5.
41. Leibovici L, Paul M. Aminoglycoside drugs in clinical practice: an evidence-based approach. J Antimicrob Chemother 2009;63(2):246–51.
42. Aarts MA, Hancock JN, Heyland D, et al. Empiric antibiotic therapy for suspected ventilator-associated pneumonia: a systematic review and meta-analysis of randomized trials. Crit Care Med 2008;36(1):108–17.
43. Elphick HE, Tan A. Single versus combination intravenous antibiotic therapy for people with cystic fibrosis. Cochrane Database Syst Rev 2005;(2):CD002007.
44. Bustamante CI, Wharton RC, Wade JC. In vitro activity of ciprofloxacin in combination with ceftazidime, aztreonam, and azlocillin against multiresistant isolates of Pseudomonas aeruginosa. Antimicrobial Agents Chemother 1990;34(9):1814–5.

45. Kanellakopoulou K, Sarafis P, Galani I, et al. In vitro synergism of beta-lactams with ciprofloxacin and moxifloxacin against genetically distinct multidrug-resistant isolates of *Pseudomonas aeruginosa*. Int J Antimicrob Agents 2008;32(1): 33–9.

46. Fish DN, Choi MK, Jung R. Synergic activity of cephalosporins plus fluoroquinolones against *Pseudomonas aeruginosa* with resistance to one or both drugs. J Antimicrob Chemother 2002;50(6):1045–9.

47. Pendland SL, Messick CR, Jung R. In vitro synergy testing of levofloxacin, ofloxacin, and ciprofloxacin in combination with aztreonam, ceftazidime, or piperacillin against *Pseudomonas aeruginosa*. Diagn Microbiol Infect Dis 2002;42(1):75–8.

48. Neu HC. Synergy and antagonism of combinations with quinolones. Eur J Clin Microbiol Infect Dis 1991;10(4):255–61.

49. Mayer I, Nagy E. Investigation of the synergic effects of aminoglycoside-fluoroquinolone and third-generation cephalosporin combinations against clinical isolates of *Pseudomonas spp*. J Antimicrob Chemother 1999;43(5): 651–7.

50. Bliziotis IA, Samonis G, Vardakas KZ, et al. Effect of aminoglycoside and beta-lactam combination therapy versus beta-lactam monotherapy on the emergence of antimicrobial resistance: a meta-analysis of randomized, controlled trials. Clin Infect Dis 2005;41(2):149–58.

51. Safdar N, Handelsman J, Maki DG. Does combination antimicrobial therapy reduce mortality in Gram-negative bacteraemia? A meta-analysis. Lancet Infect Dis 2004;4(8):519–27.

52. Paul M, Leibovici L. Combination antibiotic therapy for *Pseudomonas aeruginosa* bacteraemia. Lancet Infect Dis 2005;5(4):192–3 [discussion: 193–4].

53. Vidal L, Gafter-Gvili A, Borok S, et al. Efficacy and safety of aminoglycoside monotherapy: systematic review and meta-analysis of randomized controlled trials. J Antimicrob Chemother 2007;60(2):247–57.

54. Petrosillo N, Ioannidou E, Falagas ME. Colistin monotherapy vs. combination therapy: evidence from microbiological, animal and clinical studies. Clin Microbiol Infect 2008;14(9):816–27.

55. Falagas ME, Matthaiou DK, Bliziotis IA. The role of aminoglycosides in combination with a beta-lactam for the treatment of bacterial endocarditis: a meta-analysis of comparative trials. J Antimicrob Chemother 2006;57:639–47.

56. German guidelines for the diagnosis and management of infective endocarditis. Int J Antimicrob Agents 2007;29(6):643–57.

57. Baddour LM, Wilson WR, Bayer AS, et al. Infective endocarditis: diagnosis, antimicrobial therapy, and management of complications: a statement for healthcare professionals from the Committee on Rheumatic Fever, Endocarditis, and Kawasaki Disease, Council on Cardiovascular Disease in the Young, and the Councils on Clinical Cardiology, Stroke, and Cardiovascular Surgery and Anesthesia, American Heart Association: endorsed by the Infectious Diseases Society of America. Circulation 2005;111(23):e394–434.

58. Elliott TS, Foweraker J, Gould FK, et al. Guidelines for the antibiotic treatment of endocarditis in adults: report of the Working Party of the British Society for Antimicrobial Chemotherapy. J Antimicrob Chemother 2004;54(6):971–81.

59. Westling K, Aufwerber E, Ekdahl C, et al. Swedish guidelines for diagnosis and treatment of infective endocarditis. Scand J Infect Dis 2007;39(11-12): 929–46.

60. Bailey JA, Virgo KS, DiPiro JT, et al. Aminoglycosides for intra-abdominal infection: equal to the challenge? Surg Infect (Larchmt) 2002;3(4):315–35.

61. Matthaiou DK, Peppas G, Bliziotis IA, et al. Ciprofloxacin/metronidazole versus beta-lactam-based treatment of intra-abdominal infections: a meta-analysis of comparative trials. Int J Antimicrob Agents 2006;28(3):159–65.
62. Falagas ME, Matthaiou DK, Karveli EA, et al. Meta-analysis: randomized controlled trials of clindamycin/aminoglycoside vs. beta-lactam monotherapy for the treatment of intra-abdominal infections. Aliment Pharmacol Ther 2007; 25:537–56.
63. Wong PF, Gilliam AD, Kumar S, et al. Antibiotic regimens for secondary peritonitis of gastrointestinal origin in adults. Cochrane Database Syst Rev 2005;(2):CD004539.
64. Ostrosky-Zeichner L. Combination antifungal therapy: a critical review of the evidence. Clin Microbiol Infect 2008;14(Suppl 4):65–70.
65. Vazquez JA. Clinical practice: combination antifungal therapy for mold infections: much ado about nothing? Clin Infect Dis 2008;46(12):1889–901.
66. Meletiadis J, Stergiopoulou T, O'Shaughnessy EM, et al. Concentration-dependent synergy and antagonism within a triple antifungal drug combination against *Aspergillus* species: analysis by a new response surface model. Antimicrobial Agents Chemother 2007;51(6):2053–64.
67. Shalit I, Shadkchan Y, Samra Z, et al. In vitro synergy of caspofungin and itraconazole against *Aspergillus* spp.: MIC versus minimal effective concentration end points. Antimicrobial Agents Chemother 2003;47(4):1416–8.
68. Gafter-Gvili A, Vidal L, Goldberg E, et al. Treatment of invasive candidal infections: systematic review and meta-analysis. Mayo Clin Proc 2008;83(9):1011–21.
69. Caillot D, Thiebaut A, Herbrecht R, et al. Liposomal amphotericin B in combination with caspofungin for invasive aspergillosis in patients with hematologic malignancies: a randomized pilot study (Combistrat trial). Cancer 2007; 110(12):2740–6.
70. Groll AH, Young C, Schwerdtfeger R, et al. Randomized comparison of safety, tolerance and pharmacokinetics of caspofungin, liposomal amphotericin B and the combination of both in allogeneic hematopoietic stem cell recipients (CASLAMB trial). Presented at the 48th Annual ICAAC/IDSA 46th Annual Meeting; Washington DC, October 25–28, 2008.

Meta-analytical Studies on the Epidemiology, Prevention, and Treatment of Human Immunodeficiency Virus Infection

Paschalis I. Vergidis, MD[a], Matthew E. Falagas, MD, MSc, DSc[b,c], Davidson H. Hamer, MD[d,*]

KEYWORDS

• HIV • AIDS • Meta-analysis • Risk factors
• Epidemiology • Mother-to-child transmission
• Antiretroviral treatment

Since the description of the first acquired immunodeficiency syndrome (AIDS) cases and the identification of human immunodeficiency virus (HIV) as the cause of the disease, an abundance of studies have been conducted to evaluate its epidemiology, therapeutic options, and outcomes. Globally, there were an estimated 33 million people living with HIV infection in 2007.[1] As access to treatment has increased, the total number of deaths caused by AIDS has decreased. As research progressed, original data were combined in meta-analyses in an attempt to answer clinical questions and solidify the evidence applied into clinical practice.

[a] Boston Medical Center, Department of Medicine, Section of Infectious Diseases, One Boston Medical Center Place, Dowling 3N, Boston, MA 02118, USA
[b] Alfa Institute of Biomedical Sciences (AIBS), 9 Neapoleos Street, 151 23 Marousi, Athens, Greece
[c] Tufts University School of Medicine, Boston, MA, USA
[d] Departments of International Health and Medicine, Boston University Schools of Public Health and Medicine, Center for International Health & Development, Boston, MA, USA
* Corresponding author. Center for International Health and Development, Crosstown 3rd floor, 801 Massachusetts Avenue, Boston, MA 02118.
E-mail address: dhamer@bu.edu (D.H. Hamer).

Infect Dis Clin N Am 23 (2009) 295–308
doi:10.1016/j.idc.2009.01.013
0891-5520/09/$ – see front matter © 2009 Elsevier Inc. All rights reserved.

In this review article we summarize several meta-analyses that have been published since 2000. Searches were conducted using Medline and the Cochrane reviews database. Combinations of search terms such as HIV, AIDS, and meta-analyses were used to locate relevant literature. We focused our review on the following topics: risk factors for HIV acquisition, epidemiology in men who have sex with men (MSM), mother-to-child-transmission (MTCT), prognostic markers of disease progression, efficacy of antiretroviral treatment (ART), resistance testing, adherence, side effects of ART, and vaccine efficacy in HIV infection. Meta-analyses based on studies conducted in resource-limited settings were included in our review. Because of space limitations we have not included meta-analyses on interventions to reduce risk behavior; metabolic abnormalities; specific organ involvement (such as hematologic or gastrointestinal complications); and diagnosis, prophylaxis, and management of opportunistic infections.

RISK FACTORS FOR HIV ACQUISITION
Heterosexual Infectivity

Heterosexual infectivity estimates are heterogeneous and largely depend on several cofactors. Investigators analyzed data of 15 study populations including both longitudinal and cross-sectional data at the level of the individual and couple.[2] Infectivity differences, expressed as number of transmissions per 1000 contacts, were 8.1 (95% confidence interval [CI], 0.4–15.8) in uncircumcised versus circumcised men, and 6.0 (95% CI, 3.3–8.8) in individuals with genital ulcer disease compared with those without genital ulcers. Regarding the stage of disease, the differences in transmission were 1.9 (95% CI, 0.9–2.8) comparing late-stage to mid-stage cases, and 2.5 (95% CI, 0.2–4.9) comparing early-stage to mid-stage index cases.

Infectivity was weakly associated with age and geographic area. Limited data suggested that infectivity was higher for penile-anal versus penile-vaginal transmission. Data on viral load, viral subtype, and antiretroviral use were available in fewer than two study populations, thus these cofactors were not included in the analysis. Based on this meta-analysis, the commonly cited infectivity rate of one transmission per 1000 contacts represents serodiscordant couples with low prevalence of the aforementioned cofactors. It is noteworthy that HIV infectivity studies are difficult and costly to conduct for both logistical and ethical reasons.

In another systematic review, risk factors for HIV acquisition in sub-Saharan Africa were illustrated.[3] The analysis included 68 epidemiologic studies from 1986 to 2006 involving 17,000 infected individuals and 73,000 controls. Women who reported three or more sex partners had an odds ratio (OR) of 3.64 (95% CI, 2.87–4.62) of HIV acquisition versus women with 0-2 partners. Similarly men reporting three or more partners had an OR of 3.15 (95% CI, 2.08–4.78) compared with those with zero to two partners. The number of partners was grouped on the basis of lifetime partners or, if unavailable, on the number of partners over the last five or more years. The sexually transmitted infection (STI) most commonly associated with HIV infection was herpes simplex virus type 2 (HSV-2). The OR was 4.62 (95% CI, 2.85–7.47) in women and 6.97 (95% CI, 4.68–10.38) in men. Finally, about 7% of infected women reported having paid sex versus 3% of controls. The study showed that, even in high prevalence areas, high rates of partner change among heterosexuals (and especially paid sex) increase the risk of HIV acquisition.

Effect of Male Circumcision

The effect of male circumcision in reduction of female to male HIV transmission has been evaluated in several studies. The biologic basis of decrease in transmission risk may be explained by the high density of HIV target cells in the foreskin, mainly Langerhans cells and macrophages. In a meta-analysis of 27 studies in sub-Saharan Africa published up to April 1999 the crude relative risk (RR) of HIV infection was 0.52 (95% CI, 0.40–0.68) in circumcised versus uncircumcised men.[4] In 15 of these studies, after adjusting for confounding factors, such as age, sociodemographic factors, sexual behavior, condom use, and presence of STIs, the association was stronger with an adjusted RR of 0.42 (95% CI, 0.34–0.54). More recently, randomized controlled trials (RCTs) in Africa have confirmed that male circumcision reduces the risk of female-to-male transmission by 50% to 60%.[5–7]

The effect of male circumcision in MSM was studied in a meta-analysis of 15 observational studies that included 53,567 men, 52% of whom were circumcised.[8] The odds of being HIV infected was 14% lower among circumcised MSM compared with uncircumcised individuals, but this did not reach statistical significance (OR 0.86, 95% CI, 0.65–1.13). Similarly, there was no difference in an analysis restricted to MSM who were primarily engaged in anal insertive sex. No difference in the acquisition of other STIs was identified. Interestingly, there was a significant protective effect in studies conducted before the era of highly active antiretroviral therapy (HAART). This may be related to changes in risk behavior in the HAART era. A major limitation of this meta-analysis is that the included studies were observational in nature and most did not control for confounding variables. Thus the question of whether circumcision confers protection against HIV transmission in MSM remains open.

Role of STIs

The role of coexistent STIs in HIV acquisition has been widely studied. Eighteen cohort and nested case-control studies assessing the relationship between HIV and HSV-2 infection, as confirmed by serologic testing, were included in a meta-analysis.[9] There were 14 studies in men (nine in the general population and five among MSM) and 10 studies in women (four in the general population and 6 among high-risk sex workers). Both men and women with HSV-2 infection had an approximately threefold higher risk for HIV acquisition. Estimates were adjusted for age and sexual behavior. In the general population the adjusted RR was 2.7 for men (95% CI, 1.9–3.9) and 3.1 for women (95% CI, 1.7–5.6). All studies in men showed a positive association; however in high-risk women, RRs ranged from 0.5 to 6.3 with significant heterogeneity. Thus estimates from these studies should be interpreted with caution. In MSM the RR of HIV acquisition was lower than in the general population (RR 1.7; 95% CI, 1.2–2.4).

In a prior meta-analysis based on nine cohort and nested case-control studies with documented HSV-2 infection before HIV acquisition, the RR estimate was 2.1 (95% CI, 1.4–3.2).[10] In the same article, the investigators found in an analysis of 22 case-control and cross-sectional studies that the risk estimate was 3.9 (95% CI, 3.1–5.1), but the temporal sequence of the two infections could not be documented. These results suggested that controlling HSV-2 infection may decrease HIV transmission. However, a recent RCT showed that suppressive antiherpes therapy in HSV-2 seropositive women and MSM did not affect rates of HIV acquisition.[11]

In a meta-analysis of 23 studies, including a total of 30,739 women, bacterial vaginosis was associated with an increased risk of HIV acquisition.[12] The biologic basis of the increased risk may depend on a change in vaginal flora. Data were analyzed for the four incidence study populations and separately for the remaining 21 prevalence study populations. Studies were conducted in the United States, Thailand, and sub-Saharan Africa. The diagnosis was established using clinical criteria, Nugent's score (a Gram stain scoring system of vaginal secretions), or both. The RR of HIV acquisition was 1.61 (95% CI, 1.21–2.13) based on the HIV-incidence studies.

All but one of the prevalence studies showed a higher HIV seroprevalence in women with bacterial vaginosis, but the OR estimates were highly heterogeneous. Even though other STIs have been shown to increase the risk of HIV acquisition with a higher RR, the greater prevalence of bacterial vaginosis may result in similar attributable disease risk.

The role of the spermicide nonoxynol-9 (N-9) for prevention of STI transmission has been reviewed. In a meta-analysis of nine trials, including 5096 women, it was shown that N-9 did not confer protection against STIs.[13] Regarding HIV acquisition, a meta-analysis of four of the above RCTs demonstrated a RR of 1.12 (95% CI, 0.88–1.42) in women using the spermicide. On the other hand, the risk of genital lesions was higher among women receiving N-9 (RR 1.18, 95% CI, 1.02–1.36). Most lesions were in the vulva and their etiology was unclear. There was an association between these lesions and risk of HIV infection. Of note, the study included predominantly high-risk female sex workers and thus may not be generalizable.

HIV EPIDEMIOLOGY IN MEN WHO HAVE SEX WITH MEN

In a meta-analysis of 83 studies, which included 38 low- and middle-income countries in the Americas, Asia, Africa, and Eastern Europe, the global prevalence of HIV infection among MSM was investigated.[14] Data were stratified based on the prevalence of disease in the general population (very low prevalence, <0.5% of adults; low prevalence, 0.5%–1.0%; medium prevalence, 1.1%–5.0%; and high prevalence, >5%). In very low prevalence countries, the pooled OR for MSM transmission was 58.4 (95% CI, 56.3–60.6); in low-prevalence countries 14.4 (95% CI, 13.8–14.9); and in medium- to high-prevalence countries 9.6 (95% CI, 9.0–10.2). Because of the heterogeneity of the ORs of HIV infections across different countries, the value of the analysis lies in what it reveals about the overall trends of the epidemic. More specifically, the OR for MSM transmission in Central and Latin America was 33.3 (95% CI, 32.3–34.2); in Asia 18.7 (95% CI, 17.7–19.7); in Africa 3.8 (95% CI, 3.3–4.3) and in Eastern Europe only 1.3 (95% CI, 1.1–1.6). A limitation of the study lies in the fact that in many developing countries homosexuality is associated with social stigma and thus it may be difficult to identify the MSM population.

Investigators from the Centers for Disease Control and Prevention (CDC) attempted to explain the disparities of HIV infection among black and white MSM.[15] In a meta-analysis of 53 studies between 1980 and 2006 it was shown that behavioral risk factors do not explain the higher rates of HIV infection among black MSM. Specifically, black MSM reported fewer sex partners (OR 0.64, 95% CI, 0.45–0.92) and less overall substance use (OR 0.71, 95% CI, 0.53–0.97). No significant differences in reported unprotected anal intercourse, commercial sex work, or sex with known HIV-positive partners were identified. Of note, studies in the first decade of the epidemic demonstrated high rates of unprotected anal intercourse among black MSM.[16] This may have increased the background prevalence of HIV infection among black men. In the meta-analysis, STIs occurred more frequently among black MSM (OR 1.64, 95% CI, 1.07–2.53) and black MSM were less likely than white MSM to report taking ART (OR 0.43, 95% CI, 0.30–0.61).

MOTHER-TO-CHILD TRANSMISSION

Interventions shown to prevent MTCT include antiretroviral (ARV) prophylaxis, cesarean section, and avoiding breastfeeding. Conclusions regarding prevention of vertical transmission were drawn in a meta-analysis of 15 RCTs,[17] most of which were conducted in developing countries. In five placebo-controlled trials of zidovudine monotherapy, transmission risk was significantly reduced (pooled RR 0.57, 95% CI, 0.45–0.71). There was no significant effect on the incidence of stillbirth, premature delivery and risk of infant death. A meta-analysis of 10 RCTs conducted in Africa and published from 1999 to 2007 showed 10.6% transmission (95% CI, 8.6–13.1) at 4 to 6 weeks after birth in the setting of ARV use as compared with 21.0% transmission (95% CI, 15.5–27.7) for placebo.[18] In these trials different regimens were used ante-, intra-, or postpartum in the mother or newborn. Once the effectiveness of ARVs was established, the placebo arms of several trials were discontinued and later studies compared different regimens. Medications used included zidovudine, nevirapine, stavudine, and didanosine. The evidence is high grade as data were obtained from high-quality RCTs. Despite the heterogeneity of the studies, data regarding the treatment arms were robust.

Regarding the role of duration of membrane rupture in vertical HIV transmission, 15 prospective cohort studies conducted in Europe and North America were analyzed by the international perinatal HIV group.[19] Data for 4721 mother-child pairs with duration of ruptured membranes of 24 hours or less were analyzed. In a logistic regression model, four covariates were included: maternal CD4 count, mode of delivery (nonelective cesarean section, instrumented or noninstrumented vaginal delivery), period of ARV use (antepartum, intrapartum, neonatal, or none), and birth weight. After adjusting for these covariates, duration of ruptured membranes was significantly associated with transmission (OR 1.02, 95% CI, 1.01–1.04 for each 1-hour increment). Women with AIDS had a more pronounced increase in the risk. Of note, data on maternal HIV viral load were limited.

The risk of HIV transmission through breastfeeding was determined in a meta-analysis of nine randomized, placebo-controlled trials of 4085 children including 993 definitively infected children.[20] Of 539 children with known timing of infection, 42% had late postnatal transmission. The risk of transmission was found to be constant throughout the breastfeeding period and was associated with lower maternal CD4 count and infant male sex. Maternal age, parity, and birth weight were not associated with increased risk of postnatal transmission. The cumulative probability of transmission was 9.3% at 18 months. The overall risk was 8.9 transmissions per 100 child-years of breastfeeding. A longer duration of breastfeeding was associated with a higher probability of HIV transmission. All studies were conducted in urban settings and thus may have underestimated the risk in rural areas where breastfeeding continues for longer periods.

PROGNOSTIC MARKERS

In a meta-analysis of 16 RCTs, including 3146 participants, it was shown that both the CD4 count and viral load at 24 weeks after starting ART are significant independent prognostic markers of disease progression to AIDS or death.[21] In a meta-analysis of 30 prospective and retrospective studies, including 2370 patients, multivariate regression analysis showed that baseline CD4 count was correlated with virologic suppression at 6 and 12 months after initiating ART in treatment-naïve patients. However, baseline viral load did not correlate with virologic suppression.[22] Of note, treatment included two nucleoside reverse transcriptase inhibitors (NRTIs) plus nevirapine, indinavir, nelfinavir, or efavirenz.

Prognostic markers of disease progression in vertically infected children have been the matter of extensive research. In an international meta-analysis of eight studies, which included 574 infected children, the risk of disease progression to stage C was correlated with higher maternal viral loads at or close to delivery (OR 1.25, 95%

CI, 1.04–1.52).[23] This effect was more pronounced in the first 6 months of life. The effect on mortality was borderline (OR 1.26, 95% CI, 0.96–1.65). These effects were independent of maternal or infant treatment.

Genetic polymorphisms of chemokine and chemokine receptor genes have been studied as markers for disease progression. In an international meta-analysis of 10 studies, including 1317 children, CCR5-delta32 and CCR2-64I alleles showed a protective effect in the first years of infection.[24] The CCR5-delta32 allele was found in 4.8% of patients of European descent, and 1.4% of those of African descent. Neither of the alleles showed a significant protection for progression to AIDS overall. However, both alleles conferred time-dependent protection against death. More specifically, the CCR5-delta32 allele had a protective effect during the first 3 years of life. No protective effect was shown against death after progression to AIDS.

EFFICACY OF ANTIRETROVIRAL THERAPY
Efficacy in Treatment-Naïve Patients

Several studies have addressed the efficacy of different ARV regimens. During the past 10 to 15 years, the use of triple therapy was established as the standard of care. In an analysis of 12 randomized trials the OR for disease progression or death with triple therapy compared with double therapy was 0.62 (95% CI, 0.50–0.78).[25] Results of the immunologic and virologic response were consistent with the clinical outcomes. Another meta-analysis of multicenter RCTs addressed the outcome of treatment using two different regimens.[26] The pooled analysis showed that treatment containing two non-nucleoside reverse transcriptase inhibitors (NNRTIs) and a protease inhibitor (PI) was consistently more effective in suppressing HIV-1 viral load compared with two NRTIs alone (RR 3.44, 95% CI, 2.43–4.87). A notable limitation of the analysis was that the definition of viral suppression differed among the studies (eg, viral load <400 copies/mL, <200 copies/mL, and so forth) and individual-level data were not available.

In a meta-analysis of 23 clinical trials (published from 1994 through 2000) including 3257 treatment-naïve patients, the combination of two NRTIs with a PI, an NNRTI, or a third NRTI had comparable efficacy.[27] The most frequently used regimen was lamivudine, zidovudine, and indinavir. The percentage of patients with undetectable viral load (≤50 copies/mL) at week 48 was 46% (95% CI, 41%–52%) for the PI-based regimen, 51% (95% CI, 43%–59%) for the NNRTI-based regimen, and 45% (95% CI, 36%–54%) for the triple NRTI therapy. The weighted mean increase in CD4 count in all three regimens was 160 cells/mm^3 (95% CI, 146–175 cells/mm^3). There was a trend toward higher CD4 counts in the PI-based regimen; however, there was considerable overlap among the confidence intervals. Later studies, however, showed the inferiority of triple NRTI treatment.[28,29]

In another meta-analysis, investigators compared the initiation of treatment with an NNRTI versus a PI.[30] In 12 head-to-head RCTs, including 3337 patients, an NNRTI-based regimen was directly compared with a PI-based regimen in patients who had limited or no previous drug experience. Nine of the trials assessed efavirenz and three assessed nevirapine. Six different PIs were assessed. In three trials a ritonavir-boosted PI was assessed. In the direct meta-analysis, the NNRTI-based regimens were superior to the PI-based regimens in terms of virologic suppression (OR 1.60, 95% CI, 1.31–1.96). The difference was reduced in higher quality studies (blinded trials, trials reporting adequate allocation concealment methods, and trials with appropriate randomization), but it still favored the use of an NNRTI-based regimen. The difference was also attenuated in trials assessing the use of stavudine and didanosine, a regimen that is no longer recommended as initial treatment. There was no difference in death or disease progression (OR 0.87, 95% CI, 0.56–1.35) nor in withdrawal of treatment owing to adverse events (OR 0.68, 95% CI, 0.43–1.08). A significant limitation is that most of the trials did not include the coformulated lopinavir/ritonavir, but instead older PI-based regimens.

In this same article, an indirect comparison using 14 other trials, including 4042 patients, was conducted. Indirect estimates were calculated for ART with an NNRTI versus ART with a PI, adjusted by the results of their comparisons against a common intervention (two NRTIs). In six of these trials the use of two NRTIs was compared with the use of two NRTIs and an NNRTI. In eight trials the use of two NRTIs was compared with the use of two NRTIs and a PI. In these comparisons, the NNRTI-based regimen was associated with a worse outcome than the PI-based regimen in terms of virologic suppression (OR 0.26, 95% CI, 0.07–0.91). Most studies did not report adequate information on CD4 cell count changes. There were no differences in terms of death or disease progression (OR 1.28, 95% CI, 0.56–2.94) and withdrawals because of adverse events (OR 1.46, 95% CI, 0.66–3.24). The discrepancy between direct and indirect comparisons, presented above, is in accordance with previous studies suggesting that indirect comparisons may be unreliable for complex interventions.[31]

Notably, another indirect meta-analysis of triple-drug regimens showed that PI-based regimens were superior to NNRTI-based regimens including either delavirdine or nevirapine in terms of progression to AIDS or death as well as immunologic and virologic response in patients with advanced immunosuppression.[32] More specifically, the use of a PI-based regimen reduced clinical progression by 40% to 50%. The comparison was again indirect and the studies did not include efavirenz which is currently the most commonly used NNRTI in the developed world.

In a recent updated review of 53 trials (published from 1994 through 2004) including 14,264 patients, the combination of two NRTIs with a PI, an NNRTI, or a third NRTI were again compared.[33] Efavirenz-based regimens were most commonly used. At week 48, 64% of patients receiving an NNRTI-based or boosted-PI-based regimen had undetectable viral load (≤ 50 copies/mL). This was significantly higher than the percentage of patients with undetectable viral load receiving triple NRTI treatment (54%) or an unboosted PI (43%). The increase in CD4 count was significantly higher in patients taking a boosted PI (200 cells/mm^3). Pill count was not found to be a significant predictor of effectiveness in multivariate analyses in contrast to the previous review by the same study group.[27] This most recent analysis included more studies so the data are considered more robust.

Switching Regimen because of Side Effects

PIs are associated with metabolic abnormalities, including lipodystrophy and hyperlipidemia. In a meta-analysis of nine RCTs, 833 patients were switched from a PI-based regimen to a regimen including two NRTIs in addition to one of the following: abacavir, efavirenz, or nevirapine.[34] A total of 616 patients continued the PI. The switch to abacavir increased the risk of virologic failure compared with the PI-based regimen. Specifically, the risk ratio for virologic failure with abacavir was 2.56 (95% CI, 1.17–5.64). In the patients whose PI was changed to efavirenz, the risk ratio was 0.83 (95% CI, 0.36–1.91) and with nevirapine 0.54 (95% CI, 0.29–1.02). Of note, in patients where the PI was discontinued there was a trend toward lower cholesterol levels, but this was not significant. One of the limitations of this meta-analysis is that it included many trials, each of which had a relatively small sample size.

Efficacy of Treatment in Resource-Limited Settings

A meta-analysis of treatment efficacy, performed on 29 studies from 12 African countries, included either observational or cohort studies and involved mainly HIV-infected adults.[35] In 15 studies all patients were treatment-naïve; in nine studies, 74% were treatment-naïve; and in one study only 34% were treatment-naïve. In four papers ART status was not clear. The analyzed data included the combined results of both dual and triple regimens. At baseline the mean CD4 count was 141 cells/mm^3 and the mean viral load was 5.2log$_{10}$. This analysis provided evidence that ART increases the CD4 count from 3 months until 3 years. Most patients had an undetectable viral load (less than 400 copies/mL) at each analyzed time point (3, 6, 12, 18, 24 months, and more than 24 months). The weight of evidence in these studies was weak (III or IV). None of the studies were randomized nor did they have a control group. Nevertheless, the analysis provides evidence that ART can be used successfully in Africa. It was noted that cost of treatment and laboratory tests influenced the choice of the regimen.

Another meta-analysis of 10 observational studies addressed the efficacy of ART in resource-limited settings.[36] For the purposes of the analysis, the researchers grouped outcome data following initiation of treatment in the following intervals: months 3 to 4, 6, 12, 18, and 24. To define viral suppression, a viral load of less than 400 or 500 copies/mL was used. The mean proportion of patients with an undetectable viral load was 0.697 (95% CI, 0.582–0.812) at month 6, 0.573 (95% CI, 0.432–0.715) at month 12, and 0.634 (95% CI, 0.506–0.762) at month 18. These results are comparable to viral suppression rates in the developed world. Variability may have been introduced because these studies were conducted in different countries, mainly in Africa. In metaregression analysis, it was shown that availability of free laboratory testing did not account for significant variability in the results. However, provision of free ART accounted for the largest amount of variability. At 12 months, the mean proportion of patients with undetectable viral load was 30.5% higher in those who received free treatment compared with those who had to pay. This finding has significant implications in allocating resources in these countries.

ANTIRETROVIRAL RESISTANCE TESTING

In three meta-analytical studies the issue of resistance testing–directed therapy in treatment-experienced patients was addressed. The first meta-analysis was based on four RCTs on genotypic resistance testing (GRT), one RCT on phenotypic resistance testing (PRT), and one RCT on both genotypic and phenotypic testing.[37] The original studies were published between 1999 and 2001. The meta-analysis showed better virologic response in patients who were treated based on results of GRT. Based on four studies, at 6 months 38.8% of patients treated based on resistance testing had undetectable viral load, in contrast to only 28.7% of patients treated based on clinical decision (OR 1.6, 95% CI, 1.2–2.2). No significant benefit was shown with the use of PRT based on two studies (OR 1.1, 95% CI, 0.8–1.6). Inadequate detection of minority drug-resistant species with the assays used at the time may explain the relative lack of ability of PRT for guiding regimen change decisions.

Another meta-analysis was based on 10 RCTs published from 1999 through 2003.[38] In five studies GRT versus control was compared, and in four PRT versus control was compared. One study compared GRT with PRT. At 6 months 10% more patients treated based on GRT had undetectable viral load compared with empiric treatment (95% CI, 5%–16%). The benefit was greater for patients with higher baseline viral load. In addition, the benefit was more prominent in smaller trials, which suggests possible bias. Regarding PRT, virologic results were similar at 6 months. Of note, limited data were available regarding PRT. The authors suggested some explanations for the limited benefit of resistance testing, as shown in RCTs, despite the theoretical advantage of detecting resistance mutations or direct detection of the efficacy of ART to certain isolates. Patient adherence may be a significant confounding factor. In non-adherent patients, the benefit of testing may be lost. Variable pharmacokinetics may also affect treatment outcome. As knowledge advances, improvement in testing may offer greater benefits.

In the most recent meta-analysis, which was based on eight RCTs published between 1999 and 2002, similar results were obtained.[39] At 6 months, ART guided by resistance testing resulted in undetectable viral loads in 40.2% of patients as compared with 32.9% in patients treated empirically (pooled risk ratio 1.23, 95% CI, 1.09–1.40). Subgroup analysis showed greater benefit with GRT with expert interpretation. There was overlap among the studies used in the aforementioned analyses and the final conclusion is that GRT offers a benefit of small magnitude. There is insufficient evidence to support the use of PRT. This is in contrast to recent and older guidelines that strongly support the use of antiretroviral resistance testing in the case of virologic failure in treatment-experienced patients.

ADHERENCE TO ANTIRETROVIRAL THERAPY

Thirty-one studies from North America, with a total of 17,573 patients, and 27 studies from sub-Saharan Africa, with a total of 12,116 patients in 12 countries, were included in a meta-analysis assessing adherence to ART.[40] Different adherence threshold measurements were used in each study (ranging from 80% to 100%). The combined adherence estimate was 64%. In the North American studies published after 1998, adherence was assessed by self-report in 71% of patients and the pooled estimate of adequate adherence, variously defined in different studies, was 55% (95% CI, 49%–62%). In the African studies published after 2002, adherence was assessed by self-report in 66% of patients and the pooled estimate was 77% (95% CI, 68%–85%). The difference between the two continents may be related to the complexity of regimens used in North America. Moreover, patients included in African studies were followed early during therapy and experienced dramatic improvement in their health status, a fact that may have affected adherence.

INTERVENTIONS TO IMPROVE ADHERENCE

Several behavioral interventions have been implemented to improve ART adherence. In a meta-analysis of 19 RCTs, including 1839 patients, the efficacy of these interventions was evaluated.[41] The most common intervention was one-on-one counseling, which was usually provided by health care providers (physicians or nurses). The median number of sessions was two and the median duration of each session was 60 minutes. Participants in the intervention arm were more likely to achieve 95% adherence compared with the control group (OR 1.50, 95% CI, 1.16–1.94). Interestingly, the effect was larger in studies that included an objective measurement of adherence (eg, pill counts, electronic drug monitoring) compared with self-reported adherence. The effect was homogeneous. Regarding undetectable viral load, based on data from 14 studies, the effect of the interventions nearly reached significance (OR 1.25, 95% CI, 0.99–1.59). The authors suggested that potency of the regimens or baseline viral resistance may have played a role in the outcome despite adequate adherence.

In a prior meta-analysis of 24 intervention studies (randomized, nonrandomized, and studies using a within-group design) published between 1996 and 2004, it was shown that interventions are efficacious in improving adherence.[42] Reminder systems and counseling were most frequently used. Success varied across the studies and the effect was significantly stronger only in those with known or anticipated adherence problems. The duration of intervention did not relate to the outcome. Most importantly, intervention efficacy did not decay with time (for up to 48 weeks of follow-up).

ADVERSE EVENTS ASSOCIATED WITH ART

Nevirapine has been associated with serious hepatotoxicity, particularly in women with a CD4 count above 250 cells/mm^3 and men with a CD4 count above 400 cells/mm^3. These data were based on a retrospective study in treatment-naïve patients.[43] In a meta-analysis of four RCTs including 410 patients who were virologically suppressed and were switched to a nevirapine-based regimen, the risk of hepatotoxicity within the first 3 months was 2% in patients with low CD4 count (as defined previously) and 4% in patients with high CD4 count.[44] The combined OR for hepatotoxicity or death was 0.77 (95% CI, 0.30–1.99) at any point during the study. A major limitation of this study is its small sample size; thus, differences in toxicity among the two study arms of around 6% may not have been detected. The meta-analysis shows that regimen simplification using nevirapine may be safely implemented. This change may be helpful particularly in resource-limited settings.

The use of ART led to a substantial decrease in the rate of MTCT. At the same time it raised several concerns regarding the safety of the antiretroviral medications. In European studies, ART, and more specifically the use of PIs, has been linked to premature delivery.[45] A meta-analysis of 14 studies with a large degree of heterogeneity was conducted.[46] Most studies used a gestational age of 37 weeks as the cut-off for prematurity. Based on data from five prospective cohort studies, ART did not increase the risk of premature delivery overall (OR 1.01, 95% CI, 0.76–1.34). In subgroup analyses no significant differences were found when monotherapy was compared with no treatment, combination treatment to no treatment, and monotherapy to combination treatment. PI-based regimens conferred an increased risk of prematurity compared with combinations that did not contain a PI (OR 1.35, 95% CI, 1.08–1.71). A randomized clinical trial in pregnant women who do not require ART for their own health would help in further elucidating the issue of prematurity.

VACCINE EFFICACY IN HIV INFECTION

The efficacy of influenza vaccination in HIV-infected adults was assessed in two meta-analyses of a small number of studies. The analysis included two prospective cohort studies, one RCT, and one case-control study. These were conducted in the United States, Japan, and Italy between 1995 and 2002 and different vaccine strains were used. Follow-up ranged from 3 months to 2 years. In the first analysis,[47] which included 646 participants, the risk difference was assessed to be −0.27 (95% CI, −0.42 to −0.11). The second analysis[48] differed in that the single case-control study was not included in the pooled estimates as it did not include prospective data. The pooled RR reduction for the development of systematic disease was 66% (95% CI, 36%–82%). However, the only RCT used in the analysis showed a risk reduction of 41% (95% CI, 2%–55%) and this may represent a more accurate estimate of vaccine efficacy. Thus further research with well-conducted RCTs in both developed and developing countries is warranted. The effect of the degree of immunosuppression on the efficacy of the vaccine also needs to be assessed.

Immunogenicity of the hepatitis A vaccine was assessed in a meta-analysis of eight studies published between 1994 and 2004, including a total of 458 participants.[49] This was an intention-to-treat analysis and patients lost to follow-up were assumed to be nonresponders. It was estimated that 64% of patients responded to the vaccine (95% CI, 52%–75%). Of note, response rates among HIV-negative controls were consistently 100%. There was significant heterogeneity among the studies. One study included pediatric patients. Removing this study from the analysis did not alter the results significantly. Interestingly, there was no significant difference in the responses between the pre- and post-HAART era. CD4 counts were not available in all studies. Further research is needed to evaluate vaccination strategies for nonresponders among HIV-infected individuals.

SUMMARY

Since the beginning of the epidemic, extensive research has been conducted in the field of HIV infection. Original research and subsequent meta-analyses have contributed to a better understanding of the disease. Epidemiologic research has shown, for example, that male circumcision reduces the risk of female-to-male transmission. Nevertheless, the question whether circumcision confers protection against HIV transmission in MSM remains open. Studies have shown a positive correlation between HIV and HSV-2 infection. However, a recent RCT found that suppressive antiherpes therapy did not affect rates of HIV acquisition.

Meta-analytical studies have advanced the knowledge on the global prevalence of infection among MSM, and disparities among black and white MSM. They have also solidified the evidence that the prophylactic use of ARVs reduces the risk of MTCT. It has also been shown that prolonged ruptured of membranes increases the rates of vertical transmission, and that breastfeeding is associated with postnatal transmission. In addition, prognostic markers of disease progression have been identified.

The introduction of ART has resulted in substantial improvements in morbidity and mortality for HIV-seropositive individuals. Several studies have defined recommended and alternative regimens. In a recent meta-analysis it was shown that in treatment-naïve patients, NNRTI-based or boosted-PI-based regimens are superior to triple NRTI or unboosted PI-based regimens in terms of virologic suppression. Recent evidence has demonstrated that ART can be successfully used in Africa with better outcomes in those receiving free treatment. Regarding resistance testing in treatment-experienced patients with virologic failure, GRT offers a benefit of small magnitude and there is insufficient evidence to support the use of PRT, in contrast to current guidelines. Meta-analyses have also shown that interventions to improve adherence can be successfully implemented. Finally, the efficacy of the influenza and hepatitis vaccine in the setting of HIV infection has been analyzed. As our knowledge advances, further questions will inevitably arise and will need to be addressed in well-conducted trials.

REFERENCES

1. Joint United Nations Programme on HIV/AIDS. Available at: http://data.unaids.org/pub/GlobalReport/2008/jc1510_2008_global_report_pp29_62_en.pdf. Accessed August, 2008.
2. Powers KA, Poole C, Pettifor AE, et al. Rethinking the heterosexual infectivity of HIV-1: a systematic review and meta-analysis. Lancet Infect Dis 2008;8(9): 553–63.

3. Chen L, Jha P, Stirling B, et al. Sexual risk factors for HIV infection in early and advanced HIV epidemics in sub-Saharan Africa: systematic overview of 68 epidemiological studies. PLoS ONE 2007;2(10):e1001.

4. Weiss HA, Quigley MA, Hayes RJ. Male circumcision and risk of HIV infection in sub-Saharan Africa: a systematic review and meta-analysis. AIDS 2000;14(15): 2361–70.

5. Auvert B, Taljaard D, Lagarde E, et al. Randomized, controlled intervention trial of male circumcision for reduction of HIV infection risk: the ANRS 1265 Trial. PLoS Med 2005;2(11):1112–22.

6. Bailey RC, Moses S, Parker CB, et al. Male circumcision for HIV prevention in young men in Kisumu, Kenya: a randomised controlled trial. Lancet 2007; 369(9562):643–56.

7. Gray RH, Kigozi G, Serwadda D, et al. Male circumcision for HIV prevention in men in Rakai, Uganda: a randomised trial. Lancet 2007;369(9562):657–66.

8. Millett GA, Flores SA, Marks G, et al. Circumcision status and risk of HIV and sexually transmitted infections among men who have sex with men: a meta-analysis. JAMA 2008;300(14):1674–84.

9. Freeman EE, Weiss HA, Glynn JR, et al. Herpes simplex virus 2 infection increases HIV acquisition in men and women: systematic review and meta-analysis of longitudinal studies. AIDS 2006;20(1):73–83.

10. Wald A, Link K. Risk of human immunodeficiency virus infection in herpes simplex virus type 2-seropositive persons: a meta-analysis. J Infect Dis 2002;185(1): 45–52.

11. Celum C, Wald A, Hughes J, et al. Effect of aciclovir on HIV-1 acquisition in herpes simplex virus 2 seropositive women and men who have sex with men: a randomised, double-blind, placebo-controlled trial. Lancet 2008;371(9630):2109–19.

12. Atashili J, Poole C, Ndumbe PM, et al. Bacterial vaginosis and HIV acquisition: a meta-analysis of published studies. AIDS 2008;22(12):1493–501.

13. Wilkinson D, Tholandi M, Ramjee G, et al. Nonoxynol-9 spermicide for prevention of vaginally acquired HIV and other sexually transmitted infections: systematic review and meta-analysis of randomised controlled trials including more than 5000 women. Lancet Infect Dis 2002;2(10):613–7.

14. Baral S, Sifakis F, Cleghorn F, et al. Elevated risk for HIV infection among men who have sex with men in low- and middle-income countries 2000-2006: a systematic review. PLoS Med 2007;4(12):1901–1.

15. Millett GA, Flores SA, Peterson JL, et al. Explaining disparities in HIV infection among black and white men who have sex with men: a meta-analysis of HIV risk behaviors. AIDS 2007;21(15):2083–91.

16. Peterson JL, Coates TJ, Catania JA, et al. High-risk sexual behavior and condom use among gay and bisexual African-American men. Am J Public Health 1992; 82(11):1490–4.

17. Suksomboon N, Poolsup N, Ket-Aim S. Systematic review of the efficacy of antiretroviral therapies for reducing the risk of mother-to-child transmission of HIV infection. J Clin Pharm Ther 2007;32(3):293–311.

18. Chigwedere P, Seage GR, Lee TH, et al. Efficacy of antiretroviral drugs in reducing mother-to-child transmission of HIV in Africa: a meta-analysis of published clinical trials. AIDS Res Hum Retroviruses 2008;24(6):827–37.

19. The International Perinatal HIV group. Duration of ruptured membranes and vertical transmission of HIV-1: a meta-analysis from 15 prospective cohort studies. AIDS 2001;15(3):357–68.

20. Coutsoudis A, Dabis F, Fawzi W, et al. Late postnatal transmission of HIV-1 in breast-fed children: an individual patient data meta-analysis. J Infect Dis 2004; 189(12):2154–66.
21. HIV Surrogate Marker Collaborative Group. Human immunodeficiency virus type 1 RNA level and CD4 count as prognostic markers and surrogate end points: a meta-analysis. AIDS Res Hum Retroviruses 2000;16(12):1123–33.
22. Skowron G, Street JC, Obee EM. Baseline CD4(+) cell count, not viral load, correlates with virologic suppression induced by potent antiretroviral therapy. J Acquir Immune Defic Syndr 2001;28(4):313–9.
23. Ioannidis JP, Tatsioni A, Abrams EJ, et al. Maternal viral load and rate of disease progression among vertically HIV-1-infected children: an international meta-analysis. AIDS 2004;18(1):99–108.
24. Ioannidis JP, Contopoulos-Ioannidis DG, Rosenberg PS, et al. Effects of CCR5-delta32 and CCR2-64I alleles on disease progression of perinatally HIV-1-infected children: an international meta-analysis. AIDS 2003;17(11):1631–8.
25. Jordan R, Gold L, Cummins C, et al. Systematic review and meta-analysis of evidence for increasing numbers of drugs in antiretroviral combination therapy. BMJ 2002;324(7340):757.
26. Enanoria WT, Ng C, Saha SR, et al. Treatment outcomes after highly active anti-retroviral therapy: a meta-analysis of randomised controlled trials. Lancet Infect Dis 2004;4(7):414–25.
27. Bartlett JA, DeMasi R, Quinn J, et al. Overview of the effectiveness of triple combination therapy in antiretroviral-naive HIV-1 infected adults. AIDS 2001; 15(11):1369–77.
28. Gallant JE, Rodriguez AE, Weinberg WG, et al. Early virologic nonresponse to tenofovir, abacavir, and lamivudine in HIV-infected antiretroviral-naive subjects. J Infect Dis 2005;192(11):1921–30.
29. Gulick RM, Ribaudo HJ, Shikuma CM, et al. Triple-nucleoside regimens versus efavirenz-containing regimens for the initial treatment of HIV-1 infection. N Engl J Med 2004;350(18):1850–61.
30. Chou R, Fu R, Huffman LH, et al. Initial highly-active antiretroviral therapy with a protease inhibitor versus a non-nucleoside reverse transcriptase inhibitor: discrepancies between direct and indirect meta-analyses. Lancet 2006; 368(9546):1503–15.
31. Bucher HC, Guyatt GH, Griffith LE, et al. The results of direct and indirect treatment comparisons in meta-analysis of randomized controlled trials. J Clin Epidemiol 1997;50(6):683–91.
32. Yazdanpanah Y, Sissoko D, Egger M, et al. Clinical efficacy of antiretroviral combination therapy based on protease inhibitors or non-nucleoside analogue reverse transcriptase inhibitors: indirect comparison of controlled trials. BMJ 2004;328(7434):249.
33. Bartlett JA, Fath MJ, DeMasi R, et al. An updated systematic overview of triple combination therapy in antiretroviral-naive HIV-infected adults. AIDS 2006; 20(16):2051–64.
34. Bucher HC, Kofler A, Nuesch R, et al. Meta-analysis of randomized controlled trials of simplified versus continued protease inhibitor-based antiretroviral therapy in HIV-1-infected patients. AIDS 2003;17(17):2451–9.
35. Hammond R, Harry TC. Efficacy of antiretroviral therapy in Africa: effect on immunological and virological outcome measures—a meta-analysis. Int J STD AIDS 2008;19(5):291–6.

36. Ivers LC, Kendrick D, Doucette K. Efficacy of antiretroviral therapy programs in resource-poor settings: a meta-analysis of the published literature. Clin Infect Dis 2005;41(2):217–24.
37. Torre D, Tambini R. Antiretroviral drug resistance testing in patients with HIV-1 infection: a meta-analysis study. HIV Clin Trials 2002;3(1):1–8.
38. Panidou ET, Trikalinos TA, Ioannidis JP. Limited benefit of antiretroviral resistance testing in treatment-experienced patients: a meta-analysis. AIDS 2004;18(16): 2153–61.
39. Ena J, Ruiz de Apodaca RF, Amador C, et al. Net benefits of resistance testing directed therapy compared with standard of care in HIV-infected patients with virological failure: a meta-analysis. Enferm Infecc Microbiol Clin 2006;24(4): 232–7.
40. Mills EJ, Nachega JB, Buchan I, et al. Adherence to antiretroviral therapy in sub-Saharan Africa and North America: a meta-analysis. JAMA 2006;296(6):679–90.
41. Simoni JM, Pearson CR, Pantalone DW, et al. Efficacy of interventions in improving highly active antiretroviral therapy adherence and HIV-1 RNA viral load. A meta-analytic review of randomized controlled trials. J Acquir Immune Defic Syndr 2006;43(Suppl 1):S23–35.
42. Amico KR, Harman JJ, Johnson BT. Efficacy of antiretroviral therapy adherence interventions: a research synthesis of trials, 1996 to 2004. J Acquir Immune Defic Syndr 2006;41(3):285–97.
43. Stern JO, Robinson PA, Love J, et al. A comprehensive hepatic safety analysis of nevirapine in different populations of HIV infected patients. J Acquir Immune Defic Syndr 2003;34(Suppl 1):S21–33.
44. De LE, Leon A, Arnaiz JA, et al. Hepatotoxicity of nevirapine in virologically suppressed patients according to gender and CD4 cell counts. HIV Med 2008;9(4): 221–6.
45. Thorne C, Patel D, Newell ML. Increased risk of adverse pregnancy outcomes in HIV-infected women treated with highly active antiretroviral therapy in Europe. AIDS 2004;18(17):2337–9.
46. Kourtis AP, Schmid CH, Jamieson DJ, et al. Use of antiretroviral therapy in pregnant HIV-infected women and the risk of premature delivery: a meta-analysis. AIDS 2007;21(5):607–15.
47. Atashili J, Kalilani L, Adimora AA. Efficacy and clinical effectiveness of influenza vaccines in HIV-infected individuals: a meta-analysis. BMC Infect Dis 2006;6:138.
48. Anema A, Mills E, Montaner J, et al. Efficacy of influenza vaccination in HIV-positive patients: a systematic review and meta-analysis. HIV Med 2008;9(1):57–61.
49. Shire NJ, Welge JA, Sherman KE. Efficacy of inactivated hepatitis A vaccine in HIV-infected patients: a hierarchical Bayesian meta-analysis. Vaccine 2006; 24(3):272–9.

Meta-analyses on Behavioral Interventions to Reduce the Risk of Transmission of HIV

Paschalis I. Vergidis, MD[a], Matthew E. Falagas, MD, MSc, DSc[b,c],*

KEYWORDS

- HIV • AIDS • Meta-analysis • HIV transmission
- Behavioral intervention

HIV is usually acquired through exposure to infected body fluids. Unprotected sexual activity and needle sharing in injection drug users (IDUs) are the main modes of transmission. In an attempt to promote safe practices, several behavioral interventions have been implemented at the individual, group, and community levels. In this review article we summarize several meta-analyses that have been published since 1999. Searches were conducted using Medline and the Cochrane reviews database. Combinations of search terms such as HIV, AIDS, and meta-analyses were used to locate relevant literature. We identified meta-analyses on behavioral interventions used to reduce the risk of HIV transmission. We structured the review using data on the following populations: heterosexuals (including adolescents), minority populations (ie, African Americans and Latin/Hispanics), men who have sex with men (MSM), IDUs, and people living with HIV.

INTERVENTIONS IN HETEROSEXUALS

In a meta-analytic review of 10 studies, involving 10,008 adults, a significant effect in reducing sex-related risks was shown (OR 0.81, 95% CI 0.69–0.95).[1] The results of the studies were published between 1988 and 1996. The average age of the participants

[a] Department of Medicine, Section of Infectious Diseases, One Boston Medical Center Place, Boston Medical Center, Dowling 3N, Boston, MA 02118, USA
[b] Alfa Institute of Biomedical Sciences (AIBS), 9 Neapoleos Str & Kifisias Ave, 151 23 Marousi, Athens, Greece
[c] Department of Medicine, Tufts University School of Medicine, Boston, MA 02111, USA
* Corresponding author. Alfa Institute of Biomedical Sciences (AIBS), 9 Neapoleos Str & Kifisias Ave, 151 23 Marousi, Athens, Greece.
E-mail address: m.falagas@aibs.gr (M.E. Falagas).

Infect Dis Clin N Am 23 (2009) 309–314
doi:10.1016/j.idc.2009.02.001
0891-5520/09/$ – see front matter © 2009 Elsevier Inc. All rights reserved.

was 26. Interventions were more effective when delivered to small groups rather than on an individual basis. The studies also showed a decrease in sexually transmitted infections (STIs) (six studies; OR 0.74, 95% CI, 0.62–0.89). The authors commented that the intervention characteristics responsible for the effect are difficult to determine. In a meta-analysis of studies targeting high-risk heterosexual women, behavioral interventions had a small but significant effect.[2] Some of the studies were conducted in STI clinics and drug treatment programs. The authors suggested that combining treatment for STIs and substance abuse with behavioral interventions may be beneficial in reducing the risk of transmission.

Behavioral interventions in sexually experienced adolescents, both in and out of the classroom, showed a decrease in the risk of unprotected sex (OR 0.66, 95% CI, 0.55–0.79), but no difference in the number of partners or incident STIs.[3] Interestingly, interventions with single ethnic groups out of class were more efficacious than in-class interventions with mixed ethnic groups. Another meta-analysis of controlled trials performed in adolescents showed an overall decrease in sexual risk.[4] Nevertheless, the effect was small in the two most critical outcomes, namely condom use (mean effect size 0.07, 95% CI, 0.03–0.11) and sexual frequency (mean effect size 0.05, 95% CI, 0.02–0.09). Interventions were more successful when condoms were provided or when active condom instruction and training was included.

INTERVENTIONS IN MINORITY POPULATIONS

In the single meta-analysis published on behavioral interventions targeting heterosexual African Americans only, it was again shown that the risk of unprotected sex is reduced (OR 0.75, 95% CI 0.67–0.84).[5] The analysis was based on 35 randomized controlled trials (RCTs) including 14,682 individuals, and the average follow-up was 3 months after the intervention. The results are comparable to findings of meta-analyses including other heterosexual population groups. Greater efficacy was found for interventions that included peer education. The risk of STI transmission was marginally decreased in an analysis of 10 trials (OR 0.88, 95% CI 0.72–1.07); however the effect was significant when the study with the lowest methodological quality was removed from the analysis.

Another meta-analysis showed that intervention groups with a higher percentage of Latinos/Latin Americans increased condom use to a lesser extent than groups with a lower percentage of Latinos.[6] Interventions in groups with higher percent of Latinos were more effective when conducted by lay community members and when including threat-inducing arguments. In a meta-analysis including Latinos only it was shown that interventions targeting either males or females were more successful in reducing sexual risk behavior as compared with interventions targeting both sexes.[7] This can be explained by the fact that Latino men and women often hesitate to discuss sexual matters in each other's presence.

In black and Hispanic males attending STI clinics, behavioral interventions were proven to be efficacious in a meta-analytic review of 14 studies (reduction in unprotected sex OR 0.77, 95% CI 0.68–0.87).[8] Moreover these interventions decreased the risk of incident STIs (OR 0.85, 95% CI 0.73–0.99). The authors concluded that culturally tailored interventions from ethnically matched deliverers were successful.

INTERVENTIONS IN MEN WHO HAVE SEX WITH MEN

In a Cochrane review, 58 interventions among MSM were summarized.[9] These were included in 44 studies of 18,585 participants. In each of these studies MSM constituted at least one third of the participants. In the meta-analysis, outcomes measured closest to 12 months after the intervention were included. Most studies were conducted in the United States. Interventions were also evaluated in the United Kingdom, Australia, New Zealand, Canada, Brazil, Russia, and Bulgaria. Sixteen interventions focused on HIV-positive populations. About 70% of the individuals were white and 30% were African American, Latino, Asian, or belonged to another ethnic group.

Forty interventions were compared with minimal or no prevention intervention. Eighteen interventions were delivered in small-group format, 11 in individual-level format, and 11 in community-level format. These interventions reduced self-reported unprotected anal sex by 27% (95% CI 15%–37%). This represents a decrease from a mean of 10.1 unprotected occasions to 7.4 over a 6-month period. In subgroup analysis the reduction was 20% among individual-level interventions, and 30% among small-group and community-level interventions. Effects were quite homogeneous among study groups. Interestingly, interventions were more effective among non-gay identified MSM. Another 18 experimental interventions were measured against standard prevention and included eight small-group and 10 individual-level interventions. These reduced unprotected anal sex by 17% (95% CI 5%–27%) beyond changes observed with standard interventions. This Cochrane review showed that interventions were most effective for white populations.

In a systematic review of the literature, barriers to implement the interventions in MSM were addressed.[10] These included geographic or social isolation. Innovative approaches, such as interventions over the telephone or having peer opinion leaders disseminate messages through social networks, were implemented in an attempt to overcome the aforementioned barriers. Based on analyses of four studies on individual-level interventions there was a significant effect size on unprotected anal intercourse (OR 0.57, 95% CI 0.37–0.87, n = 4689). For community-level interventions based on analyses of 12 studies, the effect size was also found to be significant (OR = 0.73, 95% CI 0.61–0.88, n = 2480). The Internet has been increasingly used over the past several years as a means to meet sexual partners. A meta-analysis of eight studies indicated that high-risk sexual behavior was more likely among MSM who sought partners online than those who did not (OR 1.68, 95% CI 1.18–2.40).[11]

INTERVENTIONS IN INJECTION DRUG USERS

People who inject drugs have an increased risk of HIV acquisition both through needle sharing and high-risk sexual behavior. A meta-analysis of 37 RCTs evaluating 49 interventions in IDUs was conducted.[12] The study included 10,190 participants with a mean age of 35 (range: 26 to 41 years). Fifty-three percent of the participants were in drug treatment programs. Eight-eight percent of the participants reported IDU within the preceding 3 months, 46% were sharing needles, and 29% traded sex for drugs. Interventions included both sex- and drug-related risk reduction. Clean syringes were not provided. Participants reduced IDU (effect size d = 0.08, 95% CI 0.03–0.13), increased condom use (d = 0.19, 95% CI 0.11–0.26), and reduced the frequency of trading sex for drugs (d = 0.33, 95% CI 0.10–0.57). Additionally, the interventions facilitated entry into a drug treatment program. Notably, condom use tended to decay over time. The authors suggest that additional strategies, such as booster sessions, may be beneficial.

In an earlier analysis, investigators examined the effect of interventions in illegal drug users.[13] Of 33 studies, 94% enrolled IDUs and 21% crack users. Interventions had a significant effect in reducing sexual risk (OR 0.86, 95% CI 0.76–0.98). Interventions conducted within drug abuse treatment programs also had a significant effect (d = 0.31, 95% CI 0.20–0.42) as shown in a meta-analysis of 18 studies.[14] Individuals involved in drug treatment programs have a reduction in sexual risk behavior. An important conclusion of the analysis is that interventions provided within a treatment program have an impact on risk reduction further and above that produced by drug treatment alone.

INTERVENTIONS IN HIV-INFECTED INDIVIDUALS

As HIV-infected patients experience longevity with antiretroviral treatment (ART), secondary HIV prevention is of paramount importance in reducing the transmission of the virus. People diagnosed with HIV tend to reduce their sexual risk behavior as shown in a meta-analysis of 27 studies.[15] Sexual practices were assessed before and after counseling and testing for HIV in 6558 individuals. The studies included 6685 untested participants. The HIV-infected group had a weighted mean effect size indicating significant sexual risk reduction relative to untested individuals. However, HIV-negative participants did not reduce their sexual risk behavior compared to untested individuals. Of note, effect sizes were heterogeneous indicating that participants' responses to counseling are complex.

Another meta-analysis of 12 controlled trials again showed decrease in the risk of unprotected sex in HIV-infected patients (OR 0.57, 95% CI, 0.40–0.82).[16] Results from two studies showed even a decrease in the risk of acquisition of chlamydia or gonorrhea (OR 0.20, 95% CI, 0.05–0.73). In a meta-analysis of 15 RCTs, including 3,234 individuals, intervention lowered the risk on condom use (mean effect size 0.16, 95% CI, 0.08–0.25) but not for the number of sexual partners (mean effect size –0.01, 95% CI, –0.16 to 0.14).[17] Interventions were more successful if the sample included fewer MSM or younger individuals. As explained above, other meta-analyses have shown that behavioral interventions are efficacious in presumably HIV-negative MSM. None of the studies in this meta-analysis provided motivational and behavioral skills to HIV-infected MSM. Thus further research on more comprehensive risk reduction programs in HIV-infected MSM is necessary.

Many infected patients receiving appropriate ART have a substantially decreased risk of HIV transmission because their viral load is low to undetectable. At the same time, some people may engage in unprotected sex believing that HIV is a less threatening disease because of the availability of ART. Based on meta-analyses of 25 studies, the prevalence of unprotected sex was not higher among those receiving ART compared with those not receiving treatment (OR 0.92, 95% CI 0.65–1.31).[18] No difference was found between those with detectable viremia compared with those with an undetectable viral load. Interestingly, unprotected sex was more common in people who agreed that the availability of ART reduces their concerns about safe sex practices regardless of their serostatus.

SYNTHESIS OF META-ANALYSES

In a synthesis of 18 meta-analytical studies, the effect of behavioral interventions was summarized.[19] Each of these meta-analyses targeted a specific population, namely adolescents,[3,4] heterosexual adults,[1,2] Latinos,[6,7] MSM,[10,20–22] drug users,[12–14] people with severe mental illness,[23] STI clinic patients[8,24] and HIV-infected individuals.[16,17] In the synthesis of the meta-analyses examining condom use, a median effect size of 1.34 (95% CI 1.13–1.64) was found. The weakest effect was found in adolescents and the strongest in MSM. Interventions delivered to specific groups, such as single racial groups of adolescents, or same-gender Latinos, were more efficacious than nonsegmented interventions. However, the effect of segmentation in same gender group was not reproduced in all meta-analyses.

SUMMARY

Different behavioral interventions have found to be efficacious in reducing high-risk sexual activity. Interventions have been evaluated in both original research and meta-analytic reviews. Most of the studies have shown that interventions are efficacious among different study populations. In adolescents, both in- and out-of-the-classroom interventions showed a decrease in the risk of unprotected sex. In African Americans, greater efficacy was found for interventions including peer education. For Latinos, effect was larger in interventions with segmentation in the same gender. Geographic and social isolation are barriers in approaching MSM. For IDUs, interventions provided within a treatment program have an impact on risk reduction above that produced by drug treatment alone. Finally, people diagnosed with HIV tend to reduce their sexual risk behavior. However, adherence to safe sex practices for life can be challenging. Relentless efforts for implementation of behavioral interventions to decrease high-risk behavior are necessary to decrease HIV transmission.

REFERENCES

1. Neumann MS, Johnson WD, Semaan S, et al. Review and meta-analysis of HIV prevention intervention research for heterosexual adult populations in the United States. J Acquir Immune Defic Syndr 2002;30(Suppl 1):S106–17.
2. Logan TK, Cole J, Leukefeld C. Women, sex, and HIV: social and contextual factors, meta-analysis of published interventions, and implications for practice and research. Psychol Bull 2002;128(6):851–85.
3. Mullen PD, Ramirez G, Strouse D, et al. Meta-analysis of the effects of behavioral HIV prevention interventions on the sexual risk behavior of sexually experienced adolescents in controlled studies in the United States. J Acquir Immune Defic Syndr 2002;30(Suppl 1):S94–105.
4. Johnson BT, Carey MP, Marsh KL, et al. Interventions to reduce sexual risk for the human immunodeficiency virus in adolescents, 1985–2000: a research synthesis. Arch Pediatr Adolesc Med 2003;157(4):381–8.
5. Darbes L, Crepaz N, Lyles C, et al. The efficacy of behavioral interventions in reducing HIV risk behaviors and incident sexually transmitted diseases in heterosexual African Americans. AIDS 2008;22(10):1177–94.
6. Albarracin J, Albarracin D, Durantini M. Effects of HIV-prevention interventions for samples with higher and lower percents of Latinos and Latin Americans: a meta-analysis of change in condom use and knowledge. AIDS Behav 2008;12(4):521–43.
7. Herbst JH, Kay LS, Passin WF, et al. A systematic review and meta-analysis of behavioral interventions to reduce HIV risk behaviors of Hispanics in the United States and Puerto Rico. AIDS Behav 2007;11(1):25–47.
8. Crepaz N, Horn AK, Rama SM, et al. The efficacy of behavioral interventions in reducing HIV risk sex behaviors and incident sexually transmitted disease in black and Hispanic sexually transmitted disease clinic patients in the United States: a meta-analytic review. Sex Transm Dis 2007;34(6):319–32.
9. Johnson WD, Diaz RM, Flanders WD, et al. Behavioral interventions to reduce risk for sexual transmission of HIV among men who have sex with men. Cochrane Database Syst Rev 2008;(3):CD001230.
10. Herbst JH, Beeker C, Mathew A, et al. The effectiveness of individual-, group-, and community-level HIV behavioral risk-reduction interventions for adult men who have sex with men: a systematic review. Am J Prev Med 2007;32(4 Suppl):S38–67.

11. Liau A, Millett G, Marks G. Meta-analytic examination of online sex-seeking and sexual risk behavior among men who have sex with men. Sex Transm Dis 2006;33(9):576–84.
12. Copenhaver MM, Johnson BT, Lee IC, et al. Behavioral HIV risk reduction among people who inject drugs: meta-analytic evidence of efficacy. J Subst Abuse Treat 2006;31(2):163–71.
13. Semaan S, Des Jarlais DC, Sogolow E, et al. A meta-analysis of the effect of HIV prevention interventions on the sex behaviors of drug users in the United States. J Acquir Immune Defic Syndr 2002;30(Suppl 1):S73–93.
14. Prendergast ML, Urada D, Podus D. Meta-analysis of HIV risk-reduction interventions within drug abuse treatment programs. J Consult Clin Psychol 2001;69(3): 389–405.
15. Weinhardt LS, Carey MP, Johnson BT, et al. Effects of HIV counseling and testing on sexual risk behavior: a meta-analytic review of published research, 1985–1997. Am J Public Health 1999;89(9):1397–405.
16. Crepaz N, Lyles CM, Wolitski RJ, et al. Do prevention interventions reduce HIV risk behaviours among people living with HIV? A meta-analytic review of controlled trials. AIDS 2006;20(2):143–57.
17. Johnson BT, Carey MP, Chaudoir SR, et al. Sexual risk reduction for persons living with HIV: research synthesis of randomized controlled trials, 1993 to 2004. J Acquir Immune Defic Syndr 2006;41(5):642–50.
18. Crepaz N, Hart TA, Marks G. Highly active antiretroviral therapy and sexual risk behavior: a meta-analytic review. JAMA 2004;292(2):224–36.
19. Noar SM. Behavioral interventions to reduce HIV-related sexual risk behavior: review and synthesis of meta-analytic evidence. AIDS Behav 2008;12(3):335–53.
20. Herbst JH, Sherba RT, Crepaz N, et al. A meta-analytic review of HIV behavioral interventions for reducing sexual risk behavior of men who have sex with men. J Acquir Immune Defic Syndr 2005;39(2):228–41.
21. Johnson WD, Hedges LV, Ramirez G, et al. HIV prevention research for men who have sex with men: a systematic review and meta-analysis. J Acquir Immune Defic Syndr 2002;30(Suppl 1):S118–29.
22. Johnson WD, Holtgrave DR, McClellan WM, et al. HIV intervention research for men who have sex with men: a 7-year update. AIDS Educ Prev 2005;17(6): 568–89.
23. Johnson-Masotti AP, Weinhardt LS, Pinkerton SD, et al. Efficacy and cost-effectiveness of the first generation of HIV prevention interventions for people with severe and persistent mental illness. J Ment Health Policy Econ 2003;6(1):23–35.
24. Ward DJ, Rowe B, Pattison H, et al. Reducing the risk of sexually transmitted infections in genitourinary medicine clinic patients: a systematic review and meta-analysis of behavioural interventions. Sex Transm Infect 2005;81(5):386–93.

Meta-analyses on Viral Hepatitis

Lise L. Gluud, MD, DrMedSc[a,b,*], Christian Gluud, MD, DrMedSc[a]

KEYWORDS

- Viral hepatitis • Meta-analyses • Randomized trials
- Systematic reviews • Hepatitis A • Hepatitis B • Hepatitis C

Large randomized trials and systematic reviews with meta-analyses of randomized trials are the reference standard for comparisons of interventions.[1] Adequate sample size and bias control are essential for both randomized trials and meta-analyses to reduce the risk of random error and systematic errors.[2–4] To assess the quality of bias control, a number of components are important. Empiric evidence suggests that the randomization methods, assessed by the allocation sequence generation and allocation concealment, and double blinding are essential to assess the control of bias.[1,2] Trials without adequate randomization may overestimate intervention effects.[1,2] Trials without double blinding also may overestimate intervention effects, although the evidence supporting this component is less clear.[1,2] Unfortunately, large trials with adequate bias control often are unavailable. Observational studies of cohorts of published randomized trials on viral hepatitis and other hepatobiliary diseases show that most trials are small and few report adequate randomization or double blinding.[5,6] The quality of the results of a systematic review reflects the quality of bias control in the individual trials ("bias in = bias out"). Systematic reviews with meta-analyses of randomized trials, however, do offer the opportunity to analyze the potential influence of inadequate or unclear bias control in groups of trials.

Worldwide, acute and chronic hepatitis are common causes for liver disease. The prevalence and incidence of the diseases vary with the geographic region and to a large extent depend on socioeconomic factors and mode of transmission. This article describes meta-analyses on available interventions for viral hepatitis type A, B, and C. The interventions assessed include active and passive immunization (vaccines and immunoglobulins) for hepatitis A and B and treatments for hepatitis B and C. The authors focused on meta-analyses from systematic reviews with clear and reproducible methods. Searches for eligible meta-analyses were conducted in

[a] Cochrane Hepato-Biliary Group, Copenhagen Trial Unit, Centre for Clinical Intervention Research, Rigshospitalet, Copenhagen University Hospital, DK 2100 Copenhagen, Denmark
[b] Department of Internal Medicine, Gentofte University Hospital, Hellerup, DK 2900 Copenhagen, Denmark
* Corresponding author. Department of Internal Medicine, Gentofte University Hospital, Hellerup, DK 2900 Copenhagen, Denmark.
E-mail address: liselottegluud@yahoo.dk (L.L. Gluud).

Infect Dis Clin N Am 23 (2009) 315–330
doi:10.1016/j.idc.2009.01.005
0891-5520/09/$ – see front matter © 2009 Elsevier Inc. All rights reserved.

id.theclinics.com

Medline, EMBASE, and The Cochrane Library and by scanning reference lists. When the meta-analyses did not report odds ratios, risk ratios [RRs], or similar points estimated with 95% confidence intervals [CIs] and measures of intertrial heterogeneity, the authors recalculated these values using RevMan version 5 (the Nordic Cochrane Center, Copenhagen, Denmark). Intertrial heterogeneity was described as χ^2 P-values.

HEPATITIS A

Hepatitis A is the most common cause of acute viral hepatitis.[7–9] The main transmission is fecal–oral from person to person. Accordingly, patterns of hepatitis A infections correlate with hygienic and sanitary conditions.[7] Hepatitis A usually is self-limiting, rarely is associated with acute liver failure, and does not lead to chronic liver disease. The disease may be asymptomatic, especially in children. In adults, the illness typically has an abrupt onset with fever, malaise, abdominal discomfort, jaundice, and elevated liver enzymes, primarily aspartate aminotransferase (AST) and alanine aminotransferase (ALT). Symptoms generally last for less than 2 months. The diagnosis is confirmed by serologic testing with identification of hepatitis A virus surface antigen IgM antibody (anti-HAV IgM).[10,11]

Hepatitis A Vaccine and Immunoglobulins

Both active and passive immunization with vaccines and immunoglobulin given as primary and secondary prevention are recommended in certain populations at an increased risk of hepatitis A.[10,11] The vaccine provides long-term protection for immunocompetent persons. If immediate protection is necessary, the vaccine may offer some protection if administered within about 9 days. Passive immunization with immunoglobulin provides immediate, short-term protection. The authors found no systematic reviews or meta-analyses on vaccines but did find one meta-analysis on immunoglobulins for hepatitis A.[12] The meta-analysis included six randomized trials on immunoglobulins versus no intervention or placebo for primary and secondary prevention of hepatitis A. The primary outcome measure was acute viral hepatitis as defined by the authors of the included trials. The terms "infectious hepatitis," "non-B viral hepatitis," and "hepatitis A" were considered synonyms. No analyses of disease severity, illness duration, or adverse events were possible. Four of the included trials dealt with primary prevention before exposure, and two trials dealt with secondary prevention after exposure. The size of the included trials varied considerably, from 724 to 116,438 participants. The duration of follow-up was 2 to 12 months. None of the included trials reported adequate allocation sequence generation. Only one trial reported adequate allocation concealment and double blinding by use of a placebo. The remaining trials did not report adequate allocation concealment and were not blinded. The authors performed meta-analyses using random-effect models. Their analyses found that immune globulins reduced the number of patients who had hepatitis A when used as primary prevention (314 of 174,265 participants [0.2%] versus 972 of 100,623 participants [1%]; RR 0.17, 95% CI, 0.06–0.51). Subgroup analyses suggested that the beneficial effect of immune globulins primarily was found in the two Russian trials that included children (RR 0.12, 95% CI, 0.07–0.20) but not in the remaining trials that were performed in United States and Israel and included adults (RR 0.29, 95% CI, 0.06–1.43). The two trials dealing with secondary prevention that included adults and children from the United States and Israel found that immune globulin reduces the number of patients who have hepatitis A (29 of 2653 participants [1%] versus 76 of 2303 participants [3%]; RR 0.31, 95% CI, 0.20–0.47). The effect was found in a subgroup including data on children from one of the trials (RR 0.33, 95% CI, 0.15–0.72). No subgroup analysis on secondary prevention for adults was possible.

The main limitation of the meta-analysis on immune globulins for primary and secondary prevention of hepatitis A is related to the unclear control of bias in the included trials. Because of the small number of included trials, the ability to analyze the association between the results and bias control was limited. Furthermore, most of the included trials did not specify how the outcome measure (ie, hepatitis) was defined. The proportion of patients who had hepatitis in the secondary prevention trials was only 1% of treated participants and 3% of untreated participants. A recent large, randomized trial compared the effect of hepatitis A vaccine and immunoglobulin used as postexposure prophylaxis.[13] Among the randomly assigned 4524 participants, 1414 were included in a per-protocol analysis. The occurrence of acute hepatitis A was based on the detection of anti hepatitis A virus-(HAV) IgM, clinical symptoms, and elevated liver enzymes. Acute symptomatic hepatitis A was found in about 4% of those randomly assigned to vaccine and 3% of those randomly assigned to immunoglobulin. This difference was not statistically significant (RR, 1.35, 95% CI, 0.70–2.67). The low risk of developing symptomatic hepatitis A after exposure suggests that both treatment options provide protection.

HEPATITIS B

Epidemiologic studies suggest that more than 350 million persons worldwide are chronically infected with hepatitis B and that about 1 million die from hepatitis B infection each year.[14,15] The usual mode of transmission is through transfusion of blood or blood products or sexual or other intimate personal contact. The course of the infection is variable, ranging from no symptoms to acute liver failure.[16] Symptoms of acute hepatitis B occur 4 to 20 weeks after infection and include fever, jaundice, malaise, and elevated liver enzymes. Less than 1% of patients who have hepatitis B infection develop acute liver failure. The infection resolves completely in about 9 of 10 adults but often becomes chronic in young children and in adults who have immune deficiencies.[17] Persons who have a high viral load have an increased risk of chronic liver disease and hepatocellular carcinoma.[18,19]

The diagnostic criteria of hepatitis B include serologic markers, biochemical markers of liver disease (including elevated liver enzyme levels), and histologic changes in the liver. Acute hepatitis B may be diagnosed when patients present with clinical symptoms, liver enzymes elevated to at least twice the upper limit of normal values, and presence of immunoglobulin M antibodies against hepatitis core antigen (anti-HBc IgM). The diagnosis of chronic hepatitis B is more complex and is based on the detection of hepatitis B virus surface antigen (HBsAg), hepatitis B envelope antigen (HBeAg), and hepatitis B virus (HBV) DNA levels.[20] Hepatitis B infection is classified as chronic if HBsAg is detectable for at least 6 months. Some patients clear HBsAg after 6 months, but others remain infected. Patients who have chronic hepatitis B infection are classified as being healthy carriers when no signs of inflammatory liver disease are present (Table 1). These patients are HBeAg negative, have detectable anti-hepatitis B envelope antibody (anti-HBe), less than 10^6 copies of HBV DNA/mL, normal transaminases, and no histologic signs of chronic hepatitis. A few patients have an occult hepatitis B infection with detectable HBV DNA but no HBsAg.[21] The occult infection has been demonstrated in subgroups with an impaired immune response, but the clinical significance is not clear. Among patients infected with hepatitis B perinatally, an immune-tolerant phase with presence of HBsAg, HBeAg, and detectable HBV DNA may develop.[22] These patients have an increased risk of later

Table 1
Definitions and diagnostic criteria for chronic hepatitis B infection

Condition	Definition	Diagnostic criteria
Inactive HBsAg carrier state	Persistent infection with HBV and no signs of inflammatory liver disease.	Presence of HBsAg for at least 6 months No detectable HBeAg Presence of anti-HBe Serum HBV DNA levels $< 10^5$ copies/mL Normal transaminases No signs of chronic hepatitis on liver biopsy
Chronic hepatitis B	Chronic inflammatory disease of the liver caused by infection with HBV	Presence of HBsAg for at least 6 months. Presence or absence of HBeAg. HBV DNA levels at least 10^5 copies/mL. Persistent or intermittent elevation of transaminase levels. Liver biopsy showing chronic hepatitis.

developing chronic hepatitis B. Patients who are HBsAg positive for more than 6 months and who have evidence of inflammatory liver disease are classified as having chronic hepatitis B. Chronic hepatitis B is classified further based on the presence of HBeAg or anti-HBe combined with HBV DNA levels. The presence of HBeAg and high HBV DNA levels indicate a high viral load and active disease, whereas the presence of anti-HBe and low or undetectable HBV DNA levels indicate inactive disease.

Hepatitis B Vaccine and Immunoglobulin

Vertical transmission of hepatitis B from mother to infant is associated with a considerable risk of developing chronic infection.[23] A high viral load (presence of HBeAg and high HBV DNA levels) increases the risk of transmitting the infection. Active and passive immunization of infants of mothers who have hepatitis B may decrease the risk of transmission. A systematic review of randomized trials evaluated the effects of hepatitis B immunization administered to newborn infants of HbsAg-positive mothers.[24,25] The review included 29 randomized trials described in 39 references. Eighteen trials included only mothers who had HBeAg; the remaining trials included mothers with or without HBeAg or did not describe HBeAg status. The vaccine regimens assessed varied considerably. Plasma-derived or recombinant vaccines were given as repeated injections over months to obtain an effective antibody response. In some trials, hepatitis B immunoglobulins with high levels of anti-hepatitis B surface antibody (anti-HBs) were administered concurrently or alone to achieve immediate protection. The mean duration of follow-up was 19 months. Five of the included trials were classified as having adequate bias control based on an assessment of the reported allocation sequence generation, allocation concealment, and double blinding. The included trials found that, compared with placebo or no intervention, the risk of hepatitis B was reduced by vaccine (RR 0.28, 95% CI, 0.20–0.40; four trials) or immunoglobulin (RR 0.50, 95% CI, 0.41–0.60; one trial). In 10 trials, 13% of patients randomly assigned to immunoglobulin plus vaccine and 19% of patients randomly assigned to vaccine alone developed hepatitis B (RR 0.54, 95% CI, 0.41–0.73). There were no apparent differences between plasma-derived and recombinant vaccines or high-dose versus low-dose regimens.

A systematic review updated in 2001 included 21 randomized trials on the effect of hepatitis B vaccines for health care workers.[26] The trials assessed a range of regimens including plasma-derived or recombinant vaccines versus placebo or no intervention as well as different modes of administration or booster vaccination of persons who did not respond to initial regimens. None of the included trials was classified as having adequate bias control, based on the reported randomization methods or blinding. Only one trial reported adequate allocation concealment, and two trials were double blind. The primary outcome measure was occurrence of hepatitis B assessed by sero-conversion from negative to positive anti-hepatitis B core antibody (anti-HBc) or HBsAg. Four of the included trials found that plasma-derived vaccines reduced incident hepatitis B compared with no intervention (3% versus 5%; RR 0.51, 95% CI, 0.35–0.73). None of the included trials on recombinant vaccines versus no intervention reported incident hepatitis B. The number of participants without protective anti-HBs after vaccination ranged from 4% to 6% in individual trials. In two of the remaining trials, the proportion of participants who developed anti-HBs after booster vaccinations ranged from 30% to 68%. No apparent differences were seen for the regimens assessed, but the trials were small, and the risk of overlooking clinically relevant differences was considerable.

Treatment of Hepatitis B

Apart from the clinical outcomes, a number of biochemical, virologic, and histologic outcome measures may be of interest when assessing the effect of treatments for patients who have hepatitis B.[15,16,20] A biochemical response is defined as normalization of ALT or AST levels. A virologic response is defined as loss of detectable HBV DNA (in non-PCR based assays corresponding to values $< 10^5$ copies/mL). Seroconversion with loss of HBeAg is assessed also. The histologic changes in liver biopsies may be assessed using standardized scores such as the Histologic Activity Index or Metavir. The outcome measures generally are assessed during treatment (early response), at the end of treatment, or after treatment. The risk of late reactivation or relapse after treatment is present mainly during the first 12 months after treatment. A response observed 12 months after treatment is defined as sustained.

At present, no systematic reviews or meta-analyses on treatment of acute hepatitis B have been published. Two randomized trials were performed after an observational trial found that steroid therapy may be beneficial in the treatment of acute hepatitis B.[27,28] The trials were small, and the results were not statistically significant. When the results of the trials are combined in a random-effects meta-analysis, however, the results suggest that steroid therapy increases mortality compared with placebo (RR 0.41, 95% CI, 0.17–0.66). A fixed-effect meta-analysis also found increased mortality. Subsequent randomized trials on acute hepatitis B found no significant benefits of cyanidanol,[29] thymomodulin,[30] or lamivudine.[31] Accordingly, no specific treatments currently are recommended for treatment of acute hepatitis B.[15,20] The available treatments for chronic hepatitis B are interferon, lamivudine, and adefovir dipivoxil.[15,32,33]

Interferon

Interferon-alpha has both antiviral and immunomodulatory effects.[34] Interferon-alpha has been the recommended treatment for chronic hepatitis B for several years.[15,32,33]

A meta-analysis of patients who had chronic hepatitis B and HBeAg included 15 randomized trials on interferon-alpha for at least 3 months versus no intervention.[35] Only English language trials published in peer-reviewed journals were included. Fifteen trials with 837 patients were included. The patients had been HBsAg and HBeAg positive for at least 6 months, had histologic evidence of chronic hepatitis, and had persistent or intermittently elevated liver enzymes. Eight trials excluded patients who had decompensated liver disease. Loss of detectable HBeAg was the primary outcome measure in all trials. The methodological quality was assessed using elaborate composite scales based on various aspects, including design, analyses, and reporting. The maximum score was 1.00, indicating the highest quality. The scores of the individual trials ranged from 0.55 to 1.00. Eight trials were classified as reporting adequate randomization (allocation sequence generation or allocation concealment). The results of the trials were combined and presented as pooled proportions, differences in proportions, and P-values. The analyses showed that interferon increased the proportion of responders compared with placebo or no intervention as assessed by sustained loss of HBeAg (33% versus 12%, $P = .0001$), HBsAg (8% versus 2%, $P = .001$), and HBV DNA (37% versus 17%, $P = .0001$). Several serious and non-serious adverse events were reported. The most frequent were flulike symptoms. Other adverse events included depression, leucopenia, and thrombocytopenia. For several treatment responders, exacerbations in liver disease with increased liver enzyme elevations were seen. Severe exacerbations of liver disease with jaundice and liver failure were recorded. The authors reanalyzed the data in the published paper to combine the results of individual trials in meta-analysis. Results were presented as risk ratios with CIs. All trials reported loss of HBeAg. In fixed-effect meta-analysis, interferon increased the proportion of patients who had sustained loss of HBeAg compared with placebo or no intervention (risk ratio 2.91, 95% CI 2.14–3.96). There was little intertrial heterogeneity (χ^2 for heterogeneity, $P = .77$). Twelve trials reported loss of HbsAg, and 14 reported loss of HBV DNA. When the results of these trials were combined, interferon increased the proportion of patients who lost HBsAg (risk ratio 4.10, 95% CI, 2.05–8.21, χ^2 for heterogeneity, $P = .60$) as well as HBV DNA (risk ratio 3.42, 95% CI, 2.34–5.00, χ^2 for heterogeneity, $P = .76$). When the meta-analyses were recalculated using random-effect models, the overall conclusions concurred. Both models suggested that interferon has a beneficial effect on loss of HBsAg and HBV DNA.

No systematic reviews or meta-analyses have been published on the use of interferon in patients who have normal liver enzymes. One randomized trial from China[36] reported that only 10% of patients who had normal liver enzymes responded to interferon (lost HBeAg). Likewise, retrospective analyses reported in randomized trials excluding patients who had normal liver enzymes suggest that patients who lost HBeAg after interferon had higher baseline AST and ALT levels than nonresponders.[35] Similar results have been found in studies analyzing predictive factors for patients who have chronic hepatitis B who respond to interferon.[37,38] Accordingly, the use of interferon for patients who have chronic hepatitis B and normal liver enzymes is not presently recommended.[15,32,33]

To improve the effect of interferon-alpha, a pegylated form with prolonged half-life has been developed.[39] Two meta-analyses on peginterferon found only one randomized trial comparing peginterferon with conventional interferon for HBeAg-positive chronic hepatitis B.[40,41] After publication of the meta-analysis, one additional randomized trial on peginterferon versus interferon for initial treatment of HBeAg-positive chronic hepatitis B was published.[42] Both trials reported the sustained virologic response of included patients. One of the trials included 194 patients randomly assigned to one of four allocation arms comparing three doses of peginterferon and one dose of interferon.[40] Treatment response was defined as loss of HBeAg, HBV DNA suppression, and normalization of ALT. Overall, peginterferon increased the proportion of treatment responders compared with interferon (24% versus 12%, $P = .036$). None of the individual outcome measures were statistically significant when analyzed separately. The second trial included 230 patients and found that peginterferon increased the proportion of patients who achieved a sustained loss of HBeAg (24% versus 14%, $P = .04$).[42] There was no apparent difference between the two treatment arms in the proportion of patients who had a sustained loss of HbsAg or HBV DNA or normalization of ALT, whether analyzed separately or combined.

No meta-analyses or systematic reviews of the use of interferon for patients who have HBeAg-negative chronic hepatitis B have been published. Four randomized trials with a total of 170 patients have reported the proportion of patients who achieve a 12-month sustained response (defined as loss of HBV DNA and normalization of ALT) with interferon compared with no intervention.[43–46] The response rates in the individual trials vary considerably. When the results of the individual trials are combined in a fixed-effect meta-analysis, the proportion of patients who had a sustained response was 50% for patients randomly assigned to interferon, compared with 14% of untreated controls (RR 4.68, 95% CI, 2.30–9.49). A random-effect meta-analysis reached the same conclusions. The trials included in this analysis had unclear bias control as assessed by the reported randomization, blinding, and follow-up. Furthermore, cohort studies[47] suggest that relapse may occur as late as 5 years after treatment and that long-term response rates for interferon range from 15% to 25%.

Lamivudine

Lamivudine is a nucleoside reverse transcriptase inhibitor with antiviral effects. Unlike interferon, lamivudine is administered orally and has fewer adverse events.[15,32,33] There are no published systematic reviews or meta-analyses of the use of lamivudine in the treatment of chronic hepatitis B. Two double-blind, placebo-controlled, randomized trials have compared lamivudine with placebo.[48,49] One of the trials[49] reported adequate randomization (allocation sequence based on stratified random numbers [2:2:1] administered through a central independent unit). Included patients were assigned randomly to lamivudine, 25 mg daily (n = 142), lamivudine, 100 mg daily (n = 143), or placebo (n = 73). The other trial did not describe randomization methods.[48] Of 143 patients initially randomized, 137 fulfilled the inclusion criteria and are described in the published report. Among these, 66 patients were assigned randomly to lamivudine, 100 mg daily, and 71 to placebo. The treatment duration in both trials was 1 year. The primary outcome measure in both trials was improvement in histology using the Knodell index[49] or Histologic Activity Index score.[48] When the results of the two trials are combined in fixed-effect meta-analyses, lamivudine, 100 mg daily, increased the proportion of patients who had histologic improvement (55% versus 34%, RR 2.26, 95% CI, 1.63–3.12, χ^2 for heterogeneity $P = .95$). Likewise, lamivudine reduced the proportion of patients with worsening of histology scores (8% versus 25%, RR 0.33, 95% CI, 0.20–0.57, χ^2 for heterogeneity $P = .35$). Including data on patients receiving lamivudine, 25 mg, did not change the overall results. In the trial comparing two doses of lamivudine and placebo,[49] the virologic response rates (HBeAg seroconversion and normalization of ALT) at the end of treatment was not significantly different for patients receiving 25 mg lamivudine compared with placebo (13% versus 4%, $P = .08$) but were significantly higher for patients receiving lamivudine, 100 mg daily (16% versus 4%, $P = .02$). None of the included patients achieved HBsAg seroconversion. The virologic outcome measures were not reported separately. The trial comparing lamivudine, 100 mg, versus placebo found that at the end of treatment lamivudine increased the proportion of patients who had HBeAg seroconversion (32% versus 11%, $P = .003$) or sustained loss of detectable HBV DNA (44% versus 16%, $P < .001$). Both trials reported that lamivudine increased the proportion of patients who had normal ALT at the end of treatment. The sustained ALT levels are not described. Several patients experienced a flare-up in liver enzyme after termination of lamivudine, however. In both trials, few patients experienced adverse events. Adverse events included gastrointestinal symptoms (such as diarrhea, vomiting, and loss of appetite), rash, muscle pain, and depression. Both randomized and observational studies have found that a considerable proportion of patients relapse after lamivudine monotherapy and that lamivudine resistance is a common problem.[50] The long-term relapse rate after lamivudine was calculated, based on individual patient data for 42 patients from two randomized trials[51,52] comparing lamivudine and interferon alone or in combination.[53] Using Kaplan-Meier method, investigators found the 3-year cumulative relapse rate for lamivudine was 54%. High pretreatment ALT levels and low HBV DNA levels were the most important predictors for achieving a sustained response.

Adefovir

The nucleotide drug adefovir dipivoxil was launched in 2003 as an alternative to interferon or lamivudine for chronic hepatitis B.[54] The drug is converted to adefovir in plasma and tissues and works by blocking viral replication. The effect of adefovir has been evaluated in a health technology assessment including a systematic review with four randomized trials.[55] The authors were unable to combine the results of the individual trials in a meta-analysis because of clinical heterogeneity. One of the included trials compared 48 weeks of adefovir dipivoxil versus placebo for HBeAg-negative chronic hepatitis B.[56] At the end of treatment, 51% of the patients in the treatment group had undetectable HBV DNA, compared with none of patients randomly assigned to placebo ($P < .001$). Adefovir also increased the proportion of patients who achieved normal transaminase levels or improved histology. After week 48, patients who received adefovir were again assigned randomly to continue treatment for an additional 48 weeks or to switch to placebo.[57] The results showed that after discontinuation of adefovir, only 8% had undetectable HBV DNA, compared with 71% of patients who continued with adefovir treatment. Likewise, within 8 weeks of stopping adefovir therapy, ALT levels returned to pretreatment values or higher in most patients who were assigned randomly to continue with placebo. Similar results were found in a randomized trial on adefovir for HBeAg-positive chronic hepatitis B.[58] The trial included three treatment arms comparing 48 weeks of adefovir dipivoxil given at a daily dose of 10 or 30 mg versus placebo. Adefovir increased the proportion of patients with an end-of-treatment virologic, biochemical, or histologic response. The higher dose of adefovir was associated with a small increase in the proportion of responders but also with a considerably higher risk of renal and other adverse events. After 48 weeks, the trial was designed to continue with patients reassigned from adefovir, 30 mg, to continue with placebo; patients reassigned from adefovir, 10 mg, to continue with adefovir, 10 mg, or placebo; and the placebo group to continue with adefovir, 10 mg. The continuation study was terminated after 91% of included patients received at least one incorrect dose of medication because of a randomization error.

Combination treatment regimens

Combination therapy with interferon plus lamivudine or adefovir has the potential benefit of achieving additive or synergistic antiviral effects. In a meta-analysis of randomized trials, the effect of lamivudine plus interferon versus interferon monotherapy for HBeAg-positive chronic hepatitis B was assessed.[59] Eight randomized trials were included. Six trials evaluated conventional interferon, and two trials evaluated pegylated interferon administered for 6 months to 1 year. Two trials included previously untreated patients. Remaining trials included untreated patients as well as patients who had relapsed or did not respond to previous antiviral therapy. The quality of bias control was assessed using a five-point composite scale on randomization, double blinding, and follow-up. Five of the included trials were assessed as having a low-quality score of two points, whereas three trials (including the two trials of peginterferon) received four or five points. Accordingly, most trials of interferon had inadequate bias control. The proportion of patients who had at least a 6-month virologic response (defined as loss of HBV DNA) was reported in the five low-quality trials of conventional interferon (with a total of 369 patients) and both trials of peginterferon (with a total of 1177 patients). Overall, the proportion of patients who had a virologic response was higher in the combination group than in the monotherapy group (odds ratio 2.10, 95% CI, 1.30–3.30). The effect, however, was seen only in the low-quality trials of conventional interferon (odds ratio 11.7, 95% CI, 7.80–17.6). The proportion of patients who had a sustained virologic response in the two high-quality trials of peginterferon was 12% in both treatment groups (odds ratio 1.10, 95% CI, 0.50–2.30). Likewise, the proportion of patients who had normalization of ALT or improved histology was higher in the combination group than in the monotherapy group for trials of conventional interferon but not in trials of peginterferon. No differences were seen in the proportion of patients who had loss of detectable HBeAg with conventional interferon or peginterferon.

One randomized trial has compared peginterferon plus lamivudine versus peginterferon for HBeAg-negative chronic hepatitis B.[60] The trial included 48 patients who were assigned randomly (1:1.5) to open-label treatment with monotherapy (n = 19) or combination therapy (n = 29). The randomization method (allocation sequence generation or concealment) was not specified. No statistically significant differences were found between the two treatment groups regarding sustained response (8/19 versus 14/29 for biochemical response, and 7/19 versus 10/29 for loss of HBV DNA). No systematic reviews, meta-analyses, or randomized trials have assessed the effect of peginterferon plus adefovir.

Recommendations

The currently recommended guidelines for treatment of chronic hepatitis B with interferon, lamivudine, or adefovir suggest that the choice of treatment should be determined at the individual patient level.[15,32,33] Treatment has been recommended for patients who have chronic hepatitis B and marked elevation of liver enzymes (at least twice the upper normal level) or a liver biopsy showing moderate to severe hepatitis. The recommended dose of conventional interferon is 5 to 6 million units three times per week for 12 to 24 months. Longer treatment duration is recommended for patients who have HBeAg-negative hepatitis B. Treatment may be stopped after HBeAg seroconversion. The dose of peginterferon used in randomized trials of HBeAg-positive chronic hepatitis B is 180 μg once weekly for pegylated interferon alfa-2a and 100 μg once weekly for pegylated interferon alfa-2b given for 48 to 52 weeks. For conventional as well as pegylated interferon, long-term treatment is not feasible because of the risk of adverse events. The dose of lamivudine in randomized trials is 100 mg daily given for at least 1 year. Long-term lamivudine is associated with an increased risk of developing resistant viral strains. Adefovir dipivoxil at a daily dose of 10 mg seems well tolerated in some patients for up to 5 years, but the long-term development of resistant strains and adverse events remain to be established. There is no evidence to support the combination of interferon-alpha plus lamivudine or adefovir dipivoxil. Furthermore, for several of the recommended treatment regimens, additional systematic reviews and randomized trials are needed.

HEPATITIS C

Worldwide, chronic hepatitis C is one of the main causes of end-stage liver disease. In the United States and Europe, hepatitis C accounts for 40% of the cases of end-stage cirrhosis and 60% of the cases of hepatocellular carcinoma.[14,61] The virus is transmitted through intravenous drug abuse, transfusion of blood, transplantation of organs, occupational exposure to blood, and possibly through high-risk sexual behavior.[62] The acute infection usually is without symptoms, and the incidence of acute hepatitis C therefore is difficult to determine. The prevalence has declined since the late 1980s, especially since the screening of blood and blood products was introduced in 1992. Hepatitis C virus (HCV) RNA is detectable 1 to 3 weeks after exposure. Potential symptoms occur after 4 to 12 weeks. Anti-HCV is detectable in 50% to 70% of patients at the onset of symptoms, increasing to more than 90% 3 months after exposure. The acute infection may be severe, as seen in acute hepatitis B, with malaise, weakness, anorexia, and jaundice. Symptoms usually subside with a concurrent decline in ALT after several weeks. Acute liver failure is rare. At least 85% of patients develop chronic infection.[63] Among patients who have chronic hepatitis C, 5% to 20% develop cirrhosis over a period of approximately 20 to 25 years. Ten years after cirrhosis develops, about 30% of patients develop end-stage liver disease. The yearly risk of developing hepatocellular carcinoma for patients who have hepatitis C–related cirrhosis is 1% to 2%. Furthermore, patients who have chronic hepatitis C can develop extrahepatic manifestations, including rheumatoid symptoms, keratoconjunctivitis sicca, lichen planus, glomerulonephritis, lymphoma, essential mixed cryoglobulinemia, and porphyria cutanea tarda.

Guidelines on the diagnosis and management of hepatitis C suggest that testing for hepatitis C virus antibody (anti-HCV) should be the recommended approach for testing for hepatitis C in clinical practice.[64–66] The presence of anti-HCV suggests previous or ongoing infection. For patients who have anti-HCV, actual infection with hepatitis C is diagnosed subsequently by detection of HCV RNA. When acute infection is suspected or in patients who are immunosuppressed, anti-HCV may be negative. For these patients, HCV RNA should be measured to exclude hepatitis C. The infection is classified as chronic when HCV RNA is detectable for at least 6 months. Regular screening of patients who have chronic infection is advised to identify those who develop chronic hepatitis C, which is diagnosed by elevated ALT or AST for at least 6 months or by histologic changes. When patients are considered eligible for treatment, the hepatitis C genotype should be assessed. There are six major genotypes.[67] The genotype does not predict the outcome of the infection but is associated with the treatment response. Considering the protracted course of the disease, clinical trials are designed to determine the virologic response to treatment (loss of HCV RNA). Because the infection often relapses during the first 6 months after treatment, the main outcome measure in clinical trials should be the sustained virologic response, defined as loss of HCV RNA at least 6 months after treatment.

Interventions for Patients Who have Acute or Chronic Hepatitis C

In spite of concentrated efforts, no vaccine or immunoglobulins for acute or chronic hepatitis C have been developed as yet. The recommended treatments for hepatitis C are interferon-alpha, ribavirin, and peginterferon. Interferon-alpha was the first treatment to be registered. The effect of interferon for acute hepatitis C has been assessed in a systematic review of randomized trials.[68,69] The review included four randomized trials of interferon alfa-2b versus no intervention for 141 patients who had transfusion-acquired acute hepatitis C. Three trials reported the proportion of patients who had a virologic response. Fixed-effect meta-analysis of the trials showed that interferon increased the proportion of patients who had end-of-treatment and sustained virologic response (end-of-treatment response: RR 8.46, 95% CI, 2.74–26.07; sustained response: RR 6.44, 95% CI, 2.00–20.70). There was little intertrial heterogeneity in either analysis (χ^2 for intertrial heterogeneity $P = .91$ and $P = .89$, respectively). The effect of interferon-alpha versus placebo or no intervention for previously untreated patients who had chronic hepatitis C was assessed in a systematic review including 54 randomized trials.[70] Eight of the included trials reported the proportion of patients who had a virologic response. Only one of these trials reported adequate randomization assessed by the allocation concealment. A fixed-effect meta-analysis of the trials suggested that interferon reduces the proportion of patients who have a sustained virologic response (23/209 patients [11%] versus 2/200 patients [1%], RR 7.47, 95% CI, 2.88–19.4, χ^2 for heterogeneity $P = .98$). The effect was also seen at the end of treatment (RR 15.74, 95% CI, 6.56–37.8, χ^2 for heterogeneity $P = .56$).

Ribavirin is a nucleoside analogue with antiviral effects. A systematic review that included 11 randomized trials with 521 patients assessed the effect of ribavirin versus placebo or no intervention.[71] Only one trial was classified as having adequate bias control based on the randomization methods and blinding. Only 1 of 199 patients randomly assigned to ribavirin and 1 of the 154 patients in the control group achieved a sustained virologic response. Accordingly, fixed-effect meta-analyses found no apparent difference between the proportions of patients who had a sustained virologic response in the two groups (RR 1.01, 95% CI, 0.96–1.07). Likewise, ribavirin had no effect on the virologic response at the end of treatment, although there was a transient effect on liver enzymes.

A systematic review of 48 randomized trials with 6585 patients compared the effect of interferon-alpha plus ribavirin versus interferon-alpha.[72] The review included trials on previously untreated patients and patients who had a transient response (relapsers) or no response (nonresponders) to previous treatment with interferon alone or to interferon combined with ribavirin. Meta-analyses found that the combination of interferon-alpha plus ribavirin significantly decreased the proportion of previously untreated patients who did not have a sustained virologic response (RR 0.74, 95% CI, 0.70–0.78). The effect of interferon-alpha plus ribavirin also was seen for relapsers and nonresponders (relapsers: RR 0.67, 95% CI, 0.57–0.78; nonresponders: RR 0.89, 95% CI, 0.83–0.96). Combination therapy with interferon-alpha and ribavirin also improved the proportion of patients who had a histologic or biochemical response. When the review was updated, 72 randomized trials with 9991 patients were identified and included.[73] The updated review confirmed that interferon-alpha plus ribavirin improved sustained virologic response in previously untreated patients (risk ratio 0.72, 95% CI, 0.68–0.76), in relapsers (risk ratio 0.63, 95% CI, 0.54–0.73), and in nonresponders (risk ratio 0.89, 95% CI, 0.84–0.94).

The effect of pegylated interferon versus conventional interferon-alpha was assessed in a systematic review with 18 randomized trials.[74] The size of the trials varied considerably, from 48 to 1530 patients. Eleven trials did not report adequate randomization. None of the trials was double blind. The proportion of patients with a sustained virologic response was 50% for 2594 patients randomly assigned to peginterferon plus ribavirin, versus 38% for 2065 patients randomly assigned to interferon-alpha plus ribavirin (risk ratio 0.80, 95% CI, 0.74–0.88). Meta-regression analyses suggested that a low virologic load was associated with a positive response (P = .006). Twelve of the trials included previously untreated patients, one trial included previous relapsers, and two trials included nonresponders to previous treatment. The remaining trials did not report whether patients were untreated, relapsers, or nonresponders or did not report results for these patient groups separately. Subgroup analyses showed that a benefit of peginterferon plus ribavirin was seen in previously untreated patients (RR 0.77, 95% CI, 0.69–0.87) but not in relapsers (RR 0.77, 95% CI, 0.57–1.04) or nonresponders (RR 0.93, 95% CI, 0.84–1.03). The proportion of patients who had adverse events was higher in the peginterferon group than in the interferon group. Accordingly, dose reductions were necessary significantly more often during treatment with peginterferon plus ribavirin (RR 1.44, 95% CI, 1.14–1.82). The risk of neutropenia, thrombocytopenia, arthralgia, injection-site reaction, dermatologic symptoms, nausea, and coughing was increased also. The proportion of patients who had improved histology was not statistically different in the two treatment groups.

Recommendations

The current guidelines for the treatment for hepatitis C recommend peginterferon plus ribavirin.[64–66] No trials have been performed on peginterferon plus ribavirin for patients who have acute hepatitis C. It may be argued, however, that perhaps the data on chronic hepatitis C can be extrapolated to patients who have acute infection. The dose of peginterferon in randomized trials is 1.5 μg/kg once weekly for peginterferon alfa-2b or 180 μg once weekly for peginterferon alpha-2a. The dose of ribavirin is 800 to 1200 mg in most trials, depending on body weight (more or less than 75 mg). Based on the combined evidence, the recommended duration of therapy for hepatitis C genotype 2 or 3 is 6 months, whereas hepatitis C genotype 1 is treated for 12 months.

SUMMARY

This article summarizes the meta-analyses of interventions for viral hepatitis A, B, and C. Some of the interventions assessed are described in small trials with unclear bias control. Other interventions are supported by large, high-quality trials. Although attempts have been made to adjust for unclear bias control, analysis of publication bias and other biases is difficult when only few trials are available. It is possible that some of the meta-analyses presented in this article are biased. Furthermore, performing updated cumulative meta-analyses also may introduce random error.[3,4] The extent and direction of bias may vary. On average, however, bias leads to overestimated intervention benefits.[1] Accordingly, the benefit of some of the interventions suggested in this article may be exaggerated by systematic and random errors. Additional research including large, randomized trials is necessary to clarify the true intervention effects.

REFERENCES

1. Gluud LL. Bias in clinical intervention research. Am J Epidemiol 2006;163:
   493–501.

2. Wood L, Egger M, Gluud LL, et al. Empirical evidence of bias in treatment effect estimates in controlled trials with different interventions and outcomes: meta-epidemiological study. BMJ 2008;336:601–5.
3. Brok J, Thorlund K, Gluud C, et al. Trial sequential analysis reveals insufficient information size and potentially false positive results in many meta-analyses. J Clin Epidemiol 2008;61:763–9.
4. Wetterslev J, Thorlund K, Brok J, et al. Trial sequential analysis may establish when firm evidence is reached in cumulative meta-analysis. J Clin Epidemiol 2008;61:64–75.
5. Kjaergard LL, Frederiksen SL, Gluud C. Validity of randomized clinical trials in gastroenterology from 1964–2000. Gastroenterology 2002;122:1157–60.
6. Kjaergard LL, Nikolova D, Gluud C. Randomized clinical trials in hepatology: predictors of quality. Hepatology 1999;30:1134–8.
7. Shapiro CN, Margolis HS. World-wide epidemiology of hepatitis A virus infection. J Hepatol 1993;18:S11–4.
8. Bell BP, Kruszon-Moran D, Shapiro CN, et al. Hepatitis A virus infection in the United States: serologic results from the Third National Health and Nutrition Examination Survey. Vaccine 2005;23:5798–806.
9. Ansaldi F, Bruzzone B, Rota MC, et al. Hepatitis A incidence and hospital-based seroprevalence in Italy: a nation-wide study. Eur J Epidemiol 2008;23: 45–53.
10. Advisory Committee on Immunization Practices (ACIP) Centers for Disease Control and Prevention (CDC). Update: prevention of hepatitis A after exposure to hepatitis A virus and in international travelers. Updated recommendations of the Advisory Committee on Immunization Practices (ACIP). MMWR Morb Mortal Wkly Rep 2007;56:1080–4.
11. American Academy of Pediatrics Committee on Infectious Diseases. Hepatitis A vaccine recommendations. Pediatrics 2007;120:189–99.
12. Bianco E, De Masi S, Mele A, et al. Effectiveness of immune globulins in preventing infectious hepatitis and hepatitis A: a systematic review. Dig Liver Dis 2004; 36:834–42.
13. Victor JC, Monto AS, Surdina TY, et al. Hepatitis A vaccine versus immune globulin for postexposure prophylaxis. N Engl J Med 2007;357:1685–94.
14. Perz JF, Armstrong GL, Farrington LA, et al. The contributions of hepatitis B virus and hepatitis C virus infections to cirrhosis and primary liver cancer worldwide. J Hepatol 2006;45:529–38.
15. Lok AS, McMahon BJ. Chronic hepatitis B. Hepatology 2007;45:507–39.
16. Lai CL, Yuen ME. The natural history and treatment of chronic hepatitis B: a critical evaluation of standard treatment criteria and end points. Ann Intern Med 2007; 147:58–61.
17. Ganem D, Prince AM. Hepatitis B virus infection—natural history and clinical consequences. N Engl J Med 2004;350:1118–29.
18. Chen CJ, Yang HI, Su J, et al. Risk of hepatocellular carcinoma across a biological gradient of serum hepatitis B virus DNA level. JAMA 2006;295:65–73.
19. Chen G, Lin W, Shen F, et al. Past HBV viral load as predictor of mortality and morbidity from HCC and chronic liver disease in a prospective study. Am J Gastroenterol 2006;101:1797–803.
20. Hoofnagle JH, Doo E, Liang TJ, et al. Management of hepatitis B: summary of a clinical research workshop. Hepatology 2007;45:1056–75.
21. Torbenson M, Kannagai R, Astemborski J, et al. High prevalence of occult hepatitis B in Baltimore injection drug users. Hepatology 2004;39:51–7.

22. Lok AS, Lai CL. A longitudinal follow-up of asymptomatic hepatitis B surface antigen-positive Chinese children. Hepatology 1988;8:1130–3.

23. Yao JL. Perinatal transmission of hepatitis B virus infection and vaccination in China. Gut 1996;38:S37–8.

24. Lee C, Gong Y, Brok J, et al. Effect of hepatitis B immunisation in newborn infants of mothers positive for hepatitis B surface antigen: systematic review and meta-analysis. BMJ 2006;332:328–36.

25. Lee C, Gong Y, Brok J, et al. Hepatitis B immunisation for newborn infants of hepatitis B surface antigen-positive mothers. Cochrane Database Syst Rev 2006;2:CD004790.

26. Chen W, Gluud C. Vaccines for preventing hepatitis B in health-care workers. Cochrane Database Syst Rev 2005;4:CD000100.

27. Greenberg HB, Robinson WS, Knauer CM, et al. Hepatitis B viral markers in severe viral hepatitis: influence of steroid therapy. Hepatology 1981;1:54–7.

28. Gregory PB, Knauer CM, Kempson RL, et al. Steroid therapy in severe viral hepatitis. A double-blind, randomized trial of methyl-prednisolone versus placebo. N Engl J Med 1976;294:681–7.

29. Schomerus H, Wiedmann KH, Dölle W, et al. (+)-Cyanidanol-3 in the treatment of acute viral hepatitis: a randomized controlled trial. Hepatology 1984;4:331–5.

30. Galli M, Crocchiolo P, Negri C, et al. Attempt to treat acute type B hepatitis with an orally administered thymic extract (thymomodulin): preliminary results. Drugs Exp Clin Res 1985;11:665–9.

31. Kumar M, Satapathy S, Monga R, et al. A randomized controlled trial of lamivudine to treat acute hepatitis B. Hepatology 2007;45:97–101.

32. de Franchis R, Hadengue A, Lau G, et al. EASL International Consensus Conference on Hepatitis B. 13-14 September, 2002 Geneva, Switzerland. Consensus statement (long version). J Hepatol 2003;39:S3–25.

33. Lok AS, McMahon BJ. Chronic hepatitis B. Hepatology 2001;34:1225–41.

34. Tompkins WA. Immunomodulation and therapeutic effects of the oral use of interferon-alpha: mechanism of action. J Interferon Cytokine Res 1999;19:817–28.

35. Wong DK, Cheung AM, O'Rourke K, et al. Effect of alpha-interferon treatment in patients with hepatitis B e antigen-positive chronic hepatitis B. Ann Intern Med 1993;119:312–23.

36. Lok AS, Wu PC, Lai CL, et al. A controlled trial of interferon with or without prednisone priming for chronic hepatitis B. Gastroenterology 1992;102:2091–7.

37. Brook MG, Karayiannis P, Thomas HC. Which patients with chronic hepatitis B virus infection will respond to alpha-interferon therapy? A statistical analysis of predictive factors. Hepatology 1989;10:761–3.

38. Thomas HC, Karayiannis P, Brook G. Treatment of hepatitis B virus infection with interferon. Factors predicting response to interferon. J Hepatol 1991;13:S4–7.

39. Bailon P, Palleroni A, Schaffer CA, et al. Rational design of a potent, long-lasting form of interferon: a 40 kDa branched polyethylene glycol-conjugated interferon alpha-2a for the treatment of hepatitis C. Bioconjug Chem 2001;12:195–202.

40. Cooksley WG, Piratvisuth T, Lee SD, et al. Peginterferon alpha-2a (40 kDa): an advance in the treatment of hepatitis B e antigen-positive chronic hepatitis B. J Viral Hepat 2003;10:298–305.

41. Hui AY, Chan HL, Cheung AY, et al. Systematic review: treatment of chronic hepatitis B virus infection by pegylated interferon. Aliment Pharmacol Ther 2005;22:519–28.

42. Zhao H, Kurbanov F, Wan MB, et al. Genotype B and younger patient age associated with better response to low-dose therapy: a trial with pegylated/

nonpegylated interferon-alpha-2b for hepatitis B e antigen-positive patients with chronic hepatitis B in China. Clin Infect Dis 2007;44:541–8.

43. Lampertico P, Del Ninno E, Manzin A, et al. A randomized, controlled trial of a 24-month course of interferon alfa 2b in patients with chronic hepatitis B who had hepatitis B virus DNA without hepatitis B e antigen in serum. Hepatology 1997; 26:1621–5.

44. Fattovich G, Farci P, Rugge M, et al. A randomized controlled trial of lymphoblastoid interferon-alpha in patients with chronic hepatitis B lacking HBeAg. Hepatology 1992;15:584–9.

45. Hadziyannis S, Bramou T, Makris A, et al. Interferon alfa-2b treatment of HBeAg negative/serum HBV DNA positive chronic active hepatitis type B. J Hepatol 1990;11:S133–6.

46. Pastore G, Sanantonio T, Milella M, et al. Anti-HBe-positive chronic hepatitis B with HBV-DNA in the serum response to a 6-month course of lymphoblastoid interferon. J Hepatol 1992;14:221–5.

47. Papatheodoridis GV, Manesis E, Hadziyannis SJ. The long-term outcome of interferon-alpha treated and untreated patients with HBeAg-negative chronic hepatitis B. J Hepatol 2001;34:306–13.

48. Dienstag JL, Schiff ER, Wright TL, et al. Lamivudine as initial treatment for chronic hepatitis B in the United States. N Engl J Med 1999;341:1256–63.

49. Lai CL, Chien RN, Leung NW, et al. A one-year trial of lamivudine for chronic hepatitis B. Asia Hepatitis Lamivudine Study Group. N Engl J Med 1998;339: 61–8.

50. Santantonio T, Mazzola M, Iacovazzi T, et al. Long-term follow-up of patients with anti-HBe/HBV DNA-positive chronic hepatitis B treated for 12 months with lamivudine. J Hepatol 2000;32:300–6.

51. Schalm SW, Heathcote J, Cianciara J, et al. Lamivudine and alpha interferon combination treatment of patients with chronic hepatitis B infection: a randomised trial. Gut 2000;46:562–8.

52. Schiff ER, Dienstag JL, Karayalcin S, et al. Lamivudine and 24 weeks of lamivudine/interferon combination therapy for hepatitis B e antigen-positive chronic hepatitis B in interferon nonresponders. J Hepatol 2003;38:818–26.

53. van Nunen AB, Hansen BE, Suh DJ, et al. Durability of HBeAg seroconversion following antiviral therapy for chronic hepatitis B: relation to type of therapy and pretreatment serum hepatitis B virus DNA and alanine aminotransferase. Gut 2003;52:420–4.

54. Hadziyannis SJ, Papatheodoridis GV. Treatment of HBeAg negative chronic hepatitis B with new drugs (adefovir and others). J Hepatol 2003;39(Suppl 1): S172–6.

55. Shepherd J, Jones J, Takeda A, et al. Adefovir dipivoxil and pegylated interferon alfa-2a for the treatment of chronic hepatitis B: a systematic review and economic evaluation. Health Technol Assess 2006;10:iii–xiv, 1.

56. Hadziyannis SJ, Tassopoulos NC, Heathcote EJ, et al. Adefovir dipivoxil for the treatment of hepatitis B e antigen-negative chronic hepatitis B. N Engl J Med 2003;348:800–7.

57. Hadziyannis SJ, Tassopoulos NC, Heathcote EJ, et al. Long-term therapy with adefovir dipivoxil for HBeAg-negative chronic hepatitis B. N Engl J Med 2005; 352:2673–81.

58. Marcellin P, Chang TT, Lim SG, et al. Adefovir dipivoxil for the treatment of hepatitis B e antigen-positive chronic hepatitis B. N Engl J Med 2003;348: 808–16.

59. Rudin D, Shah SM, Kiss A, et al. Interferon and lamivudine vs. interferon for hepatitis B e antigen-positive hepatitis B treatment: meta-analysis of randomized controlled trials. Liver Int 2007;27:1185–93.

60. Kaymakoglu S, Oguz D, Gur G, et al. Pegylated interferon Alfa-2b monotherapy and pegylated interferon Alfa-2b plus lamivudine combination therapy for patients with hepatitis B virus E antigen-negative chronic hepatitis B. Antimicrobial Agents Chemother 2007;51:3020–2.

61. Alberti A, Vario A, Ferrari A, et al. Review article: chronic hepatitis C—natural history and cofactors. Aliment Pharmacol Ther 2005;22:74–8.

62. Alter MJ. Prevention of spread of hepatitis C. Hepatology 2002;35:S93–8.

63. Seeff LB. Natural history of hepatitis C. Am J Med 1999;107:10S–5S.

64. Consensus statement. EASL International Consensus Conference on Hepatitis C. J Hepatol 1999;30:956–61.

65. Booth JC, O'Grady J, Neuberger J. The Royal College of Physicians of London and the British Society of Gastroenterology. Clinical guidelines on the management of hepatitis C. Gut 2001;49:11–21.

66. Strader DB, Wright T, Thomas DL, et al. Diagnosis, management, and treatment of hepatitis C. Hepatology 2004;39:1147–71.

67. Simmonds P. Viral heterogeneity of the hepatitis C virus. J Hepatol 1999;31: 54–60.

68. Myers RP, Regimbeau C, Thevenot T, et al. Interferon for acute hepatitis C. Cochrane Database Syst Rev 2001;4:CD000370.

69. Poynard T, Regimbeau C, Myers RP, et al. Interferon for acute hepatitis C. Cochrane Database Syst Rev 2002;1:CD000369.

70. Myers RP, Regimbeau C, Thevenot T, et al. Interferon for interferon naive patients with chronic hepatitis C. Cochrane Database Syst Rev 2002:CD000370.

71. Brok J, Gluud LL, Gluud C. Ribavirin monotherapy for chronic hepatitis C infection: a Cochrane Hepato-Biliary Group systematic review and meta-analysis of randomized trials. Am J Gastroenterol 2006;101:842–7.

72. Kjaergard LL, Krogsgaard K, Gluud C. Interferon alfa with or without ribavirin for chronic hepatitis C: systematic review of randomised trials. BMJ 2001;323: 1151–5.

73. Brok J, Gluud LL, Gluud C. Effects of adding ribavirin to interferon to treat chronic hepatitis C infection: a systematic review and meta-analysis of randomized trials. Arch Intern Med 2005;165:2206–12.

74. Simin M, Brok J, Stimac D, et al. Cochrane systematic review: pegylated interferon plus ribavirin vs. interferon plus ribavirin for chronic hepatitis C. Aliment Pharmacol Ther 2007;25:1153–62.

Meta-analyses on the Prevention and Treatment of Respiratory Tract Infections

Ilias I. Siempos, MD[a], George Dimopoulos, MD[a,b],
Matthew E. Falagas, MD, MSc, DSc[a,c,d],*

KEYWORDS

- Ventilator-associated pneumonia • ICU
- Health-care associated pneumonia
- *Streptococcus pneumoniae* • *Staphylococcus aureus*
- *Pseudomonas aeruginosa* • *Acinetobacter baumannii*

Respiratory tract infections (RTIs) are diseases of high prevalence and considerable morbidity and economic burden. In addition, lower RTIs, in particular, are associated with mortality. Approximately one tenth of patients who have AECOPD resulting in acute hypercapnic respiratory failure die during their hospitalization.[1] CAP is among the 10 most common causes of death in the United States.[2] VAP, which complicates the course of up to one third of mechanically ventilated patients, carries approximately a 25% possibility of recurrence[3] and a 40% possibility of death.[4] These considerations motivate clinicians and investigators to improve the care of patients who have RTIs.

Researchers' intense efforts to address issues dealing with RTIs have led to a great number of high-quality studies and publications, creating a need to accumulate the available evidence, appraise it critically, and synthesize it appropriately. Systematic reviews and meta-analyses are considered a proper way to address this need; indeed, they are thought to provide the best available evidence and are used consistently for

[a] Alfa Institute of Biomedical Sciences (AIBS), 9 Neapoleos Street, 151 23 Marousi, Athens, Greece
[b] Critical Care Department, Attikon University Hospital, 1 Rimini Street, 124 62 Athens, Greece
[c] Department of Medicine, Henry Dunant Hospital, 107 Mesogion Avenue, 115 26 Athens, Greece
[d] Department of Medicine, Tufts University School of Medicine, 145 Harrison Avenue, Boston, MA 02111, USA
* Corresponding author: Alfa Institute of Biomedical Sciences (AIBS), 9 Neapoleos Street, 151 23 Marousi, Greece.
E-mail address: m.falagas@aibs.gr (M.E. Falagas).

Infect Dis Clin N Am 23 (2009) 331–353
doi:10.1016/j.idc.2009.01.006
0891-5520/09/$ – see front matter © 2009 Elsevier Inc. All rights reserved.

the formulation of clinical practice guidelines. An increasing number of meta-analyses on RTIs have been performed and published during recent years (**Fig. 1**).

In the present study, the authors sought to accumulate and evaluate meta-analyses dealing with the prevention and/or treatment of upper or lower RTIs of bacterial origin in adult immunocompetent patients.

METHODS

Two reviewers (I.I.S. and G.D.) independently performed the computerized literature search of PubMed (publications indexed up to October 2008) to retrieve potentially eligible articles. For each infection, an appropriate search phrase was used (**Table 1**). No limitations on time or language of publication were set. References of the retrieved reports were searched as well.

The authors sought meta-analyses dealing with the prevention and/or treatment of RTIs of bacterial etiology in adult immunocompetent patients. The studied infections were otitis, sinusitis, tonsillitis/tonsillopharyngitis, AECOPD, CAP, and nosocomial pneumonia (including VAP). Each of these infections was defined by clinical, laboratory, and/or imaging findings attributed to this infection by the authors of the individual meta-analyses.

Only meta-analyses of RCTs were considered for inclusion in this review. The authors omitted articles on chronic infections (such as chronic rhinosinusitis), articles on infections of etiology other than bacterial (namely, viral, fungal, or parasitic), and reports on surgical procedures for the prevention and/or treatment of infections. Meta-analyses of trials exclusively enrolling children also were excluded, although, meta-analyses involving both adults and children were considered eligible.

Although the authors attempted to accumulate all available meta-analyses that fulfilled their inclusion criteria, they present only a selected proportion of them here. When more than one meta-analysis on the same issue has been published, the authors discuss the most recent meta-analysis or the one with the methodologically most rigorous analysis. For each infection, the authors pose several clinically relevant questions and then present concisely the meta-analyses that attempted to address them.

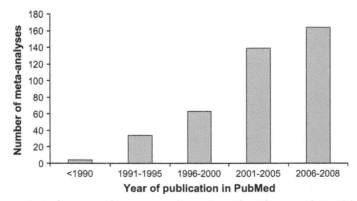

Fig. 1. The number of meta-analyses on RTIs (regardless of etiology, study participants, and study focus) indexed in PubMed up to November 2008. These meta-analyses were retrieved by using the search phrase "respiratory tract infection" and the limit "meta-analysis" in PubMed for the specific time intervals (ie, before 1990, 1991–1995, 1996–2000, 2001–2005, and 2006–2008).

Table 1
Search strategy followed to identify eligible meta-analyses for this article

Respiratory Tract Infection	Search Phrase used in PubMed	Number of Articles Initially Retrieved
Otitis	Otitis AND (prevention OR treatment OR therapy) AND (meta-analysis OR "systematic review")	127
Sinusitis	(Sinusitis OR rhinosinusitis) AND (prevention OR treatment OR therapy) AND (meta-analysis OR "systematic review")	72
Tonsillitis/ tonsillopharyngitis	(Tonsillitis OR tonsillopharyngitis) AND (prevention OR treatment OR therapy) AND (meta-analysis OR "systematic review")	28
Acute exacerbation of chronic obstructive pulmonary disease	(Chronic bronchitis OR chronic obstructive pulmonary disease OR COPD) AND exacerbation AND (prevention OR treatment OR therapy) AND (meta-analysis OR "systematic review")	61
Community-acquired pneumonia	Community-acquired pneumonia AND (prevention OR treatment OR therapy) AND (meta-analysis OR "systematic review")	49
Nosocomial pneumonia	(Nosocomial pneumonia OR hospital acquired pneumonia OR health care associated pneumonia) AND (prevention OR treatment OR therapy) AND (meta-analysis OR "systematic review")	76
Ventilator-associated pneumonia	Ventilator-associated pneumonia OR VAP AND meta-analysis OR "systematic review"	60

META-ANALYSES ON OTITIS
Is Administration of Antimicrobials Justified for the Treatment of Patients who have Acute Otitis Externa?

A meta-analysis of RCTs assessed the effectiveness of topical antimicrobials for the treatment of patients who had acute otitis externa.[5] It revealed that antimicrobials, as opposed to placebo, increased clinical success by 46% (95% confidence interval [CI], 29%–63%) and bacteriologic eradication by 61% (95% CI, 46%–76%).[5]

What is the Antimicrobial Regimen of Choice for the Treatment of Patients who have Otitis?

Ciprofloxacin-based otic suspension for acute otitis externa
A meta-analysis of two RCTs comparing the clinical outcome of patients receiving topical ciprofloxacin/dexamethasone versus polymyxin B/neomycin/hydrocortisone otic suspension for the treatment of acute otitis externa found that time to cure was significantly less with the ciprofloxacin-based regimen.[6]

Quinolones for acute otitis externa
A meta-analysis of RCTs showed that quinolone drops did not alter clinical cure rates but improved bacteriologic eradication by 8% (95% CI, 1%–16%) compared with non-quinolone antibiotics in patients who had acute otitis externa.[5]

Ofloxacin for acute suppurative otitis media
A meta-analysis of comparative trials (mainly RCTs) showed that ofloxacin otic solution, compared with other topical or systemic antimicrobials, was associated with higher clinical success (odds ratio [OR] 2.67, 95% CI, 2.04–3.50) and higher bacteriologic eradication (OR 3.86, 95% CI, 2.54–5.87) when administered in patients (both adults and children) who have acute suppurative otitis media.[7]

Azithromycin for acute otitis media
A meta-analysis of RCTs comparing 3 to 5 days of azithromycin versus other antibiotics for the treatment of patients who had acute otitis media reported no difference between the compared regimens with regard to clinical failure (OR 1.12, 95% CI, 0.81–1.54).[8]

META-ANALYSES ON SINUSITIS
Is Administration of Antimicrobials Justified for the Treatment of Patients who have Sinusitis?

Several meta-analyses assessed the putative therapeutic role of antimicrobial agents in patients who have acute sinusitis.[9–13] A meta-analysis of 17 RCTs revealed that in such patients antibiotics (mainly amoxicillin) were associated with higher rates of clinical success (OR 1.82, 95% CI, 1.34–2.46) and more adverse events (OR 1.87, 95% CI, 1.21–2.90) than placebo.[9] Interestingly, compared groups did not differ with respect to disease complications or recurrence.[9]

Another research group performed a meta-analysis on the same topic by using individual patients' data from 2547 adults enrolled in nine RCTs.[10] It was found that 15 patients who had symptoms commonly attributed to sinusitis would have to be given antibiotics before an additional patient was cured.[10] The authors of this contribution inferred that common clinical signs (eg, purulent discharge in the pharynx) are not reliable indicators of bacterial infection in patients who have sinusitis.[10]

What is the Antimicrobial Regimen of Choice for the Treatment of Patients who have Sinusitis?

Quinolones
A meta-analysis of eight RCTs compared the effectiveness and safety of quinolones (moxifloxacin, levofloxacin, and gatifloxacin) and β-lactams for the treatment of patients who have acute bacterial sinusitis.[14] It was found that administration of quinolones confers no benefit over β-lactams in terms of clinical success (OR 1.09, 95% CI, 0.85–1.39) or adverse events (OR 1.17, 95% CI, 0.86–1.59) in such patients.[14]

Azithromycin
A meta-analysis of RCTs comparing 3 to 5 days of azithromycin with other antimicrobials for the treatment of patients who have sinusitis reported no difference between the compared regimens with regard to clinical failure (OR 0.91, 95% CI, 0.60–1.39).[8]

Amoxicillin
A meta-analysis of data from 1553 patients showed that amoxicillin was clinically as effective as other antimicrobials (relative risk [RR] 0.54, 95% CI, 0.37–0.79) for the initial treatment of patients who have acute sinusitis.[15]

What is the Usefulness of Non-Antimicrobial Therapies in Patients who have Sinusitis?

Corticosteroids
A meta-analysis of four RCTs reported that administration of intranasal corticosteroids resulted in higher rates of clinical success (RR 1.11, 95% CI, 1.04–1.18) than placebo in patients who have acute sinusitis.[16]

Herbal medicines
Meta-analysis of a few RCTs showed that herbal medicines (namely, Sinupret and bromelain) may improve some symptoms of patients who have acute sinusitis.[17]

META-ANALYSES ON TONSILLITIS/TONSILLOPHARYNGITIS
What is the Antimicrobial Regimen of Choice for the Treatment of Patients who have Tonsillitis/Tonsillopharyngitis?

Azithromycin
A meta-analysis of RCTs demonstrated that a 3-day regimen of azithromycin at a dosage of 500 mg/d was more effective than 5-day regimens of other antimicrobials in terms of clinical success and bacteriologic eradication for the treatment of adult patients who have group A β-hemolytic streptococcal tonsillopharyngitis.[18] Similarly, another meta-analysis on the same topic noted that a 3- or 5-day regimen of azithromycin was as effective as longer courses of other antimicrobials in terms of clinical success (OR 1.07, 95% CI, 0.59–1.94) and bacteriologic eradication in patients who have tonsillopharyngitis.[8]

Cephalosporins
A meta-analysis of nine RCTs that compared cephalosporins with penicillin for the treatment of adult patients who had group A β-hemolytic streptococcal tonsillopharyngitis showed superiority of cephalosporins in terms of clinical success (OR 2.29, 95% CI, 1.61–3.28) and bacteriologic eradication (OR 1.83, 95% CI, 1.37–2.44).[19]

What is the Optimal Duration of Antimicrobial Treatment in Patients who have Tonsillitis/Tonsillopharyngitis?

The authors' research group conducted a meta-analysis of 11 RCTs involving patients of any age that compared short-duration ($\leq$ 7 days) versus long-duration ($\geq$ 2 days' difference) therapy for group A β-hemolytic streptococcal tonsillopharyngitis, using the same antimicrobial agent (with the same dosage and same route of administration) but given for different periods of time.[20] The administered antibiotics were penicillin V, oral or intramuscular cephalosporins, and clindamycin.[20] Compared with long-duration regimens, short-duration antimicrobial regimens were associated with lower rates of clinical success (OR 0.49, 95% CI, 0.25–0.96) and reduced bacterlologic eradication (OR 0.49, 95% CI, 0.32–0.74).[20]

In contrast, in another meta-analysis of five RCTs comparing 5 days of cephalosporins (namely, cefpodoxime, cefuroxime, cefotiam, and cefdinir) versus 10 days of penicillin for adult patients who had group A β-hemolytic streptococcal tonsillopharyngitis, no difference was found between the compared regimens regarding bacteriologic eradication (OR 1.46, 95% CI, 0.96–2.22).[21] The latter meta-analysis[21] differed from the previous meta-analysis[20] in that it involved only adults (instead of patients of any age), and it included RCTs that compared both different treatment durations and different antimicrobial agents (ie, cephalosporins versus penicillin).

META-ANALYSES ON ACUTE EXACERBATIONS OF CHRONIC OBSTRUCTIVE PULMONARY DISEASE
Do Vaccinations Against Pneumococcus and Influenza Protect From Acute Exacerbations of Chronic Obstructive Pulmonary Disease?

Vaccination against pneumococcus
A meta-analysis assessed the effects of injectable pneumococcal vaccine as a means to prevent exacerbations in patients who have chronic obstructive pulmonary disease (COPD).[22] By including data from four RCTs (two trials using a 14-valent vaccine and

two using a 23-valent vaccine), this meta-analysis showed that pneumococcal vaccination was not associated with fewer exacerbations (OR 1.43, 95% CI, 0.31–6.69), fewer episodes of pneumonia (OR 0.89, 95% CI, 0.58–1.37), or reduced all-cause mortality (OR 0.94, 95% CI, 0.67–1.33) in patients who have COPD.[22]

Vaccination against influenza

A meta-analysis assessed the effects of influenza vaccination as a means to prevent exacerbations in subjects who had COPD.[23] Eleven RCTs comparing live or inactivated virus vaccines with placebo were included.[23] Inactivated vaccine against influenza, as opposed to placebo, was associated with fewer exacerbations per patient (weighted mean difference [WMD] −0.37, 95% CI, −0.64 to −0.11).[23]

Does Administration of Antimicrobials Prevent Acute Exacerbations of Chronic Obstructive Pulmonary Disease?

A meta-analysis of nine RCTs examined whether the use of prophylactic antibiotics may lead to fewer AECOPDs.[24] It was found that administration of prophylactic antimicrobials, as opposed to placebo or no treatment, was not associated with fewer exacerbations per patient per year (WMD −0.15, 95% CI, −0.34–0.04) but resulted in more adverse events.[24] These findings, combined with concerns about the possible emergence of antimicrobial resistance, seem to argue against the prescription of antibiotics as prophylaxis for individuals who have COPD.

Is Administration of Antimicrobial Agents Justified for the Treatment of Patients who have Acute Exacerbations of Chronic Obstructive Pulmonary Disease?

So far three meta-analyses of RCTs examined the effect of antimicrobial treatment on clinical outcomes of patients who have AECOPD.[25–27] In general, the studies agreed that antibiotics, regardless of choice, may be valuable in patients who have AECOPD with increased cough and sputum purulence.[25–27] In detail, the most recent relevant meta-analysis, which included 13 RCTs, showed that administration of antibiotics was associated with fewer treatment failures (OR 0.25, 95% CI, 0.16–0.39) and lower mortality (OR 0.20, 95% CI, 0.06–0.62) than placebo in patients who have severe exacerbations requiring hospitalization.[25] In contrast, antibiotics did not reduce treatment failures in outpatients who had mild-to-moderate AECOPD (OR 1.09, 95% CI, 0.75–1.59).[25] The authors of this meta-analysis[25] concluded that, although antimicrobials do not provide any advantage in nonsevere AECOPD,[28] their administration in inpatients who have severe exacerbations results in lower mortality than seen with placebo.

What is the Antimicrobial Regimen of Choice for the Treatment of Patients who have Acute Exacerbations of Chronic Obstructive Pulmonary Disease?

Traditional antimicrobials

Penicillins (amoxicillin, ampicillin, and pivampicillin), trimethoprim/sulfamethoxazole (TMP/SMX), and doxycycline traditionally have been used for the management of patients who have AECOPD without risk factors for treatment failure. A meta-analysis of five RCTs showed equivalence between penicillins and trimethoprim-based regimens with regard to clinical success (OR 1.68, 95% CI, 0.91–3.09) and the number of drug-related adverse events (OR 0.37, 95% CI, 0.11–1.24) in such patients.[29]

Advanced versus traditional antimicrobials

A meta-analysis of 12 RCTs examined the comparative effectiveness and safety of traditional (amoxicillin, ampicillin, pivampicillin, TMP/SMX, and doxycycline) and advanced antimicrobials (macrolides, quinolones, amoxicillin/clavulanic acid [A/C], and second- or third-generation cephalosporins) for the treatment of patients who have AECOPD.[30] It was found that use of traditional, as opposed to advanced, antibiotics was associated with lower rates of clinical success (OR 0.51, 95% CI, 0.34–0.75) but not with lower mortality (OR 0.64, 95% CI, 0.25–1.66) or more adverse events (OR 0.75, 95% CI, 0.39–1.45).[30]

Macrolides, quinolones, and amoxicillin/clavulanic acid

A meta-analysis of 19 RCTs representing 7405 individuals and comparing macrolides (clarithromycin, azithromycin, dirithromycin, roxithromycin) with quinolones (levofloxacin, moxifloxacin, gemifloxacin), A/C with quinolones, and A/C with macrolides in patients who had AECOPD was conducted.[31] No difference in treatment success was found between macrolides recipients and quinolones recipients (OR 0.94, 95% CI, 0.73–1.21), between A/C recipients and quinolones recipients (OR 0.86, 95% CI, 0.55–1.34), or between A/C recipients and macrolides recipients (OR1.70, 95% CI, 0.72–4.03).[31] Compared with quinolones, however, macrolides were associated with lower effectiveness in microbiologically evaluable patients (OR 0.47, 95% CI, 0.31–0.69) and with more recurrences of AECOPD, whereas A/C was associated with more adverse events (mainly diarrhea) than quinolones (OR 1.36, 95% CI, 1.01–1.85).[31]

Azithromycin

A meta-analysis of RCTs comparing azithromycin with amoxicillin or A/C for the treatment of patients who have lower RTIs (including AECOPD) showed equivalence between the comparators in treatment failure (RR 1.09, 95% CI, 0.64–1.85) and bacteriologic eradication (RR 0.95, 95% CI, 0.87–1.03).[32]

What is the Optimal Duration of Antimicrobial Treatment in Patients who have Acute Exacerbations of Chronic Obstructive Pulmonary Disease?

Two meta-analyses evaluated the comparative effectiveness of short- versus long-duration antimicrobial treatment of patients who have AECOPD.[33,34] The more recent meta-analysis included seven RCTs that compared regimens with the same antimicrobial agent, in the same daily dosages, given for different time periods (5 days versus 7–10 days).[33] The agents studied were cefixime, moxifloxacin, levofloxacin, grepafloxacin, gatifloxacin, and clarithromycin.[33] There was no difference between the compared arms with regard to clinical success rates (RR 0.99, 95% CI, 0.95–1.03), but short-duration treatment was safer than long-duration treatment in terms of drug-related adverse events (RR 0.84, 95% CI, 0.72–0.97).[33]

What is the Usefulness of Non-Antimicrobial Therapies in Patients who have Acute Exacerbations of Chronic Obstructive Pulmonary Disease?

Inhaled bronchodilators

A meta-analysis of RCTs demonstrated that inhaled short-acting β-agonists and anticholinergic agents were comparable regarding short-duration changes in forced expiratory volume in 1 second (FEV1).[35] Similarly, the combination of a short-acting β-agonist and ipratropium had no greater effect on FEV1 than either used alone.[35]

Methylxanthines

A meta-analysis of four RCTs examined the usefulness of intravenous methylxanthines (such as aminophylline) for the treatment of patients who have AECOPD.[36] It was found that methylxanthines did not improve lung function but did cause more episodes of nausea and vomiting (OR 4.6, 95% CI, 1.7–12.6) than comparators when administered in such patients.[36]

Systemic corticosteroids

So far two meta-analyses have assessed the effectiveness of systemic corticosteroids in subjects who have AECOPD.[37,38] The more recent meta-analysis included 10 RCTS and demonstrated that corticosteroids (either parenteral or oral) were associated with fewer treatment failures (RR 0.54, 95% CI, 0.41–0.71) and shorter hospital stay than placebo.[37] The use of corticosteroids, however, carried a higher risk for hyperglycemia than placebo (RR 5.88, 95% CI, 2.40–14.41).[37]

Mycolytics

A meta-analysis of RCTs comparing oral mucolytics (such as domiodol, bromhexine, ambroxol, S-carboxymethylcysteine, and potassium chloride) with placebo showed equivalence in terms of duration of symptoms.[39]

Noninvasive mechanical ventilation

Several meta-analyses examined the usefulness of noninvasive mechanical ventilation (NIMV) in treating patients who had acute respiratory failure caused by AECOPD.[37,40–44] The most recent of meta-analysis included 14 RCTs and revealed that use of NIMV was associated with lower in-hospital mortality, fewer intubations, and shorter hospital stay than standard management of patients who have AECOPD and respiratory acidosis.[37]

META-ANALYSES ON COMMUNITY-ACQUIRED PNEUMONIA
Is Atypical Coverage Needed in Patients who have Nonsevere Community-Acquired Pneumonia?

A meta-analysis of 18 RCTs was conducted to examine whether monotherapy with a β-lactam (namely, penicillin or cephalosporin) is as effective as monotherapy with a antibiotic active against atypical pathogens (eg, quinolone, macrolide, or ketolide) for the treatment of patients who have mild-to-moderate CAP.[45] No difference was found between the compared regimens in terms of clinical failure (RR 0.97, 95% CI, 0.87–1.07) or all-cause mortality (RR 1.20, 95% CI, 0.84–1.71).[45] In the subgroup analysis of data from 10 patients who had CAP caused by *Legionella pneumophilae*, however, the clinical success rates for β-lactams were lower than those for agents active against atypical pathogens (RR 0.40, 95% CI, 0.19–0.85).[45] Given that *Legionella pneumophilae* is an uncommon cause of CAP, the authors of that meta-analysis recommended monotherapy with β-lactams for the empiric treatment of patients who have nonsevere CAP.[45] Their conclusions, although in concordance with British Thoracic Society guidelines,[46] contradicted the relevant Infectious Diseases Society of America/American Thoracic Society consensus guidelines, which promote atypical coverage in patients who have CAP of any severity.[47]

Is Atypical Coverage Needed in Patients who have Community-Acquired Pneumonia Requiring Hospitalization?

So far two meta-analyses performed by the same research group have examined the need of ensuring antibiotic coverage for atypical pathogens in patients who have CAP requiring hospitalization.[48,49] The more recent of these two meta-analyses[48,49] included 25 RCTs and revealed no difference between the atypical arm and the non-atypical arm regarding mortality (RR 1.15, 95% CI, 0.85–1.56), clinical success, bacteriologic eradication, or adverse events.[48] For CAP caused by *Legionella pneumophilae*, however, the clinical success rate was higher in the atypical than in the non-atypical arm.[48] It should be noted that none of the RTCs included in the meta-analysis compared β-lactam monotherapy versus combination therapy using a β-lactam and an atypical antibiotic.[48] Like the authors of the meta-analysis on nonsevere CAP,[45] the authors of the meta-analysis on severe CAP[48] concluded that initial atypical coverage does not afford any benefit in patients who have CAP.

Which is the Antimicrobial Regimen of Choice for the Treatment of Patients who have Community-Acquired Pneumonia?

Several classes of antimicrobials for nonsevere community-acquired pneumonia

A meta-analysis examined the comparative effectiveness of different antimicrobial regimens for the treatment of outpatients who have CAP.[50] It accumulated data from 13 RCTs, and in patients who had mild-to-moderate CAP it found no difference in clinical success rates or mortality between macrolides and fluoroquinolones (five trials), between macrolides and β-lactams (three trials), between quinolones and β-lactams (three trials), or between cephalosporins and β-lactams/β-lactamase inhibitors (two trials).[50]

Quinolones

Several meta-analyses examined the role of quinolones in treating patients who have CAP.[51–57] Recently, the authors' research group conducted a meta-analysis of 23 RCTs to examine whether the administration of respiratory quinolones (namely, levofloxacin, moxifloxacin, and gemifloxacin) is more effective than macrolides and/or β-lactams for the treatment of patients (either inpatients or outpatients) who have CAP.[51] Although mortality was not different among the compared regimens (OR 0.85, 95% CI, 0.65–1.12), quinolones performed better than comparators in terms of clinical success (OR 1.17, 95% CI, 1.00–1.36).[51] This finding also held true for the subgroup of patients who had severe CAP (OR 1.84, 95% CI, 1.02–3.29) or those requiring hospital admission (OR = 1.30, 95% CI, 1.30 to 1.61).[51] The fact that a significant proportion of the RCTs included in the this meta-analysis[51] were open label and were sponsored by the industry should be taken into account when interpreting its results.

Azithromycin

A meta-analysis of 18 RCTs examining the comparative effectiveness of azithromycin and other antibacterials for the treatment of patients who had CAP was performed.[8] Azithromycin was associated with fewer clinical failures than comparators (OR 0.63, 95% CI, 0.41–0.95).[58] Again, most of the included RCTs were open label and thus potentially were susceptible to bias.

Does Initial Discordant Treatment with β-lactams Affect the Outcome of Patients who have Pneumococcal Community-Acquired Pneumonia?

A meta-analysis of six prospective studies (two RCTs) that compared the clinical effectiveness of concordant (active in vitro) β-lactam monotherapy with discordant (inactive in vitro) monotherapy with the same β-lactam in patients who had pneumococcal pneumonia was conducted to clarify the effect of initial therapy with discordant β-lactam antibiotics on the outcomes of such patients.[59] It revealed that initial treatment with concordant and discordant β-lactam antibiotics for pneumococcal CAP did not differ in clinical success rates (OR 2.57, 95% CI, 0.46–14.34), mortality (risk difference −0.05, 95% CI, −0.23–0.12), or bacteriologic eradication (risk difference −0.18, 95% CI, −0.79–0.42).[59]

What is the Optimal Duration of Antimicrobial Treatment in Patients who have Community-Acquired Pneumonia?

The optimal duration of antimicrobial treatment of patients who have CAP was the subject of two meta-analyses.[60,61] The more recent of these studies included seven RCTs (five involving adults and two involving children) that compared short-duration (≤ 7 days) versus long-duration (≥ 2 days' difference) therapy with the same antimicrobial agent in the same daily dosages.[60] The antibiotics administered in adults were amoxicillin, cefuroxime, ceftriaxone, telithromycin, and gemifloxacin.[60] No differences were found between short- and long-duration regimens in clinical success rates (OR 0.89, 95% CI, 0.74–1.07), mortality (OR 0.57, 95% CI, 0.23–1.43), or adverse events (OR 0. 90, 95% CI, 0.72–1.13).[60] No differences were found regarding these outcomes in the subgroup analysis of adults.[60] This meta-analysis included RCTs that enrolled patients who had mild-to-moderate CAP;[60] caution is merited in extrapolating these findings to patients who have severe CAP.

When Should one Switch From Intravenous to Oral Antimicrobial Therapy?

Based on the findings of a meta-analysis of six RCTs, an early switch from intravenous to oral as opposed to conventional intravenous treatment for the whole duration of therapy of inpatients who had moderate-to-severe CAP did not affect clinical success rates (OR 0.76, 95% CI, 0.36–1.59), mortality (OR 0.81, 95% CI, 0.49–1.33), or pneumonia recurrence (OR 1.81, 95% CI, 0.70–4.72).[62] In addition, length of hospital stay was shorter (WMD −3.34 days, 95% CI, −4.42 to −2.25), and drug-related adverse events were fewer (OR 0.65, 95% CI, 0.48–0.89) in the early-switch group.[62] These findings corroborated those of a previous meta-analysis[63] and further supported the relevant Infectious Diseases Society of America/American Thoracic Society consensus guidelines, which state that "patients should be switched from intravenous to oral therapy as soon as they are hemodynamically stable and improving clinically, and have a normally functioning gastrointestinal tract."[47]

What is the Usefulness of Non-Antimicrobial Therapies in Patients who Have Community-Acquired Pneumonia?

Corticosteroids

Two meta-analyses evaluated the effectiveness of corticosteroids as an adjunct to antimicrobial treatment in immunocompetent adult patients who have severe bacterial CAP.[64,65] The more meta-analysis included four RCTs that enrolled 189 subjects who had CAP.[64] Administration of corticosteroids in such patients was associated with lower all-cause in-hospital mortality than seen with placebo (OR 0.21, 95% CI, 0.05–0.83).[64] All included trials had small sample sizes, and most of them did not provide any information about the adrenal function of enrolled patients before treatment (information that is crucial, because it has been reported that the potential benefits of corticosteroids may be valid only for patients who have adrenal insufficiency); these limitations should be taken into consideration when evaluating the findings of this meta-analysis.[64]

META-ANALYSES ON NOSOCOMIAL PNEUMONIA / VENTILATOR-ASSOCIATED PNEUMONIA
What is the Value of Nonpharmacologic Measures in Preventing Nosocomial Pneumonia/Ventilator-Associated Pneumonia?

Early tracheostomy

A meta-analysis of five RCTs attempted to examine whether early tracheostomy is associated with better clinical outcomes than late tracheostomy or prolonged endotracheal intubation in mechanically ventilated patients.[66] It was found that early tracheostomy, as opposed to comparators, did not reduce the incidence of VAP (RR 0.90, 95% CI, 0.66–1.21) or all-cause in-hospital mortality (RR 0.79, 95% CI 0.45–1.39);[66] however, it shortened both the duration of mechanical ventilation (WMD −8.5 days, 95% CI, −15.3 to −1.7) and the length of ICU stay (WMD −15.3 days, 95% CI, −24.6 to −6.1).[66]

Rotational bed therapy
Two meta-analyses addressed the use of rotational bed therapy.[67,68] The more recent included 12 RCTs comparing rotational bed therapy with standard management of mechanically ventilated patients.[67] Rotational bed therapy, although associated with a lower incidence of VAP (OR 0.40, 95% CI, 0.27–0.58) than standard care, failed to reduce all-cause in-hospital mortality (OR 1.02, 95% CI, 0.77–1.34), duration of mechanical ventilation (WMD −1.06, 95% CI, −2.86–0.74), or length of ICU stay (WMD −0.90, 95% CI, −2.82–1.01).[67]

Prone positioning
Several meta-analyses examined the effectiveness of prone positioning on outcomes of patients who had acute respiratory failure (including patients who had acute respiratory distress syndrome);[69–72] among the outcomes tested was the incidence of VAP. The three meta-analyses that included only RCTs[70–72] agreed that prone positioning was not associated with lower incidence of VAP (WMD 0.78%, 95% CI, 0.40–1.51), lower all-cause ICU mortality (OR 0.79, 95% CI, 0.45–1.39), or shorter duration of mechanical ventilation (WMD −0.42 days, 95% CI, −1.56–0.72).[72]

Closed versus open tracheal suction systems
Six meta-analyses have examined whether closed tracheal suction systems protect against VAP.[73–78] Analysis of data from nine RCTs showed that patients managed with closed versus open tracheal suction systems did not differ in the incidence of VAP (OR 0.96, 95% CI, 0.72–1.28), all-cause mortality (OR 1.04, 95% CI, 0.78–1.39), or length of ICU stay.[73] The use of closed systems, however, resulted in more prolonged duration of mechanical ventilation (WMD 0.65 days, 95% CI, 0.28–1.03) and higher rates of colonization of the respiratory tract (OR 2.88, 95% CI, 1.50–5.52) than the use of open ones.[73]

Passive (heat-and-moisture exchangers) versus active humidifiers
Several meta-analyses addressed the use of passive humidifiers (heat-and-moisture exchangers) versus active humidifiers.[79–82] Old meta-analyses of six[82] and eight[81] trials noted that passive humidifiers were superior to active humidifiers in reducing the incidence of VAP, but those meta-analyses did not examine the effect of humidification on other important clinical outcomes.[81,82] Thus far, the most comprehensive meta-analysis on the topic included 13 RCTs, which enrolled 2580 patients receiving mechanical ventilation.[79] It found no difference between patients managed with passive versus active humidifiers with respect to the incidence of VAP (OR 0.85, 95% CI, 0.62–1.16), all-cause mortality (OR 0.98, 95% CI, 0.80–1.20), length of ICU stay (WMD −0.68 days, 95% CI, −3.65–2.30), duration of mechanical ventilation (WMD 0.11 days, 95% CI, −0.90–1.12), or episodes of airway occlusion (OR 2.26, 95% CI, 0.55–9.28).[79] This meta-analysis[79] further supported the relevant guidelines by the American Thoracic Society/Infectious Diseases Society of America[83] and those of the Centers for Disease Control and Prevention,[84] which state no preference for the use of passive or active humidifiers to prevent VAP in mechanically ventilated patients.

Subglottic secretion drainage

A meta-analysis of five RCTs examined the effectiveness of subglottic secretion drainage in preventing VAP.[85] It found that this intervention, as opposed to standard care of mechanically ventilated patients, was associated with a lower incidence of VAP (RR 0.51, 95% CI, 0.37–0.71), shorter duration of mechanical ventilation (WMD 2 days, 95% CI, 1.7–2.3 days), and shorter length of ICU stay (WMD 3 days, 95% CI, 2.1–3.9 days).[85]

Noninvasive mechanical ventilation

A meta-analysis of three RCTs showed that the use of NIMV, as opposed to invasive mechanical ventilation, decreased the incidence of VAP (RR 0.24, 95% CI, 0.08–0.73).[86]

On the other hand, two meta-analyses performed by the same research group examined whether early extubation with immediate application of NIMV is more effective than invasive positive pressure ventilation weaning in preventing VAP in endotracheally intubated patients.[87,88] It was reported that, compared with invasive ventilation weaning, NIMV weaning was associated with a lower incidence of VAP (RR 0.28, 95% CI, 0.09–0.85), lower mortality (RR 0.41, 95% CI, 0.22–0.76), and shorter duration of mechanical ventilation (WMD −7.33 days, 95% CI, −11.45 to −3.22 days).[87]

Postpyloric feeding

Two meta-analyses examined the potential of early postpyloric feeding in reducing the incidence of nosocomial pneumonia/VAP.[89,90] These meta-analyses agreed that postpyloric feeding of ICU patients did not carry any advantage over gastric feeding in terms of incidence of aspiration pneumonia (RR 1.28, 95% CI, 0.91–1.80), mortality (RR 1.01, 95% CI, 0.76–1.36), or length of ICU stay (WMD −1.46 days, 95% CI, −3.74–0.82).[89,90]

What is the Value of Pharmacologic Measures in Preventing Nosocomial Pneumonia/Ventilator-Associated Pneumonia?

Stress ulcer prophylaxis

Numerous meta-analyses examined the impact of medications given for stress ulcer prophylaxis (eg, sucralfate, antacids, and histamine$_2$-receptor antagonists) on the incidence of pneumonia in ICU patients.[91–96] Interestingly, the two most recent of these analyses[91,92] attempted to accumulate the evidence derived from the previous meta-analyses.[93–96] It was found that the use of histamine$_2$-receptor antagonists, as opposed to no prophylaxis, was not associated with a higher incidence of nosocomial pneumonia (OR 1.25, 95% CI, 0.78–2.00).[92] Sucralfate was not better than antacids (OR 0.80, 95% CI, 0.56–1.15) or than histamine$_2$-receptor antagonists (OR 0.77, 95% CI, 0.60–1.01) in terms of incidence of nosocomial pneumonia.[92]

Oral decontamination with chlorhexidine

Four meta-analyses have examined the effect of oral decontamination with antiseptics (mainly chlorhexidine) on the incidence of nosocomial pneumonia (including VAP).[97–100] Most of them agreed that topical chlorhexidine was associated with a lower incidence of nosocomial pneumonia (RR 0.74, 95% CI, 0.56–0.96) but not with lower mortality than placebo or no treatment.[97–99]

Prophylactic administration of antimicrobials (other than inhaled) for selective digestive decontamination

A comprehensive meta-analysis of 36 RCTs was performed to evaluate the effectiveness of the prophylactic administration of antimicrobials, given systemically and/or topically (but not through inhalation or endotracheal instillation), in ICU patients.[101] It was found that a combination of topical and systemic antibiotics was associated with fewer episodes of pneumonia (OR 0.35, 95% CI, 0.29–0.41) and lower all-cause mortality (OR 0.78, 95% CI, 0.68–0.89) than placebo or no treatment.[101] In addition, topical antimicrobials (alone or in combination with systemic antibiotics), as compared with placebo or no topical treatment (alone or in combination with systemic antibiotics), reduced the incidence of pneumonia (OR 0.52, 95% CI, 0.43–0.63) but not all-cause mortality (OR 0.97, 95% CI, 0.81–1.16).[101]

On the other hand, other meta-analyses focused directly on the administration of antimicrobials to achieve selective decontamination of the digestive tract in surgical and medical ICU patients[102] or in medical patients alone.[103] Compared with standard care, selective digestive decontamination reduced the incidence of pneumonia in both subsets of patients (ie, surgical and medical).[102,103] The intervention was associated with lower mortality in surgical patients (OR 0.7, 95% CI, 0.52–0.93) but not in medical patients (OR 0.91, 95% CI, 0.71–1.18).[102,103]

Prophylactic administration of inhaled antimicrobials
A meta-analysis of five RCTs examined the effect of prophylactic antibiotics administered via the respiratory tract on the development of nosocomial pneumonia/VAP.[104] It found that in ICU patients the administration of inhaled antimicrobials (namely, gentamicin, tobramycin, polymyxin, and ceftazidime) as prophylaxis was associated with fewer episodes of pneumonia (OR 0.49, 95% CI, 0.32–0.76) but not with lower mortality (OR 0.86, 95% CI, 0.55–1.32) than standard care.[104] An update of this meta-analysis, with the inclusion of an additional RCT, confirmed that prophylactic inhaled antimicrobials reduce the incidence of pneumonia (OR 0.47, 95% CI, 0.24–0.91).[105]

Probiotics
A meta-analysis of eight RCTs comparing enteral feeding plus pre-, pro-, or synbiotics versus standard enteral feeding alone in ICU patients reported no benefit for these agents in terms of the incidence of nosocomial pneumonia, in-hospital mortality, or length of ICU stay.[106]

Pharmaco-nutrients and enriched diets
A meta-analysis of RCTs noted that in ICU patients receiving enteral nutrition the administration of diets enriched with pharmaco-nutrients, as opposed to nonenriched diets, resulted in fewer episodes of nosocomial pneumonia (OR 0.54, 95% CI, 0.35–0.84), shorter duration of mechanical ventilation (WMD 2.25 days, 95% CI, 0.5–3.9), and shorter length of ICU stay (WMD 1.6 days, 95% CI, 1.9–1.2) but not in lower mortality (OR 1.10, 95% CI, 0.85–1.42).[107]

META-ANALYSES ON THE TREATMENT OF NOSOCOMIAL PNEUMONIA / VENTILATOR-ASSOCIATED PNEUMONIA
What is the Antimicrobial Regimen of Choice for Patients who have Nosocomial Pneumonia/Ventilator-Associated Pneumonia?

Comparison of several classes of antimicrobials for ventilator-associated pneumonia
A meta-analysis of 41 RCTs evaluated 29 empiric parenteral antibiotic regimens for adult patients who had clinically suspected VAP.[108] There was no evidence that any particular regimen improved survival.[108] With respect to clinical success, the combination of ceftazidime/aminoglycoside was found to be inferior to meropenem (RR 0.70, 95% CI, 0.53–0.93).[108]

Monotherapy versus combination therapy of ventilator-associated pneumonia

On the basis of the findings of the meta-analysis cited in the previous section,[108] monotherapy of patients who had VAP was not inferior to combination therapy in terms of clinical failure (RR 0.88, 95% CI, 0.72–1.07) or mortality (RR 0.94, 95% CI, 0.76–1.16). Patients at risk for multidrug-resistant organisms, who would be expected to benefit the most from empiric combination therapy, were poorly represented in this meta-analysis,[108] and this fact should be taken into consideration in the present era of increased antimicrobial resistance.

Carbapenems

The comparative effectiveness and safety of carbapenems versus other β-lactams and quinolones for the empiric treatment of patients who have nosocomial pneumonia (including VAP) was examined in a recent meta-analysis of 12 RCTs.[109] Carbapenems, alone or in combination with aminoglycosides, were associated with lower mortality than quinolones or β-lactams (OR 0.72, 95% CI, 0.55–0.95).[109] Interestingly, the compared regimens did not differ in clinical success rates (OR 1.08, 95% CI, 0.91–1.29) or number of drug-related adverse events (OR 0.81, 95% CI, 0.46–1.43).[109] In addition, in patients who had pneumonia caused by *Pseudomonas aeruginosa*, carbapenems (mainly imipenem/cilastatin) had lower clinical success rates (OR 0.42, 0.22–0.82) than the comparators.[109]

Quinolones

A meta-analysis of five RCTs compared quinolones with other antimicrobial agents (ie, imipenem/cilastatin and ceftazidime) for the treatment of patients who had nosocomial pneumonia.[110] No difference was found among the compared groups in clinical success rates (OR 1.12, 95% CI, 0.80–1.55), mortality, or bacteriologic eradication.[110]

Linezolid

A meta-analysis of five RCTs comparing linezolid with glycopeptides or β-lactams for the treatment of patients who had nosocomial pneumonia (including patients who had VAP) showed that linezolid was not associated with higher clinical success rates (OR 1.05, 95% CI, 0.75–1.46).[111]

Is there a Place for Inhaled Antimicrobials in Treating Patients who have Nosocomial Pneumonia/Ventilator-Associated Pneumonia?

The authors' research group performed a meta-analysis of five RCTs to investigate whether the administration of antimicrobials via the respiratory tract (either inhaled or endotracheally instilled) as an adjunct to systemic antibiotics was associated with better clinical success rates (OR 2.39, 95% CI, 1.29–4.44) than seen with systemic antibiotics alone.[112] Compared regimens did not differ in all-cause mortality (OR 0.84, 95% CI, 0.43–1.64) or toxicity (OR 0.34, 95% CI, 0.04–2.53).[112] Interestingly, there also is evidence that monotherapy with inhaled antibiotics might be considered in selected (rare) patients who have nosocomial pneumonia and for whom the administration of systemic antibiotics is discouraged (ie, because of toxicity).[113]

COMMENTS

Appropriately performed meta-analyses (especially those consisting of RCTs) are at the top of the hierarchy of evidence in evidence-based medicine, because they "faithfully summarize the evidence from all relevant studies on the topic of interest, and they do so concisely and transparently."[114] Meta-analyses are not a panacea, however, and their results should be viewed with caution. Indeed, the simple pooling of data (even if the pooling increases study size and thus decreases random error) is not suffi-cient to decrease systematic error; therefore it does not assure the internal validity and the generalizability of the findings of a meta-analysis.[115]

A considerable number of meta-analyses on RTIs were devoted to comparisons among several classes of antimicrobial agents. Quinolones, azithromycin, and β-lac-tams were the most consistently examined antibacterials. When interpreting the results of such contributions, one should remember that the results were based mainly on non-inferiority trials; thus, it may be anticipated that such meta-analyses fail to reveal the putative superiority of one antibacterial class over another. In addition to the results of meta-analyses, clinicians should incorporate local surveillance data on antimicrobial resistance in their decision-making process.

Meta-analyses examined the need (if any) for administering antimicrobial treatment in patients who have otitis, sinusitis, and AECOPD, a topic of hot debate. Although the overuse of antibiotics for these conditions has been blamed for development of anti-microbial resistance, the demonization of antibiotic prescription for RTIs may lead to increased mortality among patients requiring but not receiving antimicrobials.[116] Indeed, a very recent study from United Kingdom showed that antibiotic prescription on the day of diagnosis of AECOPD (or another lower RTI) was associated with lower mortality (hazard ratio 0.31, 95% CI, 0.26–0.37).[117]

Several meta-analyses assessed the optimal duration of antimicrobial treatment of patients who had RTIs (**Fig. 2**). It was found that short-duration regimens (up to 7 days) may be as effective as long-duration ones ($\geq$ 2 days' difference) for AECOPD and CAP; but this equivalence seems not to hold true for tonsillitis/tonsillopharyngitis. Shortening the duration of antimicrobial treatment may be an effective way to reduce total antibiotic exposure and thus delay the emergence of antimicrobial resistance. Interestingly, there is no adequate evidence regarding the optimal duration of antimi-crobial treatment in nosocomial pneumonia/VAP.[118]

Finally, numerous meta-analyses have examined the putative effectiveness of several measures (either nonpharmacologic or pharmacologic) to prevent nosocomial

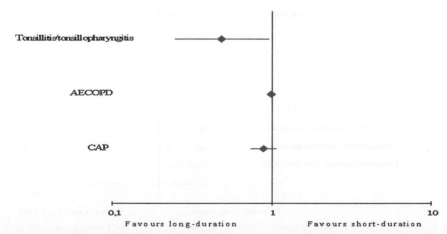

Fig. 2. Comparison antimicrobial treatment of long ($\geq$ 2 days difference) versus short (up to 7 days) duration with regard to clinical success in patients who had tonsillitis/tonsillophar-yngitis, AECOPD, and CAP. The vertical line indicates the point of no difference between the compared groups. Diamonds indicate the pooled OR (or RR) for each infection. Hori-zontal lines indicate the 95% confidence interval.

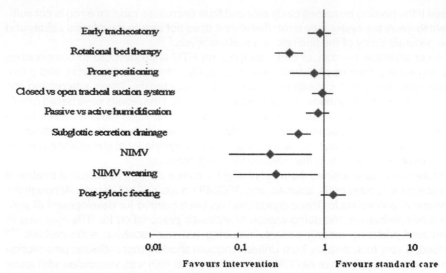

Fig. 3. Comparison of several nonpharmacologic measures ("intervention") versus standard care (or specified comparator) with regard to the incidence of nosocomial pneumonia/ VAP. The vertical line indicates the point of no difference between the compared groups. Diamonds indicate the pooled OR (or RR) for each infection. Horizontal lines indicate the 95% confidence interval. NIMV, noninvasive mechanical ventilation.

pneumonia (including VAP) (**Figs. 3** and **4**). Almost none of analyses (even those that found an advantage in the incidence of VAP) found that implementing such preventive measures conferred a survival benefit. This result may fuel the controversy regarding the mortality attributable to VAP.

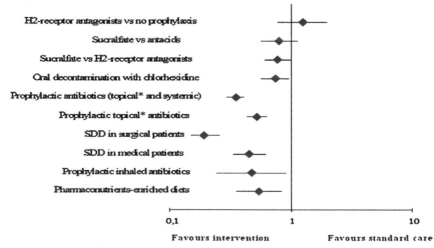

Fig. 4. Comparison of several pharmacologic measures ("intervention") versus standard care (or specified comparator) with regard to the incidence of nosocomial pneumonia/VAP. The vertical line indicates the point of no difference between the compared groups. Diamonds indicate the pooled OR (or RR) for each infection. Horizontal lines indicate the 95% confidence interval. *, Other than inhaled; H, histamine; SDD, selective digestive decontamination.

SUMMARY

The authors have endeavored to provide an overview of meta-analyses on the prevention and treatment of RTIs. Meta-analyses are useful tools to address clinically relevant questions; however, their inherent limitations should be taken into consideration when interpreting their findings.

REFERENCES

1. Connors AF Jr, Dawson NV, Thomas C, et al. Outcomes following acute exacerbation of severe chronic obstructive lung disease. The SUPPORT investigators (Study to Understand Prognoses and Preferences for Outcomes and Risks of Treatments). Am J Respir Crit Care Med 1996;154(4 Pt 1):959–67.
2. National Centre for Health Statistics. Health, United States, 2006, with chartbook on trends in the health of Americans. Available at: http://www.cdc.gov/nchs/data/hus/hus07.pdf#highlights. Assessed November 28, 2008.
3. Siempos II, Athanassa Z, Falagas ME. Frequency and predictors of ventilator-associated pneumonia recurrence: a meta-analysis. Shock 2008;30(5):487–95.
4. Chastre J, Fagon JY. Ventilator-associated pneumonia. Am J Respir Crit Care Med 2002;165(7):867–903.
5. Rosenfeld RM, Singer M, Wasserman JM, et al. Systematic review of topical antimicrobial therapy for acute otitis externa. Otolaryngol Head Neck Surg 2006; 134(4 Suppl):S24–48.
6. Rahman A, Rizwan S, Waycaster C, et al. Pooled analysis of two clinical trials comparing the clinical outcomes of topical ciprofloxacin/dexamethasone otic suspension and polymyxin B/neomycin/hydrocortisone otic suspension for the treatment of acute otitis externa in adults and children. Clin Ther 2007;29(9): 1950–6.
7. Abes G, Espallardo N, Tong M, et al. A systematic review of the effectiveness of ofloxaxin otic solution for the treatment of suppurative otitis media. ORL J Otorhinolaryngol Relat Spec 2003;65(2):106–16.
8. Ioannidis JP, Contopoulos-Ioannidis DG, Chew P, et al. Meta-analysis of randomized controlled trials on the comparative efficacy and safety of azithromycin against other antibiotics for upper respiratory tract infections. J Antimicrob Chemother 2001;48(5):677–89.
9. Falagas ME, Giannopoulou KP, Vardakas KZ, et al. Comparison of antibiotics with placebo for treatment of acute sinusitis: a meta-analysis of randomised controlled trials. Lancet Infect Dis 2008;8(9):543–52.
10. Young J, De Sutter A, Merenstein D, et al. Antibiotics for adults with clinically diagnosed acute rhinosinusitis: a meta-analysis of individual patient data. Lancet 2008;371(9616):908–14.
11. Ahovuo-Saloranta A, Borisenko OV, Kovanen N, et al. Antibiotics for acute maxillary sinusitis. Cochrane Database Syst Rev 2008;(2):CD000243.
12. Rosenfeld RM, Singer M, Jones S. Systematic review of antimicrobial therapy in patients with acute rhinosinusitis. Otolaryngol Head Neck Surg;137(3 Suppl): S32–45.
13. de Bock GH, Dekker FW, Stolk J, et al. Antimicrobial treatment in acute maxillary sinusitis: a meta-analysis. J Clin Epidemiol 1997;50(8):881–90.
14. Karageorgopoulos DE, Giannopoulou KP, Grammatikos AP, et al. Fluoroquinolones compared with beta-lactam antibiotics for the treatment of acute bacterial sinusitis: a meta-analysis of randomized controlled trials. CMAJ 2008;178(7): 845–54.

15. de Ferranti SD, Ioannidis JP, Lau J, et al. Are amoxycillin and folate inhibitors as effective as other antibiotics for acute sinusitis? A meta-analysis. BMJ 1998; 317(7159):632–7.

16. Zalmanovici A, Yaphe J. Steroids for acute sinusitis. Cochrane Database Syst Rev 2007;(2):CD005149.

17. Guo R, Canter PH, Ernst E. Herbal medicines for the treatment of rhinosinusitis: a systematic review. Otolaryngol Head Neck Surg 2006;135(4):496–506.

18. Casey JR, Pichichero ME. Higher dosages of azithromycin are more effective in treatment of group A streptococcal tonsillopharyngitis. Clin Infect Dis 2005; 40(12):1748–55.

19. Casey JR, Pichichero ME. Meta-analysis of cephalosporins versus penicillin for treatment of group A streptococcal tonsillopharyngitis in adults. Clin Infect Dis 2004;38(11):1526–34.

20. Falagas ME, Vouloumanou EK, Matthaiou DK, et al. Effectiveness and safety of short-course vs long-course antibiotic therapy for group a beta hemolytic streptococcal tonsillopharyngitis: a meta-analysis of randomized trials. Mayo Clin Proc 2008;83(8):880–9.

21. Pichichero ME, Casey JR. Bacterial eradication rates with shortened courses of 2nd- and 3rd-generation cephalosporins versus 10 days of penicillin for treatment of group A streptococcal tonsillopharyngitis in adults. Diagn Microbiol Infect Dis 2007;59(2):127–30.

22. Granger R, Walters J, Poole PJ, et al. Injectable vaccines for preventing pneumococcal infection in patients with chronic obstructive pulmonary disease. Cochrane Database Syst Rev 2006;(4):CD001390.

23. Poole PJ, Chacko E, Wood-Baker RW, et al. Influenza vaccine for patients with chronic obstructive pulmonary disease. Cochrane Database Syst Rev 2006;(1):CD002733.

24. Black P, Staykova T, Chacko E, et al. Prophylactic antibiotic therapy for chronic bronchitis. Cochrane Database Syst Rev 2003;(1):CD004105.

25. Puhan MA, Vollenweider D, Latshang T, et al. Exacerbations of chronic obstructive pulmonary disease: when are antibiotics indicated? A systematic review. Respir Res 2007;8:30.

26. Ram FS, Rodriguez-Roisin R, Granados-Navarrete A, et al. Antibiotics for exacerbations of chronic obstructive pulmonary disease. Cochrane Database Syst Rev 2006;(2):CD004403.

27. Saint S, Bent S, Vittinghoff E, et al. Antibiotics in chronic obstructive pulmonary disease exacerbations. A meta-analysis. JAMA 1995;273(12):957–60.

28. Puhan MA, Vollenweider D, Steurer J, et al. Where is the supporting evidence for treating mild to moderate chronic obstructive pulmonary disease exacerbations with antibiotics? A systematic review. BMC Med 2008;6:28.

29. Korbila IP, Manta KG, Siempos II, et al. Penicillins vs trimethoprim based regimens for acute bacterial exacerbations of chronic bronchitis: a meta-analysis of randomized controlled trials. Can Fam Physician 2009;55:60–7.

30. Dimopoulos G, Siempos II, Korbila IP, et al. Comparison of first-line with second-line antibiotics for acute exacerbations of chronic bronchitis: a metaanalysis of randomized controlled trials. Chest 2007;132(2):447–55.

31. Siempos II, Dimopoulos G, Korbila IP, et al. Macrolides, quinolones and amoxicillin/clavulanate for chronic bronchitis: a meta-analysis. Eur Respir J 2007; 29(6):1127–37.

32. Panpanich R, Lerttrakarnnon P, Laopaiboon M. Azithromycin for acute lower respiratory tract infections. Cochrane Database Syst Rev 2008;(1):CD001954.

33. Falagas ME, Avgeri SG, Matthaiou DK, et al. Short- versus long-duration antimicrobial treatment for exacerbations of chronic bronchitis: a meta-analysis. J Antimicrob Chemother 2008;62(3):442–50.
34. El Moussaoui R, Roede BM, Speelman P, et al. Short-course antibiotic treatment in acute exacerbations of chronic bronchitis and COPD: a meta-analysis of double-blind studies. Thorax 2008;63(5):415–22.
35. McCrory DC, Brown CD. Anti-cholinergic bronchodilators versus beta2-sympathomimetic agents for acute exacerbations of chronic obstructive pulmonary disease. Cochrane Database Syst Rev 2002;(4):CD003900.
36. Barr RG, Rowe BH, Camargo CA Jr. Methylxanthines for exacerbations of chronic obstructive pulmonary disease: meta-analysis of randomised trials. BMJ 2003;327(7416):643.
37. Quon BS, Gan WQ, Sin DD. Contemporary management of acute exacerbations of COPD: a systematic review and metaanalysis. Chest 2008;133(3):756–66.
38. Wood-Baker RR, Gibson PG, Hannay M, et al. Systemic corticosteroids for acute exacerbations of chronic obstructive pulmonary disease. Cochrane Database Syst Rev 2005;(1):CD001288.
39. Poole PJ, Black PN. Oral mucolytic drugs for exacerbations of chronic obstructive pulmonary disease: systematic review. BMJ 2001;322(7297):1271–4.
40. Ram FS, Picot J, Lightowler J, et al. Non-invasive positive pressure ventilation for treatment of respiratory failure due to exacerbations of chronic obstructive pulmonary disease. Cochrane Database Syst Rev 2004;(3):CD004104.
41. Keenan SP, Sinuff T, Cook DJ, et al. Which patients with acute exacerbation of chronic obstructive pulmonary disease benefit from noninvasive positive-pressure ventilation? A systematic review of the literature. Ann Intern Med 2003; 138(11):861–70.
42. Lightowler JV, Wedzicha JA, Elliott MW, et al. Non-invasive positive pressure ventilation to treat respiratory failure resulting from exacerbations of chronic obstructive pulmonary disease: Cochrane systematic review and meta-analysis. BMJ 2003;326(7382):185.
43. Keenan SP, Gregor J, Sibbald WJ, et al. Noninvasive positive pressure ventilation in the setting of severe, acute exacerbations of chronic obstructive pulmonary disease: more effective and less expensive. Crit Care Med 2000;28(6):2094–102.
44. Keenan SP, Kernerman PD, Cook DJ, et al. Effect of noninvasive positive pressure ventilation on mortality in patients admitted with acute respiratory failure: a meta-analysis. Crit Care Med 1997;25(10):1685–92.
45. Mills GD, Oehley MR, Arrol B. Effectiveness of beta lactam antibiotics compared with antibiotics active against atypical pathogens in non-severe community acquired pneumonia: meta-analysis. BMJ 2005;330(7489):456.
46. British Thoracic Society Standards of Care Committee. BTS guidelines for the management of community acquired pneumonia in adults. Thorax 2001; 56(Suppl 4):IV1–64.
47. Mandell LA, Wunderink RG, Anzueto A, et al. Infectious Diseases Society of America; American Thoracic Society. Infectious Diseases Society of America/American Thoracic Society consensus guidelines on the management of community-acquired pneumonia in adults. Clin Infect Dis 2007;44(Suppl 2):S27–72.
48. Robenshtok E, Shefet D, Gafter-Gvili A, et al. Empiric antibiotic coverage of atypical pathogens for community acquired pneumonia in hospitalized adults. Cochrane Database Syst Rev 2008;(1):CD004418.

49. Shefet D, Robenshtok E, Paul M, et al. Empirical atypical coverage for inpatients with community-acquired pneumonia: systematic review of randomized controlled trials. Arch Intern Med 2005;165(17):1992–2000.
50. Maimon N, Nopmaneejumruslers C, Marras TK. Antibacterial class is not obviously important in outpatient pneumonia: a meta-analysis. Eur Respir J 2008;31(5):1068–76.
51. Vardakas KZ, Siempos II, Grammatikos A, et al. Respiratory fluoroquinolones for the treatment of community-acquired pneumonia: a meta-analysis of randomized controlled trials. CMAJ 2008;179(12):1269–77.
52. Mittmann N, Jivarj F, Wong A, et al. Oral fluoroquinolones in the treatment of pneumonia, bronchitis and sinusitis. Can J Infect Dis 2002;13(5):293–300.
53. Salkind AR, Cuddy PG, Foxworth JW. Fluoroquinolone treatment of community-acquired pneumonia: a meta-analysis. Ann Pharmacother 2002;36(12):1938–43.
54. Fogarty C, Torres A, Choudhri S, et al. Efficacy of moxifloxacin for treatment of penicillin-, macrolide- and multidrug-resistant *Streptococcus pneumoniae* in community-acquired pneumonia. Int J Clin Pract 2005;59(11):1253–9.
55. Hoeffken G, Talan D, Larsen LS, et al. Efficacy and safety of sequential moxifloxacin for treatment of community-acquired pneumonia associated with atypical pathogens. Eur J Clin Microbiol Infect Dis 2004;23(10):772–5.
56. Tennenberg AM, Davis NB, Wu SC, et al. Pneumonia due to *Pseudomonas aeruginosa*: the levofloxacin clinical trials experience. Curr Med Res Opin 2006;22(5):843–50.
57. Bru JP, Leophonte P, Veyssier P. [Levofloxacine for the treatment of pneumococcal pneumonia: results of a meta-analysis]. Rev Pneumol Clin 2003;59(6): 348–56 [in French].
58. Contopoulos-Ioannidis DG, Ioannidis JP, Chew P, et al. Meta-analysis of randomized controlled trials on the comparative efficacy and safety of azithromycin against other antibiotics for lower respiratory tract infections. J Antimicrob Chemother 2001;48(5):691–703.
59. Falagas ME, Siempos IInd, Bliziotis IA, et al. Impact of initial discordant treatment with β-lactam antibiotics on clinical outcomes in adults with pneumococcal pneumonia: a systematic review. Mayo Clin Proc 2006;81(12):1567–74.
60. Dimopoulos G, Matthaiou DK, Karageorgopoulos DE, et al. Short- versus long-course antibacterial therapy for community-acquired pneumonia: a meta-analysis. Drugs 2008;68(13):1841–54.
61. Li JZ, Winston LG, Moore DH, et al. Efficacy of short-course antibiotic regimens for community-acquired pneumonia: a meta-analysis. Am J Med 2007;120(9): 783–90.
62. Athanassa Z, Makris G, Dimopoulos G, et al. Early switch to oral treatment in patients with moderate to severe community-acquired pneumonia: a meta-analysis. Drugs 2008;68(17):2469–81.
63. Rhew DC, Tu GS, Ofman J, et al. Early switch and early discharge strategies in patients with community-acquired pneumonia: a meta-analysis. Arch Intern Med 2001;161(5):722–7.
64. Siempos IInd, Vardakas KZ, Kopterides P, et al. Adjunctive therapies for community-acquired pneumonia: a systematic review. J Antimicrob Chemother 2008; 62(4):661–8.
65. Salluh JI, Póvoa P, Soares M, et al. The role of corticosteroids in severe community-acquired pneumonia: a systematic review. Crit Care 2008;12(3):R76.
66. Griffiths J, Barber VS, Morgan L, et al. Systematic review and meta-analysis of studies of the timing of tracheostomy in adult patients undergoing artificial ventilation. BMJ 2005;330(7502):1243.

67. Goldhill DR, Imhoff M, McLean B, et al. Rotational bed therapy to prevent and treat respiratory complications: a review and meta-analysis. Am J Crit Care 2007;16(1):50–61.
68. Delaney A, Gray H, Laupland KB, et al. Kinetic bed therapy to prevent nosocomial pneumonia in mechanically ventilated patients: a systematic review and meta-analysis. Crit Care 2006;10(3):R70.
69. Sud S, Sud M, Friedrich JO, et al. Effect of mechanical ventilation in the prone position on clinical outcomes in patients with acute hypoxemic respiratory failure: a systematic review and meta-analysis. CMAJ 2008;178(9):1153–61.
70. Abroug F, Ouanes-Besbes L, Elatrous S, et al. The effect of prone positioning in acute respiratory distress syndrome or acute lung injury: a meta-analysis. Areas of uncertainty and recommendations for research. Intensive Care Med 2008; 34(6):1002–11.
71. Tiruvoipati R, Bangash M, Manktelow B, et al. Efficacy of prone ventilation in adult patients with acute respiratory failure: a meta-analysis. J Crit Care 2008; 23(1):101–10.
72. Alsaghir AH, Martin CM. Effect of prone positioning in patients with acute respiratory distress syndrome: a meta-analysis. Crit Care Med 2008;36(2): 603–9.
73. Siempos II, Vardakas KZ, Falagas ME. Closed tracheal suction systems for prevention of ventilator-associated pneumonia. Br J Anaesth 2008;100(3): 299–306.
74. Subirana M, Solà I, Benito S. Closed tracheal suction systems versus open tracheal suction systems for mechanically ventilated adult patients. Cochrane Database Syst Rev 2007;(4):CD004581.
75. Niël-Weise BS, Snoeren RL, van den Broek PJ. Policies for endotracheal suctioning of patients receiving mechanical ventilation: a systematic review of randomized controlled trials. Infect Control Hosp Epidemiol 2007;28(5):531–6.
76. Peter JV, Chacko B, Moran JL. Comparison of closed endotracheal suction versus open endotracheal suction in the development of ventilator-associated pneumonia in intensive care patients: an evaluation using meta-analytic techniques. Indian J Med Sci 2007;61(4):201–11.
77. Jongerden IP, Rovers MM, Grypdonck MH, et al. Open and closed endotracheal suction systems in mechanically ventilated intensive care patients: a meta-analysis. Crit Care Med 2007;35(1):260–70.
78. Vonberg RP, Eckmanns T, Welte T, et al. Impact of the suctioning system (open vs. closed) on the incidence of ventilation-associated pneumonia: meta-analysis of randomized controlled trials. Intensive Care Med 2006;32(9):1329–35.
79. Siempos II, Vardakas KZ, Kopterides P, et al. Impact of passive humidification on clinical outcomes of mechanically ventilated patients: a meta-analysis of randomized controlled trials. Crit Care Med 2007;35(12):2843–51.
80. Niël-Weise BS, Wille JC, van den Broek PJ. Humidification policies for mechanically ventilated intensive care patients and prevention of ventilator-associated pneumonia: a systematic review of randomized controlled trials. J Hosp Infect 2007;65(4):285–91.
81. Kola A, Eckmanns T, Gastmeier P. Efficacy of heat and moisture exchangers in preventing ventilator-associated pneumonia: meta-analysis of randomized controlled trials. Intensive Care Med 2005;31(1):5–11.
82. Hess DR, Kallstrom TJ, Mottram CD, et al. American Association for Respiratory Care. Care of the ventilator circuit and its relation to ventilator-associated pneumonia. Respir Care 2003;48(9):869–79.

83. American Thoracic Society. Infectious Diseases Society of America. Guidelines for the management of adults with hospital-acquired, ventilator-associated, and healthcare-associated pneumonia. Am J Respir Crit Care Med. 2005;171(4): 388–416.

84. Tablan OC, Anderson LJ, Besser R, et al. Healthcare Infection Control Practices Advisory Committee. Guidelines for preventing health-care–associated pneumonia, 2003: recommendations of CDC and the Healthcare Infection Control Practices Advisory Committee. MMWR Recomm Rep 2004;53(RR-3):1–36.

85. Dezfulian C, Shojania K, Collard HR, et al. Subglottic secretion drainage for preventing ventilator-associated pneumonia: a meta-analysis. Am J Med 2005; 118(1):11–8.

86. Hess DR. Noninvasive positive-pressure ventilation and ventilator-associated pneumonia. Respir Care 2005;50(7):924–9.

87. Burns KE, Adhikari NK, Meade MO. A meta-analysis of noninvasive weaning to facilitate liberation from mechanical ventilation. Can J Anaesth 2006;53(3):305–15.

88. Burns KE, Adhikari NK, Meade MO. Noninvasive positive pressure ventilation as a weaning strategy for intubated adults with respiratory failure. Cochrane Database Syst Rev 2003;(4):CD004127.

89. Ho KM, Dobb GJ, Webb SA. A comparison of early gastric and post-pyloric feeding in critically ill patients: a meta-analysis. Intensive Care Med 2006; 32(5):639–49.

90. Marik PE, Zaloga GP. Gastric versus post-pyloric feeding: a systematic review. Crit Care 2003;7(3):R46–51.

91. Messori A, Trippoli S, Vaiani M, et al. Bleeding and pneumonia in intensive care patients given ranitidine and sucralfate for prevention of stress ulcer: meta-analysis of randomised controlled trials. BMJ 2000;321(7269):1103–6.

92. Cook DJ, Reeve BK, Guyatt GH, et al. Stress ulcer prophylaxis in critically ill patients. Resolving discordant meta-analyses. JAMA 1996;275(4):308–14.

93. Cook DJ, Reeve BK, Scholes LC. Histamine-2-receptor antagonists and antacids in the critically ill population: stress ulceration versus nosocomial pneumonia. Infect Control Hosp Epidemiol 1994;15(7):437–42.

94. Cook DJ, Laine LA, Guyatt GH, et al. Nosocomial pneumonia and the role of gastric pH. A meta-analysis. Chest 1991;100(1):7–13.

95. Tryba M. Sucralfate versus antacids or H2-antagonists for stress ulcer prophylaxis: a meta-analysis on efficacy and pneumonia rate. Crit Care Med 1991; 19(7):942–9.

96. Tryba M. Prophylaxis of stress ulcer bleeding. A meta-analysis. J Clin Gastroenterol. 1991;13(Suppl 2):S44–55.

97. Chlebicki MP, Safdar N. Topical chlorhexidine for prevention of ventilator-associated pneumonia: a meta-analysis. Crit Care Med 2007;35(2):595–602.

98. Chan EY, Ruest A, Meade MO, et al. Oral decontamination for prevention of pneumonia in mechanically ventilated adults: systematic review and meta-analysis. BMJ 2007;334(7599):889.

99. Siempos II, Falagas ME. Oral decontamination with chlorhexidine reduces the incidence of nosocomial pneumonia. Crit Care 2007;11(1):402.

100. Pineda LA, Saliba RG, El Solh AA. Effect of oral decontamination with chlorhexidine on the incidence of nosocomial pneumonia: a meta-analysis. Crit Care 2006;10(1):R35.

101. Liberati A, D'Amico R, Pifferi, et al. Antibiotic prophylaxis to reduce respiratory tract infections and mortality in adults receiving intensive care. Cochrane Database Syst Rev. 2004;(1):CD000022.

102. Nathens AB, Marshall JC. Selective decontamination of the digestive tract in surgical patients: a systematic review of the evidence. Arch Surg 1999;134(2): 170–6.
103. Kollef MH. The role of selective digestive tract decontamination on mortality and respiratory tract infections. A meta-analysis. Chest 1994;105(4):1101–8.
104. Falagas ME, Siempos II, Bliziotis IA, et al. Administration of antibiotics via the respiratory tract for the prevention of ICU-acquired pneumonia: a meta-analysis of comparative trials. Crit Care 2006;10(4):R123.
105. Falagas ME, Siempos II. Prevention of ventilator-associated pneumonia: possible role of antimicrobials administered via the respiratory tract. Eur Respir J 2008;31(5):1138–9.
106. Watkinson PJ, Barber VS, Dark P, et al. The use of pre- pro- and synbiotics in adult intensive care unit patients: systematic review. Clin Nutr 2007;26(2): 182–92.
107. Montejo JC, Zarazaga A, López-Martínez J, et al. Spanish Society of Intensive Care Medicine and Coronary Units. Immunonutrition in the intensive care unit. A systematic review and consensus statement. Clin Nutr 2003; 22(3):221–33.
108. Aarts MA, Hancock JN, Heyland D, et al. Empiric antibiotic therapy for suspected ventilator-associated pneumonia: a systematic review and meta-analysis of randomized trials. Crit Care Med 2008;36(1):108–17.
109. Siempos II, Vardakas KZ, Manta KG, et al. Carbapenems for the treatment of immunocompetent adult patients with nosocomial pneumonia. Eur Respir J 2007;29(3):548–60.
110. Shorr AF, Susla GB, Kollef MH. Quinolones for treatment of nosocomial pneumonia: a meta-analysis. Clin Infect Dis 2005;40(Suppl 2):S115–22.
111. Falagas ME, Siempos II, Vardakas KZ. Linezolid versus glycopeptide or beta-lactam for treatment of gram-positive bacterial infections: meta-analysis of randomised controlled trials. Lancet Infect Dis 2008;8(1):53–66.
112. Ioannidou E, Siempos II, Falagas ME. Administration of antimicrobials via the respiratory tract for the treatment of patients with nosocomial pneumonia: a meta-analysis. J Antimicrob Chemother 2007;60(6):1216–26.
113. Falagas ME, Agrafiotis M, Athanassa Z, et al. Administration of antibiotics via the respiratory tract as monotherapy for pneumonia. Expert Rev Anti Infect Ther 2008;6(4):447–52.
114. Cook DJ, Mulrow CD, Haynes RB. Systematic reviews: synthesis of best evidence for clinical decisions. Ann Intern Med 1997;126(5):376–80.
115. Tobin MJ, Jubran A. Meta-analysis under the spotlight: focused on a meta-analysis of ventilator weaning. Crit Care Med 2008;36(1):1–7.
116. Siempos II, Michalopoulos A, Falagas ME. Treatment of acute bacterial exacerbations of chronic bronchitis. Expert Opin Pharmacother [in press].
117. Winchester CC, Macfarlane T, Thomas M, et al. Antibiotic prescribing and outcomes of lower respiratory tract infection in UK primary care. Chest 2008, in press.
118. Grammatikos AP, Siempos II, Michalopoulos A, et al. Optimal duration of antimicrobial treatment of ventilator-acquired pneumonia. Expert Rev Anti Infect Ther 2008;6:861–6.

Meta-analyses in Prevention and Treatment of Urinary Tract Infections

Philip Masson, MBChB, BA (Hons), MA (Oxon), MRCP (UK)[a],*,
Sandra Matheson, BSc (Hons), MPH[b],
Angela C. Webster, MBBS, MM (Clin Epi), PhD, MRCP (UK)[c],
Jonathan C. Craig, MBChB, DCh, MM (Clin Epi), PhD, FRACP[c]

KEYWORDS

- Urinary tract infection • Treatment of urinary tract infection
- Prevention of urinary tract infection • Meta-analysis
- Systematic review

Urinary tract infections (UTI) are common among all age groups and are among the most frequent medical conditions requiring outpatient treatment. Complications ensuing from persistent and repeated infections result in more than 1 million hospital admissions per year in the United States alone. Apart from the youngest children, females are more vulnerable than males in all age groups; adult women are at 50 times higher risk than men, and up to 30% of women experience a symptomatic UTI in their lifetime. Because most UTI arise from the ascending route, the increased risk in women is hypothesized to arise from the anatomically shorter female urethra. In children, the incidence is more common among boys until the age of 12 months, but overall, 8.4% of girls and 1.7% of boys have suffered at least one UTI episode by the age of 7 years. Transient renal impairment is seen in up to 40% of children who have UTI, and permanent kidney damage occurs in approximately 5%. Among institutionalized individuals, UTI is the most common form of bacterial infection, with 12% to 30% of this population experiencing one episode per year. UTI occurs in 17% to 20% of pregnancies and is associated with premature membrane rupture, labor, and delivery, chorioamnionitis, and postpartum maternal and neonatal infection. Asymptomatic bacteriuria affects between 2% and 10% of pregnancies, with up to 30% of these women developing pyelonephritis. Mechanical ureteric compression causing hydroureter and hydronephrosis, as well as progesterone-induced smooth muscle relaxation are proposed mechanisms for this susceptibility.

[a] Department of Renal Medicine, Royal Infirmary of Edinburgh, EH16 4SA, Scotland, UK
[b] Centre for Kidney Research, The Children's Hospital, Westmead, NSW 2045, Australia
[c] School of Public Health, University of Sydney, Sydney, NSW 2006, Australia
* Corresponding author.
E-mail address: philip.masson@luht.nhs.scot.uk (P. Masson).

Infect Dis Clin N Am 23 (2009) 355–385
doi:10.1016/j.idc.2009.01.001
0891-5520/09/$ – see front matter © 2009 Published by Elsevier Inc.

UTI are defined by the presence of bacteria in the urine, with the usual threshold for defining UTI set at greater than 100,000 bacterial colony-forming units per milliliter (cfu/mL). The spectrum of UTI spans cystitis (bacteria in the bladder), urethral syndrome (symptoms despite sterile urine or bacterial growth < 100,000 cfu/mL), and pyelonephritis. Associated signs and symptoms include urgency, frequency, dysuria, cloudy urine, lower back pain, fevers, hematuria, and often pyuria (a urine white cell count > 10,000/mL). Pyelonephritis occurs most commonly as a result of cystitis, particularly in the presence of transient or persistent vesico-ureteric reflux. Asymptomatic bacteriuria is defined by the presence of more than 100,000 cfu/mL in the absence of signs or symptoms.

INTERVENTIONS TO PREVENT URINARY TRACT INFECTIONS

Cranberries long have been advocated for the prevention and treatment of UTI. Cranberries contain mallic acid, citric acid, quinic acid, fructose, and glucose. It is thought that fructose and proancanthocyanidins inhibit adherence of type 1 and α-galactose–specific fimbriated *Escherichia coli* to the uroepithelial cell lining of the bladder. A role for urinary hippuric acid excretion has been somewhat discredited, with several studies showing cranberry to have no or only an extremely transient effect in lowering urinary pH. Vitamin C is cited similarly as acidifying urine, but the lack of evidence that vitamin C significantly lowers urinary pH and the theoretical risk of calcium oxalate stone formation have limited its clinical application. Among elderly women, postmenopausal hormonal changes lead to changes in vaginal bacterial flora. This observation has led to interest in the role of topical estrogen creams and ring pessaries in preventing UTI. Other probiotic interventions such as Lactobacillus drinks have been proposed to maintain vaginal pH in its usual acidic range of pH 4 to 4.5, thereby inhibiting bacterial growth, with supportive observational data. No adequately sized randomized, controlled trial (RCT) for this or any other urinary antiseptic intervention other than cranberry product has been published, however.

The most commonly used non-antiseptic strategy for preventing UTI is the prescription of long-term antibiotics. Antibiotics are used most commonly for pregnant women and children because of the correlation between recurrent UTI and the development of acute pyelonephritis, low-birth-weight babies, acute renal impairment, and renal scarring. It is unclear, however, which antibiotic schedule, class, or duration of treatment is optimal for antibiotic prophylaxis, and there is little understanding of the incidence of adverse events, recurrence of infections, and development of resistant organisms after the prophylaxis ceases.

INTERVENTIONS TO TREAT URINARY TRACT INFECTION

A range of antibiotics, with different rates of cure and varying side-effect profiles, are used in the treatment of UTI. It is unclear whether short-course therapies are as effective as longer-course regimens in inducing cure and in preventing relapse and also whether the route of administration affects these outcomes or the incidence of side effects. It also is unknown whether antibiotic class, treatment duration, and route of delivery affect treatment adherence and whether compliance in turn affects clinical and microbiologic outcomes, including the subsequent development of bacterial resistance.

This overview presents the current literature, specifically evidence summarized by systematic reviews and meta-analyses, for the prevention and treatment of UTI in adults and children and comments on the quality of this evidence and its applicability to different patient groups in clinical practice.

METHODS OF LITERATURE REVIEW

In September 2008 the authors searched databases of the Cochrane Library and MEDLINE for systematic reviews of RCTs for the prevention and treatment of UTI in any patient population. Sensitive search strategies were devised by combining medical subject headings (MeSH) with text words for UTI, including "urinary tract infection," "bacteriuria," and "pyuria." Terms specific for prevention interventions included "beverages," "fruit," "cranberries," "vaccinium macrocarpon," "vaccinium oxycoccus," "vaccinium vitis-idaea," "antibiotic prophylaxis," "antibiotics," and "urinary anti-infective agents." The search terms for treatment interventions included "antibiotics," "anti-infective agents," "quinolones," "beta-lactams," "trimethoprim-sulfamethoxazole," and "nitrofurantoin," and terms for treatment delivery were "short-term," "long-term," "duration," "oral," "intravenous," and "parenteral," The results of each search strategy then were limited using terms to identify only systematic reviews and meta-analyses.

All systematic reviews of RCTs identified by the searches were assessed, and details of methodological quality and quantitative outcome data were abstracted. All systematic reviews are summarized in the tables, but only reviews that included meta-analysis are discussed in the text.

PREVENTION OF URINARY TRACT INFECTIONS IN WOMEN

One systematic review including meta-analysis of four RCTs evaluated the effectiveness of either cranberry juice or another cranberry product versus placebo in diverse populations (**Table 1**).[1] Of these, two RCTs exclusively enrolled women who had recurrent UTI; the other RCTs included elderly people aged over 60 years and patients who had at least a 12-month history of spinal cord injury and neurogenic bladder. The primary outcome of UTI was defined variably among trials and included symptomatic UTI, symptoms plus single-organism growth greater than 10^4 cfu/mL or detection of asymptomatic or symptomatic bacteriuria greater than 10^6 cfu/mL on monthly urine culture. Meta-analysis of all four RCTs evaluating 665 patients concluded that cranberry products significantly reduced the incidence of UTI by 34% at 12 months compared with control/placebo (relative risk [RR] 0.66, 95% confidence interval [CI], 0.47–0.92, $P = .01$). When results from the RCTs in women who had recurrent UTI were synthesized, the reduction in the number experiencing at least one symptomatic UTI was even more marked, with a 39% reduction at 12 months (two RCTs, n = 244, RR 0.61, 95% CI, 0.40–0.91).

Of the four cranberry-product RCTs that were combined in the meta-analysis, three had adequate allocation concealment, three were double blinded, and two reported results by intention-to-treat (ITT) principles (see **Table 4**). RCTs varied in duration (from 6 months to 1 year of active treatment), in population (from sexually active women to patients 1 year after spinal cord injury), and dosage (30–300 mL/d cranberry juice or cranberry capsules containing an unquantified concentration of active cranberry product). Despite these differences, estimates of treatment effect were similar among synthesized RCTs, with no significant heterogeneity observed among population subgroups. Estimates of effect were statistically significant for women who had uncomplicated recurrent UTI (narrower 95% CI, 0.40–0.91). All RCTs examined direct, un-confounded comparisons of cranberry product versus placebo or no treatment.

One meta-analysis assessed the effectiveness of prophylactic antibiotics versus placebo or no treatment in the prevention of UTI and included 11 RCTs of 430 nonpregnant women over 14 years of age who had a history of at least two

Table 1
Systematic review and meta-analysis literature identified for prophylaxis and treatment of UTI in pregnant and nonpregnant women[a]

Study	Description	Participants	Interventions	Outcomes	Results
Prevention: cranberry products					
Griffiths 2003	Overview of systematic reviews and RCT	All patient populations	Cranberries versus no treatment or standard treatment	Symptomatic/ asymptomatic UTI	No additional meta-analysis
Jepson 2008	Systematic review	All patient populations	Cranberry juice or capsules versus placebo or no treatment	Symptomatic/ asymptomatic UTI Side effects	Fewer symptomatic UTI at 12 months (4 RCTs, all populations, n = 665, RR 0.66, 95% CI 0.47–0.92, P = .01; for women only: 2 RCTs, n = 244, RR 0.61, 95% CI 0.40–0.91). Bacteriuria in elderly women: no meta-analysis, results reported for individual RCT only. No significant differences for side effects (no data).
Prevention: prophylactic antibiotics					
Albert 2004	Systematic review	Nonpregnant women over 14 years of age with a history of uncomplicated UTI	Antibiotics versus placebo, 6–12 months treatment duration	Symptomatic/ asymptomatic UTI Side effects	Fewer asymptomatic UTI during antibiotic prophylaxis versus placebo (11 RCTs, n = 372, RR 0.21, 95% CI 0.13–0.34, P < .00001). No significant differences after prophylaxis ceased (RR 0.82, 95% CI 0.44–1.53). Fewer symptomatic UTI during antibiotic prophylaxis versus placebo (7 RCTs, n = 257, RR 0.15, 95% CI 0.08–0.28, P < .00001). No studies assessed symptomatic UTI after prophylaxis ceased No significant differences in severe side effects (11 RCTs, n = 420, RR 1.58, 95% CI 0.47–5.28), mild side effects reported more frequently for antibiotic group (RR 1.78, 95% CI 1.06–3.00)
Smaill 2007	Systematic review	Pregnant women with asymptomatic bacteriuria	Any antibiotic versus placebo or no treatment	Pyelonephritis Birth weight	Reduced pyelonephritis (11 RCTs, n = 1955, RR 0.23, 95% CI 0.13–0.41, P < .00001). Reduced low birth weight (< 2500 g) for antibiotic group (7 RCTs, n = 1502, RR 0.66, 95% CI 0.49–0.89, P = .006).

Treatment: class of antibiotic

Vazquez 2006	Systematic review	Pregnant women with symptomatic UTI	1 RCT cephazolin versus ampicillin + gentamicin and ceftriaxone versus ampicillin + gentamicin. 1 RCT ampicillin versus nitrofurantoin. 1 RCT fosfomycin versus ceftibuten	Symptomatic/asymptomatic UTI Recurrence	No meta-analysis. Results reported for individual RCTs only.

Treatment: duration of antibiotic treatment

Milo 2005	Systematic review	Women with uncomplicated UTI	Short course (< 3 days) versus long course (7–10 days). 19 RCTs tested the same antibiotic; 14 RTCs tested different antibiotics	Symptomatic/asymptomatic UTI Pyelonephritis Side effects	No differences in symptomatic UTI within 2–15 days (24 RCTs, n = 8752, RR 1.06, 95% CI 0.88–1.28) or within 4–10 weeks (8 RTCs, n = 3141, RR 1.09, 95% CI 0.94–1.27). Subgroup analyses showed similar results for RCTs testing the same antibiotic across groups and those testing different antibiotics across groups. Fewer asymptomatic UTI for long course within 2–15 days (31 RCTs, n = 5368, RR 1.19, 95% CI 0.98–1.44, P = .08) and within 4–10 days (18 RCTs, n = 3715, RR 1.31, 95% CI 1.08–1.60, P = .006). Subgroup analyses showed this finding held only for RCTs testing same antibiotic in RCT arms (2–15 days: 18 RCTs, n = 3146, RR 1.37, 95% CI 1.07–1.74, P = .01; 4–10 weeks: 13 RCTs, n = 2502, RR 1.43, 95% CI 1.19–1.73, P = .0002). No significant differences for RCTs testing different antibiotics (2–15 days: 13 RCTs, n = 2222, RR 0.96, 95% CI 0.68–1.35, P = 0.80; 4–10 weeks: 5 RCTs, n = 1213, RR 1.13, 95% CI 0.73–1.77). No significant differences for the development of pyelonephritis (5 RCTs, n = 582, RR 3.04, 95% CI 0.32–28.93) or adverse events (29 RCTs, n = 7617, RR 0.83, 95% CI 0.74–0.93)

(continued on next page)

Table 1
(continued)

Study	Description	Participants	Interventions	Outcomes	Results
Vazquez 2006	Systematic review, 1 RCT for this comparison	Pregnant women with symptomatic UTI	1 RCT single-versus multiple-dose gentamicin	Symptomatic/ asymptomatic UTI	No meta-analysis: results reported for individual RCT
Villar 2000	Systematic review	Pregnant women with asymptomatic UTI	Single dose versus short course (4–7 days)	Recurrent asymptomatic UTI Pyelonephritis Side effects	No significant differences for "no cure" rate (10 RCTs, n = 568, RR 1.25, 95% CI 0.93–1.67), recurrent asymptomatic UTI (7 RCTs, n = 336, RR 1.14, 95% CI 0.77–1.67), pyelonephritis (2 RCTs, n = 102, RR 3.09, 95% CI 0.54–17.55). For RCTs assessing the same antibiotic for different durations, no significant differences for "no cure" (6 RCTs, n = 353, RR 1.22, 95% CI 0.84–1.76), recurrence (6 RCTs, n = 353, RR 1.08, 95% CI 0.70–1.66), or pyelonephritis (2 RCTs, n = 102, RR 3.09, 95% CI 0.54–17.55). Fewer mild side effects for single dose (9 RCTs, n = 507, R 052, 95% CI 0.32–0.85, P = .009).

Treatment: route of administration

Study	Type	Population	Interventions	Outcomes	Results
Pohl 2007	Systematic review	Mostly women with symptomatic UTI	6 RCTs switch (IV or IM then oral) versus 4–14 days parenteral. 5 RCTs oral versus 10–14 days switch. 2 RCTs single-dose parenteral plus oral versus switch, both 10 days. 1 RCT oral versus parenteral, both 7 days. 1 RCT single IM plus oral versus oral alone.	Symptomatic/asymptomatic UTI Re-infection Recurrence Side effects	Parenteral versus oral: no meta-analysis; results reported for 1 RCT only. Switch versus parenteral: no significant differences for asymptomatic (2 RCTs, n = 76 RR 1.11, 95% CI 0.90–1.36) or symptomatic cure (2 RCTs, n = 137, RR 1.01, 95% CI 0.94–1.10) or for both combined (4 RCTs, n = 294, RR 0.99, 95% CI 0.93–1.06) or after an interval (3 RCTs, n = 219, RR 0.99, 95% CI 0.86–1.13). No significant differences in re-infection after an interval (4 RCTs, n = 239, RR 0.76, 95% CI 0.30–1.90), recurrence after an interval (3 RCTs, n = 203, RR 2.79, 95% CI 0.30–25.67), or adverse events (4 RCTs, n = 292, RR 0.85, 95% CI 0.19–3.83). Heterogeneity for adverse events was explored via subgroup analyses of pediatric studies (RR 0.67, I^2 0%, 95% CI 0.30–1.53) and adult studies (RR 0.85, 95% CI 0.19–3.83). Oral versus switch: no significant differences for asymptomatic or symptomatic cure (3 RCTs, n = 599, RR 1.04, 95% CI 0.97–1.12), after an interval (3 RCTs, n = 493, RR 0.97, 95% CI 0.93–1.01), for re-infection after an interval (2 RCTs, n = 341, RR 0.64, 95% CI 0.29–1.42), or adverse events (2 RCTs, n = 506, RR 0.96, 95% CI 0.06–15.02). Single shot plus oral versus switch: no significant differences for symptomatic cure (2 RCTs, n = 225, RR 0.93, 95% CI 0.85–1.02), or adverse events (2 RCTs, n = 225, RR 4.00, 95% CI 0.46–34.75).
Vazquez 2006	Systematic review	Pregnant women with symptomatic UTI	1 RCT compared IV followed by oral versus IV. 1 RCT compared IM ceftriaxone versus IV ampicillin + gentamicin. 1 RCT IM ceftriaxone versus IV cephazolin.	Symptomatic/asymptomatic UTI Recurrence	No meta-analysis: results reported for each RCT.

a Symptomatic and asymptomatic UTI (bacteriuria) is defined as clinical and/or bacteriologic cure. Re-infection is defined as re-infection of a different bacterial strain. Recurrence is defined as recurrence of the same bacterial strain.

uncomplicated UTIs in the previous year.[2] Outcome measures included microbiologic recurrence (positive urine culture of > 100,000 bacteria/mL with isolation of a responsible agent, not necessarily the same as that causing original infection, or pyuria >10,000 bacteria/mL plus symptoms) or clinical recurrence (dysuria and/or urinary frequency) both during and after the prophylaxis period had ceased. Side effects, when recorded, were classified as severe (requiring withdrawal of treatment) or mild (not requiring withdrawal of treatment). Antibiotic prophylaxis regimens of at least 6 months' duration versus placebo were synthesized, showing that during the active treatment phase, antibiotics significantly reduced the risk of microbiologic recurrence by 79% (11 RCTs, n = 372, RR 0.21, 95% CI, 0.13–0.34, $P <$ .00001), and clinical recurrence by 85% (seven RCTs, n = 257, RR 0.15, 95% CI, 0.08–0.28, $P <$ .00001). No significant advantage was seen among the antibiotic-treated group once prophylactic treatment had ceased, however. Antibiotic-treated subjects were 58% more likely to describe severe side effects (11 RCTs, n = 420, RR 1.58, 95% CI, 0.47–5.28) and 78% more likely to describe mild side effects than those taking placebo (RR 1.78, 95% CI, 1.06–3.00).

Of the 11 RCTs included in this meta-analysis, all implied that randomization methods were used, but the precise method of allocation concealment was not reported adequately in any; thus randomization was judged unclear by review authors, although 10 RTCs were double blinded. Among the included RCTs no heterogeneity of results (I^2) was demonstrated. Data were derived from large sample sizes and gave precise estimates of effect, with narrow 95% CIs of 0.13–0.34 (for microbiologic recurrence) and 0.008–0.28 (for clinical recurrence) for risk reduction during active prophylaxis.

TREATMENT OF URINARY TRACT INFECTIONS IN WOMEN

The authors identified no meta-analyses that compared different classes of antibiotics for treatment of UTI in women.

One systematic review investigated the optimal duration of antibiotic therapy for nonpregnant women under 65 years old and included 33 RCTs of 9605 women between the ages of 18 and 65 years who had uncomplicated UTI (see **Table 1**).[3] RCTs compared short-course (3 days) with longer-course (5 to 10 days) antibiotics, although not all RCTs reported all outcomes of interest. Meta-analyses were stratified by subgrouping RCTs using different antibiotics across each intervention arm and those using the same antibiotics in each arm. Outcome measures were defined as short- or long-term failure (within 2 or 8 weeks) for symptomatic or bacteriologic criteria (positive urine culture). Overall, the rate of short-term symptomatic failure was not significantly different in the short- and longer-course groups (24 RCTs, n = 8752, RR 1.06, 95% CI, 0.88–1.28, $P =$ .52). In the 14 RCTs using the same antibiotic in each trial arm, the RR was 1.15, and the 95% CI was 0.95 to 1.39. For the 10 RCTs using different antibiotics across trial arms, the RR was 0.90, and the 95% CI was 0.62 to 1.29. Long-term symptomatic failure was reported by eight RCTs, with no significant difference between short- and long-course treatment (n = 3141, RR 1.09, 95% CI, 0.94–1.27). Short-term bacteriologic failure (30 RCTs, 5368 participants) suggested a possible advantage of longer-duration treatment, although the difference was not statistically significant (RR 1.19, 95% CI, 0.98–1.44, $P =$ .08). The 18 RCTs comparing the same antibiotic across RCT arms showed a significantly improved rate of bacteriologic cure with a longer-duration course (n = 3146, RR 1.37, 95% CI, 1.07–1.74, $P =$ .01), but this finding was not evident in the RCT using different agents in each arm (13 RCTs, n = 2222, RR 0.96, 95% CI, 0.68–1.35, $P =$ .8). Overall, long-term bacteriologic failure was significantly higher in the short-duration group than in the longer-treatment arm (18 RCTs, n = 3715, RR 1.31, 95% CI, 1.08–1.60, P = .006). Subgroup analysis showed this finding to hold true for RCTs with the same drug in each allocation arm (13 RCTs, n = 2502, RR 1.43, 95% CI, 1.19–1.73, P = .0002), and no difference was seen when different drugs were used (five RCTs, n = 1213, RR 1.13, 95% CI, 0.73–1.77).

Of the 33 RCTs contributing to the meta-analysis of UTI treatment duration, 12 reported adequate methods of allocation concealment. The remainder used unclear allocation methods (see **Table 4**).[3] Nine were double blinded, and only three RCTs analyzed by ITT. Precise estimates of effect were derived giving narrow confidence intervals, because results of many RCTs were combined. Comparisons of short versus long courses of antibiotics were direct, although the antibiotics investigated varied widely among RCTs.

Another systematic review compared different routes of antibiotic administration and included 15 RCTs.[4] Class of antimicrobial agent and duration of therapy varied among the RCTs that contributed to the meta-analysis. Participants in the RCTs were predominantly nonpregnant women, although one RCT included pregnant women, and nine RCTs included both women and children who had symptomatic UTI. Meta-analysis results combined all RCTs, and did not report results separately by patient population. Relevant outcome measures were cure rate (clinical, microbiologic, and combined), re-infection rate (new pathogen in urine), relapse rate (initial pathogen in urine), and adverse effects. In six studies of 373 patients comparing "switch" therapy, defined as initial parenteral administration (more than one dose delivered by either the intramuscular [IM] or intravenous [IV] route) followed by oral therapy, versus continued parenteral therapy, the clinical cure rates (in two RCTs, n = 137, RR 1.01, 95% CI, 0.94–1.10) and the re-infection rates after an interval (in four RCTs, n = 239, RR 0.76, 95% CI, 0.30–1.90) were not significantly different between groups. No significant difference was seen for any other outcome. Switch versus oral therapy was evaluated in five RCTs (n = 1040), and there was no significant difference in the rates of bacteriologic or clinical cure (three RCTs, n = 493, RR 0.97, 95% CI, 0.93–1.01).

Eight of 15 RCTs in the review of the route of antibiotic administration used adequate allocation concealment, six with blinded outcome assessors, and three reported by ITT. Six studies had a dropout rate of more than 10%. Moderate heterogeneity for adverse event outcomes was seen among RCTs comparing switch versus parenteral therapy. Subgroup analysis suggested that this heterogeneity might be explained by the age of the RCT participants, with pediatric studies having an RR of 0.67 (95% CI, 0.30–1.53, I^2 0%), and adult studies having an RR of 0.85 (95% CI, 0.19–3.83). All other outcome results showed consistent findings. Comparisons between routes of administration were direct, although overall comparisons were confounded by the use of different classes of antibiotics across RCT arms and by differing durations of treatment.

PREVENTION OF URINARY TRACT INFECTIONS IN PREGNANT WOMEN

One meta-analysis synthesized results from 11 RCTs comparing antibiotic prophylaxis versus placebo in pregnant women who had asymptomatic bacteriuria, and all 11 RCTs reported the development of pyelonephritis as an outcome (see **Table 1**).[5] Among contributing RCTs, the duration of prophylaxis varied from a single dose to continuation of antibiotics until 6 weeks postpartum. A 77% reduction in the incidence of pyelonephritis was seen in the group receiving prophylactic antibiotics as compared with placebo (11 RCTs, n = 1955, RR 0.23, 95% CI, 0.13–0.41). A significant reduction in incidence of low-birth-weight babies also was seen among antibiotic-treated women (seven RCTs, n = 1502, RR 0.66, 95% CI, 0.49–0.89, P = .006).

Of these 11 RCTs, none clearly reported the method of allocation concealment, three were quasi-randomized, two were described as double blind, and an additional five RTCs used placebo in the control arm (suggesting they blinded both participants and investigators) (see **Table 4**). The magnitude of the treatment effect was inconsistent among RCTs (I^2 64% for pyelonephritis); review authors thought this inconsistency might be explained by study quality, but the direction of effect was consistent, showing benefit from prophylactic antibiotics. Estimates of effect were precise, with 95% CIs of 0.14 to 0.48 for the reduction in the incidence of asymptomatic bacteriuria and 0.13 to 0.41 for the reduction in the incidence of pyelonephritis.

TREATMENT OF URINARY TRACT INFECTIONS IN PREGNANT WOMEN

The authors identified one systematic review that examined the effect of antibiotic class on UTI cure and recurrence rates in pregnant women who had symptomatic UTI, including nine RCTs with a total of 997 participants (see **Table 1**).[6] Only four RCTs compared different antibiotic classes and reported outcomes of interest. Although each RCT used the same route of administration across RCT arms, and most RCTs used comparable durations of treatment, the interventions were varied, with different classes of antibiotics and different routes of administration, and a diversity of definitions was used to report varied outcomes, so no meta-analysis was undertaken. This same review also investigated the route of administration of antibiotics and identified three relevant RCTs. These RCTs made direct comparisons of IV versus other routes of antibiotic administration but used different antibiotics in each arm of the trial and for varying durations, thereby confounding the comparisons. Thus no data could be combined in meta-analysis for outcomes relevant to pregnant women, and individual RCTs were underpowered to report any significant difference of effect.

Another meta-analysis compared the effect of varying durations of antibiotic administration in the treatment of pregnant women who had asymptomatic bacteriuria.[7] Some RCTs evaluated different durations of the same antibiotic in unconfounded comparisons, whereas others compared different antibiotics and different durations of treatment. Ten RCTs enrolling 568 women who had asymptomatic bacteriuria compared 1-day treatment and 7-day treatment. The "no cure" rate was not different between groups (RR 1.25, 95% CI, 0.93–1.67) in RCTs comparing different durations of different antibiotics. The incidence of recurrent bacteriuria was similar between groups (seven RCTs, n = 336, RR 1.14, 95% CI, 0.77–1.67). These findings did not change when only the six RCTs that compared different durations of the same antibiotic were considered: there were no significant differences in the "no cure" rate (RR 1.22, 95% CI, 0.84–1.76) or recurrent bacteria (RR 1.08, 95% CI, 0.70–1.66). Rates of pyelonephritis were similar in the short- and long-duration treatment arms (two RCTs, n = 102, RR 3.09, 95% CI, 0.54–17.55). Review authors judged allocation concealment to be adequate in one of the 10 RCTs, the implied allocation concealment to be adequate in another five, and allocation concealment to be unclear in the remaining four RCTs in which the details of allocation method were not described at all (see **Table 4**). One RCT described blinded outcome assessment, nine gave no details, and participants were aware of their treatment allocation in all 10 RCTs. Interventions were applied in direct comparisons of single-dose versus short-course treatment, which gave precise outcome estimates of effect for both benefits and harms of therapy, with narrow 95% CIs of 0.32 to 0.85 for side effects.

PREVENTION OF URINARY TRACT INFECTIONS IN ELDERLY PEOPLE AND OTHER SPECIFIC POPULATIONS

There was no meta-analysis of prevention strategies including only elderly people or other populations. Of the four RCTs included in the meta-analysis of cranberry juice/cranberry product for the prophylaxis of UTI, one large RCT specifically recruited men and women over 60 years of age.[1] The result of the meta-analysis of the four RCTs combined (n = 665) significantly favored the cranberry group (RR 0.66, 95% CI, 0.47–0.92, P = .01) (Table 2). Results for the RCT reporting only elderly people had results consistent with the other three RCTs, with no measurable heterogeneity (I^2 0%), but results were imprecise when this RCT was considered alone, so the effect was not significant. One other RCT specifically recruited patients who had neuropathic bladders; this RTC also found no significant advantage for the group given cranberry product.

The authors identified one other systematic review that examined the use of prophylactic antibiotics in elderly patients resident in extended-care facilities.[8] This review identified five RCTs examining the role of prophylactic antibiotics in patients who had indwelling urinary catheters but did not include a meta-analysis. The review concluded that there was a potential role for antibiotics in reducing the rate of UTI among patients who had short-duration urinary catheters (3–14 days), on the basis of reduced rate of bacteriuria in three RCTs. This review did not report systematically the methodological quality of the five RCTs, and these five RCTs enrolled a diverse cohort of catheterized patients, varying from incontinent stroke patients to surgical candidates requiring short-term perioperative catheterization. The RCTs made a direct comparison of antibiotic therapy versus placebo, but among RCTs different antibiotics of varying doses and routes of administration were used, with different periods of active prophylactic treatment. Although results across RCTs were consistent, there was no formal measure of heterogeneity (see Table 4).

TREATMENT OF URINARY TRACT INFECTIONS IN ELDERLY PEOPLE AND OTHER SPECIFIC POPULATIONS

One systematic review examined the effect of short- versus long-duration antibiotic treatment in elderly women (> 65 years old) who had uncomplicated UTI.[9] The review identified 15 RCTs including a total of 1644 participants (see Table 2). Five RCTs compared single-dose versus short-course (3–6 days) antibiotic treatment. Persistent UTI was less common in the short-course group up to 2 weeks after treatment (n = 356, RR 2.01, 95% CI, 1.05–3.54, P = .034). This advantage was not sustained in the longer-term (> 2 weeks) follow-up, although fewer RCTs reported this outcome (three RCTs, n = 95, RR 1.18, 95% CI, 0.59–2.32). Six RCTs compared single-dose with long-course treatment (7–14 days), finding a significant decrease in persistent UTI for long-course compared with single-dose therapy in the short term (n = 628, RR 1.93, 95% CI, 1.01–3.70, P = .047) but not in long-term follow-up (RR 1.28, 95% CI, 0.89–1.84). Six RCTs compared short-course and long-course treatments. Persistent UTI at short- and long-term follow-up was not significantly different in either group (three RCTs; short-term: n = 431 RR 0.85, 95% CI, 0.29–2.47; long-term: n = 470, RR 0.85, 95% CI, 0.54–1.32). Two RCTs compared the same antibiotic across RCT arms, again with no difference seen for persistent UTI at short-term (n = 208, RR 1.00, 95% CI, 0.12–8.57) or long-term follow-up (RR 1.18, 95% CI, 0.50–2.81). Clinical failure was not significantly different in either short-term (five RCTs, n = 395, RR 0.98, 95% CI, 0.62–1.54) or long-term follow-up (one RCT only).

Table 2

Systematic review and meta-analysis literature identified for prophylaxis and treatment of UTI for elderly persons and other populations[a]

Study	Description	Participants	Interventions	Outcomes	Results
Prevention: cranberry products					
Griffiths 2003	Overview of systematic reviews and RCT	All patient populations	Cranberries versus no treatment or standard treatment	Symptomatic/ asymptomatic UTI	No additional meta-analysis
Jepson 2008	Systematic review	All patient populations	Cranberry juice or capsules versus placebo or no treatment	Symptomatic/ asymptomatic UTI Side effects	Fewer symptomatic UTI at 12 months (4 RCTs, n = 665, RR 0.66, 95% CI 0.47–0.92, $P = .01$); results less marked for elderly people than for women. Bacteriuria in elderly women: no meta-analysis. Results reported for individual RCT only. No significant differences for side effects (no data).
Regal 2006	Systematic review	Institutionalized elderly men and women	Cranberry juice versus none or placebo	Symptomatic/ asymptomatic UTI	No additional meta-analysis
Prevention: prophylactic antibiotics					
Regal 2006	Systematic review	Institutionalized elderly men and women	Various antibiotics versus none	Symptomatic/ asymptomatic UTI	No additional meta-analysis

Treatment: duration of antibiotic treatment

Lutters 2002	Systematic review	Elderly patients with uncomplicated UTI	Short course (3–6 days) versus long course (7–14 days), single dose versus short and long course	Symptomatic UTI Re-infection Any adverse events	Short course versus single dose: fewer persistent symptomatic UTI for up to 2 weeks after treatment (5 RCTs, n = 356, RR 2.01, 95% CI 1.05–3.84, P = .034), not over 2 weeks (3 RCTs, n = 95, RR 1.18, 95% CI 0.59–2.32). Re-infections: no meta-analysis; results reported for individual RCT only. Long course versus single dose: fewer persistent symptomatic UTI for up to 2 weeks after treatment (6 RCTs, n = 628, RR 1.93, 95% CI 1.01–3.70, P = .047) but not over 2 weeks (3 RCTs, n = 95 RR 1.28, 95% CI 0.89–1.84). No differences in adverse events (3 RCTs, n = 595, RR 0.80, 95% CI 0.45–1.41) Long versus short course: no significant differences for persistent UTI short term (3 RCTs, n = 431, RR 0.85, 95% CI 0.29–2.47) or long term (3 RCTs, n = 470, RR 0.85, 95% CI 0.54–1.32). No differences in re-infection long term (2 RCTs, n = 405, RR 1.30, 95% CI 0.42–4.01). Adverse events: no meta-analysis; results reported for individual RCT only. Two RCTs comparing the same antibiotic across RCT arms reported no difference for persistent UTI at short-term (n = 208, RR 1.00, 95% CI 0.12–8.57) or long-term follow-up (n = 247, RR 1.18, 95% CI 0.50–2.81). Clinical failure was not significantly different in short-term follow-up (5 RCTs, n = 395, RR 0.98, 95% CI 0.62–1.54) and long-term follow-up (no meta-analysis; results reported for individual RCT only). Single versus short/long course combined: no differences on any outcome.

[a] Symptomatic and asymptomatic UTI (bacteriuria) is defined as clinical and/or bacteriologic cure. Re-infection is defined as re-infection of a different bacterial strain. Recurrence is defined as recurrence of the same bacterial strain.

Five of the 15 RCTs reported adequate allocation concealment; details were unclear in nine; and one used inadequate methods. Only 3 of 15 were double blinded (see **Table 4**).[9] Evidence was direct, with exclusive enrollment of the elderly in contributing RCTs, although antibiotics varied among studies, and the duration of therapy was defined by a range, with a "short" course ranging from 3 to 6 days, and a "long" course from 7 to 14 days. Less precise estimates of effect were seen than in other subgroups, with fewer RCTs (five RCTs, n = 356) and with wider CIs for all significant outcomes.

PREVENTION OF URINARY TRACT INFECTIONS IN CHILDREN

Although some RCTs in the review of cranberry products included children together with adults, there was no separate analysis of data for children.[1]

One meta-analysis investigated antibiotic prophylaxis in children and included six RCTs with a total of 388 participants, predominantly girls younger than 14 years of age, who were identified as being at risk of recurrent UTI but without a predisposing anatomic or neurologic abnormality (**Table 3**).[10] RCTs investigated a range of antibiotic classes, and members of those classes, with a variety of dosages, dosing schedules, and durations of treatment. Four RCTs compared antibiotic versus placebo with the duration of antibiotic treatment varying from 10 weeks to 12 months. The primary outcome was the number of symptomatic UTIs confirmed by bacterial growth in urine. Compared with placebo, the four studies that reported that the incidence of microbiologic recurrence was reduced in the antibiotic-treated group, although with a wide range (21%–69%) in the recurrence of repeat positive cultures (n = 388, RR 0.44, 95% CI, 0.19–1.00, relative difference [RD] −30%, 95% CI, −56% to −4%). Of these four RCTs, two reported adequate allocation concealment methods, one implied randomization but gave no details, and one used inadequate methods (**Table 4**). Only one RCT was double blinded. Results were inconsistent; the heterogeneity of findings demonstrated (I^2 75%) was not explained completely by the use of different antibiotic regimens among RCTs. Although sample sizes were large, results were imprecise with wide CIs. When analysis was limited to high-quality studies, results were not statistically significant. This review also identified two RCTs that compared antibiotic classes in prophylaxis of UTI (nitrofurantoin versus trimethoprim, and nitrofurantoin versus cefixime). Nitrofurantoin was found to be superior to trimethoprim but no different from cefixime in reducing the incidence of recurrent repeat-positive urine cultures. Nitrofurantoin was three times more likely to be discontinued because of the side effects of nausea, vomiting, or stomachache.

TREATMENT OF URINARY TRACT INFECTIONS IN CHILDREN

The authors identified four systematic reviews that investigated antibiotic class, duration of therapy, and route of antibiotic administration in the treatment of UTI in children (see **Table 3**).[11–14]

One systematic review included a meta-analysis of six RCTs enrolling 523 children aged 2 weeks to 16 years who had a diagnosis of microbiologically proven UTI and clinical acute pyelonephritis.[11] These RCTs made head-to-head comparisons of different classes of antibiotics. Reported outcomes were persistence of bacteriuria at 48 to 72 hours, resolution of clinical symptoms, symptomatic recurrence, and adverse effects. Three RCTs compared third-generation cephalosporins with other antibiotics, including co-amoxicav and co-trimoxazole. There was no difference in the reduction of persistent bacteriuria at 48 hours (two RCTs, RR 5.5, 95% CI, 0.30–01.28), recurrent or persistent UTI 5 to 10 days after the end of therapy (three

RCTs, RR 0.42, 95% CI, 0.03–6.23), or the incidence of gastrointestinal side effects (three RCTs, n = 108, RR 0.55, 95% CI, 0.10–3.16). These three RCTs did not describe trial methodology in detail, so quality assessment was unclear. Results were consistent, with no measurable heterogeneity of results. Other comparisons with single-RCT data included only third- versus fourth-generation cephalosporins, ceftriaxone versus cefotaxime, and the aminoglycosides isepamicin versus amikacin. There was no significant difference in any outcome in these RCTs.

This same meta-analysis also investigated RCTs of the duration and route of antibiotic administration.[11] The review identified six RCTs investigating the optimal duration of treatment. The only data synthesized in meta-analysis were for two RCTs comparing single-dose IV versus 7- to 10-day oral treatment, with different antibiotics across trial arms. There was no difference for asymptomatic UTI 1 to 2 days after treatment (two RCTs, n = 35, RR 1.73, 95% CI, 0.18–16.30). Both RCTs contributing data had unclear or inadequate randomization and allocation concealment (see **Table 4**). No other data synthesis was possible for other comparisons or outcomes beyond the results of the individual RCT. The review identified 12 RCTs investigating the route of antibiotic administration in children under 18 years of age who had acute pyelonephritis, defined as urinary bacterial overgrowth (> 10^8 cfu/mL) plus one symptom or sign of systemic illness such as fever, loin pain, or toxicity. RCTs investigated different antibiotics and for different time periods and also included children who had known urinary tract abnormalities such as previous UTI or vesico-ureteric reflux. Five RCTs compared short IV plus oral treatment versus continued IV for the same duration and reported no difference in asymptomatic UTI (four RCTs, n = 305, RR 0.78, 95% CI, 0.24–2.55), or re-infection within 6 months (four RCTs, n = 445, RR 1.15, 95% CI, 0.52–2.51). Three RCTs compared IV plus oral administration versus oral administration alone and also reported no difference in hours to fever resolution (two RCTs, n = 808, weighted mean difference [WMD] 2.05, 95% CI, −0.84–4.94). Two RCTs compared single IV administration versus oral administration and found no difference in persistent bacteriuria 1 to 2 days after treatment (two RCTs, n = 35, RR 1.72, 95% CI, 0.18–16.30) or relapse or re-infection within 6 weeks (two RCTs, n = 35, RR 0.24, 95% CI, 0.03–1.97). All other comparisons and outcomes were reported only in single RCTs and were not significantly different among treatment groups.

A second meta-analysis investigated the optimal duration of treatment in children who had UTI, excluding children who had previous UTI and those who had acute pyelonephritis or known renal tract abnormalities. This meta-analysis identified 10 RCTs involving 652 children.[13] The effectiveness of short-duration (2–4 days) and standard-duration (7–14 days) treatment with the same antibiotic was evaluated for the outcomes of persisting clinical symptoms, significant bacteriuria (> 10,000 cfu/mL urine) at completion of therapy, and recurrent UTI 1 month after completing treatment. No significant difference was seen in the frequency of bacteriuria at 0 to 10 days after completing treatment (eight RCTs, n = 423, RR 1.06, 95% CI, 0.64–1.76) or in recurrence of UTI within 1 to 3 months (six RCTs, n = 269, RR 0.83, 95% CI, 0.46–1.47) 3 to 15 months after completing therapy (four RCTs, n = 238, RR 1.05, 95% CI, 0.73–1.52), or 1 to 15 months after cessation of therapy (10 RCTs, n = 507, RR 0.95, 95% CI, 0.70–1.29). When data were subgrouped and analyzed by antibiotic class, no significant difference was seen in the rate of UTI recurrence between sulphonamide (five RCTs, RR 0.96, 95% CI, 0.64–1.44) and other agents (four RCTs, RR 0.93, 95% CI, 0.53–1.61). There also was no significant difference in the number of children found to have urinary pathogens resistant to the treating antibiotic on in vitro testing in those who had persistent bacteriuria or recurrent UTI (three RCTs, n = 46, RR 0.39, 95% CI, 0.12–1.29). The 10 RCTs in this review used variable criteria for treatment

Table 3
Systematic review and meta-analysis literature identified for prophylaxis and treatment of UTI in children[a]

Study	Description	Participants	Interventions	Outcomes	Results
Prevention: cranberry products					
Griffiths 2003	Overview of systematic reviews and RCTs	All patient populations	Cranberries versus no treatment or standard treatment	Symptomatic/ asymptomatic UTI	No additional meta-analysis
Jepson 2008	Systematic review	2 of 10 RCTs included children with neuropathic bladders	Cranberry juice or capsules versus placebo or no treatment	Symptomatic/ asymptomatic UTI Side effects	No synthesized data provided
Prevention: prophylactic antibiotics					
Williams 2006	Systematic review	Mostly females < 14 years at risk of re-infection	4 RCTs of antibiotics versus placebo/no treatment; 2 RCTs comparing different antibiotics	Symptomatic/ asymptomatic UTI Re-infection Side effects	Fewer repeat positive urine cultures (4 RCTs, n = 388, RR 0.44, 95% CI 0.19–1.00; RD −30%, 95% CI −56% to −4%). Other outcomes: no meta-analysis; results reported for individual RCT only. Stratified analysis showed studies with adequate allocation concealment had a RR of 0.66 (95% CI 0.30–1.39) for repeat positive urine culture; studies without adequate allocation concealment had a RR of 0.14 (95% CI 0.01–1.95). One double-blinded study gave a RR of 0.97 (95% CI 0.56–1.67); nonblinded studies gave a RR of 0.33 (95% CI 0.16–0.71). This finding demonstrates the inflated treatment effect when the study design is poor.

Treatment: class of antibiotic

Hodson 2007	Systematic review	Age 2 weeks to 16 years with acute pyelonephritis	6 RCTs tested different antibiotics; 3 RCTs compared third-generation cephalosporins versus amoxicillin or trimethoprim/sulphasoxazole. 3 RCTs had different comparisons.	Symptomatic/asymptomatic UTI Recurrence Side effects	Only pooled outcome was gastrointestinal side effects, which showed no differences between third-generation cephalosporins and either amoxicillin or trimethoprim/sulphasoxazole (3 RCTs, n = 130, RR 0.55, 95% CI 0.10–3.16). Other outcomes: only 1RCT contributed data for each outcome, although other RCTs were included in the comparison.

Treatment: duration of antibiotic treatment

Hodson 2007	Systematic review	Age 2 weeks to 16 years with acute pyelonephritis	2 RCTs: single dose versus 7–10 days treatment 1 RCT 10 days versus 42 days 1 RCT 2 weeks versus 3 weeks	Symptomatic/asymptomatic UTI Re-infection	Single-dose IV versus 7–10 days oral treatment: no differences for asymptomatic UTI 1–2 days after treatment (2 RCTs, n = 35, RR 1.73, 95% CI 0.18–16.30). Other comparisons: results reported for individual RCTs only; no meta-analysis.
Keren 2002	Systematic review	Age < 18 years with symptomatic UTI	Single-dose (or 1 day) and/or short-course (≤ 3 days) versus long-course (7 to 14 days) antibiotics	Symptomatic UTI Re-infection	Single dose/short course versus long course: higher risk of symptomatic UTI with single dose (16 RCTs, n = not reported, RR 1.94, 95% CI 1.19–3.15, no p-value reported). No differences for re-infection (16 RCTs, RR 0.76, 95% CI 0.39–1.17). Single dose versus long course: subgrouping of these RCTs reported less symptomatic UTI for long course (number of RTCs not reported, n = not reported, RR 2.73, 95% CI 1.38–5.40, p-value not reported). No differences for re-infection (RR 0.37, 95% CI 0.12–1.8). Short versus long course: no differences for symptomatic UTI (RR 1.36, 95% CI 0.68–2.72), or re-infection (RR 0.99, 95% CI 0.46–2.13). Results were not different when quality of RCT was used as a covariate.

(continued on next page)

Table 3
(continued)

Study	Description	Participants	Interventions	Outcomes	Results
Michael 2003	Systematic review	Age 3 months to 18 years with culture-proven UTI	Short course (2–4 days) versus longer course (7–14 days) of the same oral antibiotic	Symptomatic/asymptomatic UTI Recurrence Side effects	No differences for asymptomatic UTI at end of treatment (8 RCTs, n = 423, 95% CI 0.64–1.76) at 1–3 months (6 RCTs, n = 269, RR 0.83, 95% CI 0.46–1.47), at 3–15 months (4 RCTs, n = 238, RR 1.05, 95% CI 0.73–1.52), at 1–15 months (10 RCTs, n = 507, RR 0.95, 95% CI 0.70–1.29), or for recurrence (3 RCTs, n = 46, RR 0.39, 95% CI 0.12–1.29). Other outcomes: no meta-analysis.
Tran 2001	Systematic review	Age < 18 years with asymptomatic UTI	Single dose/short course (≤ 3 days) versus long course (7–14 days)	Symptomatic/asymptomatic UTI	Higher cure rate for longer treatment course (22 RCTs, n not reported, overall difference, 6.38%, 95% CI 1.88%–10.89%, p-value not reported). Results were similar when only studies comparing the same agents were synthesized (17 RCTs, overall difference, 7.92%, 95% CI 2.09%–13.8%)
Treatment: route of administration					
Hodson 2007	Systematic review	Age 2 weeks to 16 years with acute pyelonephritis	5 RCTs tested IV (3–4 days) + oral versus IV alone, both for 14 days; 3 RTCs tested IV + oral versus oral alone; 2 RTCs tested single-dose IV versus 7–10 days oral treatment; 1 RTC tested suppositories versus oral treatment; 1 RTC tested single-dose IM versus oral treatment	Symptomatic/asymptomatic UTI Recurrence	IV + oral versus IV: no difference in asymptomatic UTI (2 of 5 RCTs contributed data, n = 305, RR 0.78, 95% CI 0.24–2.55) or re-infection within 6 months (4 RCTs, n = 445, RR 1.15, 95% CI 0.52–2.51). IV + oral versus oral: no difference in symptomatic UTI (fever resolution in hours: 2 of 3 RCTs contributed data, n = 808, WMD 2.05, 95% CI −0.84–4.94). No difference in recurrence (1 RCT). Single IV versus oral: no difference in persistent bacteriuria 1–2 days after treatment (2 RCTs, n = 35, RR 1.72, 95% CI 0.18–16.30) or relapse or re-infection within 6 weeks (2 RCTs, n = 35, RR 0.24, 95% CI 0.03–1.97). Other comparisons: 1 RCT only; no meta-analysis.

[a] UTI (bacteriuria) is defined as clinical and/or bacteriologic cure. Re-infection is defined as re-infection of a different bacterial strain. Recurrence is defined as recurrence of the same bacterial strain.

durations ranging from 2 to 4 days in the short arm and from 7 to 14 days in the standard arm, but all related specifically to children who had lower urinary tract UTIs. The quality of individual RCTs varied, two of the 10 having adequate concealment; eight had implied randomization, but no further details were reported.

A third systematic review investigated single-dose, short-course ($\leq$ 4 days) and standard course ($\geq$ 5 days) antibiotic regimens in children under 18 years of age who had asymptomatic UTI.[14] This review identified 22 RCTs, including 1279 participants, comparing either the same or different antimicrobial agents in each treatment-duration group. Bacteriologic criteria for infection were uniform among RCTs, with treatment failure defined as relapse with the same organism at less than 30 days after therapy. The cure rate was significantly higher in the standard-duration ($\geq$ 5 days) treatment groups for comparisons between all classes of antibiotics (22 RCTs, overall difference 6.38%, 95% CI, 1.88%–10.89%) and for RCTs comparing the same agents across RCT arms (17 RCTs, overall difference 7.92%, 95% CI, 2.09%–13.8%). None of the 22 RCTs in this review reported details about the method of allocation concealment; one study was double blinded; and 12 were analyzed by ITT. The heterogeneity of results was explained partly by use of different drug classes across different-duration RCT arms.

The fourth meta-analysis investigated the duration of treatment for acute UTI in children aged up to 18 years but excluded RCTs restricted to children who had recurrent UTI or asymptomatic bacteriuria. This meta-analysis identified 16 RCTs comparing short-course ($\leq$ 3 days) and long-course (7–14 days) antibiotic therapy.[12] The risk of persistent UTI was higher with short-course antibiotic treatment (16 RCTs, RR 1.94, 95% CI, 1.19–3.15), but there was no difference in the re-infection rate (RR 0.76, 95% CI, 0.39–1.17). Subgroup analysis separating out RCTs using single doses versus long-course treatments also showed a higher risk of persistent UTI in the single-dose group (RR 2.73, 95% CI, 1.38–5.40) and no difference in risk of re-infection (RR 0.37, 95% CI, 0.12–1.8). RCTs comparing short (2–3 days) versus long courses of treatment reported no differences for symptomatic UTI (RR 1.36, 95% CI, 0.68–2.72) or re-infection (RR 0.99, 95% CI, 0.46–2.13). This review was available only in abstract form and so did not provide details about the quality of the included RCTs, stating only that quality was assessed before inclusion.

FROM EVIDENCE TO TREATMENT RECOMMENDATIONS
Prevention of Urinary Tract Infections

For women who have recurrent UTIs, daily intake of cranberry juice or capsules can reduce the incidence of symptomatic UTI compared with no use of cranberry product, based on consistent, direct, precise, high-quality evidence. Based on the one RCT in the meta-analysis that included only elderly patients, there is some evidence that cranberry products may be beneficial for the prevention of UTI in people over age 60 years. No meta-analysis exists to support the use of cranberry product in the prophylaxis of UTI in children.

Prophylactic antibiotics reduce the risk of symptomatic and asymptomatic UTI in women during the period when antibiotics are being administered, with only mild side effects observed (nausea, diarrhea, and candidiasis). For pregnant women who have asymptomatic bacteriuria, the use of antibiotic prophylaxis reduces the frequency of development of pyelonephritis and decreases the incidence of low-birth-weight babies. There is no evidence from meta-analysis to support the prophylactic use of antibiotics in elderly people, and the recommendation for the use of

Table 4
Considerations in using evidence from meta-analysis in clinical practice[a]

Intervention	Study	Design	Quality	Consistency	Directness	Precision	Other	Overall
Women								
Cranberry products	Griffiths 2003	Systematic overview	Randomized RCT mostly low quality (unclear allocation concealment, most not blinded)	Consistent, no measure of heterogeneity	Direct comparisons for cranberry products (juice, capsules) versus none. Direct evidence for women and elderly people. Indirect for other populations.	No meta-analysis	High number of dropouts; reporting bias may be evident.	Strong recommendation for use of cranberry products for women
	Jepson 2008	Cochrane review	3 of 4 synthesized studies had adequate randomization and allocation concealment and were double blinded; 2 ITT analyses	Consistent, no significant heterogeneity	Direct comparisons for cranberry products (juice, capsules) versus none. Direct evidence for women for and elderly people for outcomes and time periods reported. Indirect for other populations.	Precise for women, less precise for elderly men and women	Considerable variation in dropout rate, in part because of cranberry product intolerance	—

Prophylactic antibiotics	Albert 2004	Cochrane review	11 of 11 RCTs implied randomization; 10 were double blinded	Consistent evidence	Direct for the particular antibiotic dose and duration in each RCT versus placebo/none. Direct for nonpregnant women for outcomes and time periods reported. Indirect for other populations. Different antibiotics in each arm, dose and duration a possible confounder for synthesized data.	Precise for nonpregnant women	—	Strong recommendation for prophylactic antibiotics for women during the prophylactic period only
	Smaill 2007	Cochrane review	7 of 11 RCTs implied randomization; 4 had inadequate randomization; 3 were double blinded	Inconsistent results, significant heterogeneity partly explained by study quality and differing definitions of persistent bacteriuria among RCTs	Direct for particular antibiotic dose and duration in each RCT versus placebo/none. Direct for pregnant women for outcomes and time periods reported. Indirect for other populations. Different antibiotics in each arm, dose and duration a possible confounder for synthesized data.	Precise for pregnant women	Precise results for higher incidence of birth weight < 2500 g	Moderate recommendation for pregnant women for prevention of pyelonephritis

(continued on next page)

Table 4
(continued)

Intervention	Study	Design	Quality	Consistency	Directness	Precision	Other	Overall
Class of antibiotic	Vazquez 2006	Cochrane review	2 RCTs had adequate randomization and allocation concealment; 1 was unclear	Judgment not possible because data were not synthesized[a]	Direct for class of antibiotic tested in each RCT. Direct for route of administration (oral) and duration. Direct for pregnant women for outcomes and time periods reported. Indirect for other populations.	No data could be synthesized	—	No recommendation can be made favoring one drug class over another
Antibiotic duration	Milo 2005	Cochrane review	12 of 33 RCTs had adequate randomization and allocation concealment; the remainder implied randomization; 9 were double blind; 3 used ITT analysis	Consistent	Direct for short course versus long course. Direct for women for outcomes and time periods reported. Indirect for other populations and type of antibiotic in each RCT arm a possible confounder in RCTs with different antibiotic types in trial arms.	Precise, very large samples	Based on evidence from top-quality RCT	Strong recommendation for 10-day antibiotic treatment over 3-day or single-dose treatment for women

| Vazquez 2006 | Cochrane review | 1 RCT with adequate randomization and allocation concealment | Judgment not possible because data not synthesized | Direct for single versus multiple doses. Direct for pregnant women for outcomes and time periods reported. Indirect for other populations. | No data could be synthesized | — |
| Villar 2000 | Cochrane review | 1 of 10 RCTs had adequate randomization and allocation concealment; 5 implied randomization; 4 were inadequate or unclear; none were blinded | Consistent | Direct for single dose versus short course. Direct for pregnant women for outcomes and time periods reported. Indirect for other populations and type of antibiotic in each RCT arm a possible confounder in RCT that vary antibiotic type between trial arms. | Large samples | Inconsistent, moderate quality evidence of fewer mild side effects for single dose |

(continued on next page)

Table 4
(continued)

Intervention	Study	Design	Quality	Consistency	Directness	Precision	Other	Overall
Route of administration	Pohl 2007	Cochrane review	8 of 15 RCTs had adequate randomization and allocation concealment; 6 had blinded outcome assessors; 3 reported ITT	Consistent, heterogeneity explored through subgroup analysis of age	Direct for parenteral versus oral, although varying durations a possible confounder. Direct for women for outcomes and time periods reported. Indirect for other populations. Duration of treatment a possible confounding factor.	Imprecise small samples	—	Low recommendation for IV or IM over oral therapy for adults who have acute pyelonephritis
	Vazquez 2006	Cochrane review	2 of 3 RCTs with adequate randomization and allocation concealment	Consistent	Direct for IV versus IV and IM versus IV. Direct for pregnant women. Indirect for other populations and type of antibiotics varied among RCTs.	No data could be synthesized	—	—

Elderly people

Cranberry products							
Griffiths 2003	Systematic overview	Randomized RCTs, mostly low quality (unclear allocation concealment, most not blinded)	Consistent	Direct comparisons for cranberry products (juice, capsules) versus none. Direct evidence for women and elderly people. Indirect for other populations	No meta-analysis	High number of drop-outs; reporting bias may be evident	Moderate recommendation for cranberry products for elderly women
Jepson 2008	Cochrane review	Of the 4 RCTs contributing data in the meta-analysis, the 1 including elderly people was quasi-randomized, not blinded, and not ITT	No synthesized data for elderly people or people with spinal cord injury	Direct comparisons for cranberry products (juice, capsules) versus none. Direct evidence for women and elderly people for outcomes and time periods reported. Indirect for other populations	No data could be synthesized	Considerable variation in drop-out rate; some dropped out because of cranberry product intolerance	—
Regal 2006	Systematic review	1 RCT had adequate randomization/allocation concealment, double blind; 1 implied randomization, double blind; 1 was quasi-random, not blind; 2 were not randomized or blind	Consistent, no measure of heterogeneity	Direct comparisons for cranberry products (juice, capsules) versus none. Direct for elderly men and women. Indirect for other populations	No meta-analysis	—	—

(continued on next page)

Table 4 *(continued)*

Intervention	Study	Design	Quality	Consistency	Directness	Precision	Other	Overall
Prophylactic antibiotics	Regal 2006	Systematic review	Unclear reporting of RCT quality	Consistent results across RCT (no measure of heterogeneity)	Direct for elderly people. Direct for particular antibiotic dose and duration in each RCT versus placebo/none. Indirect for other populations.	No data could be synthesized	—	No recommendation for prophylactic antibiotics for elderly people
Antibiotic duration	Lutters 2002	Cochrane review	5 of 15 RCTs had adequate randomization and allocation concealment; 9 implied randomization; 1 was inadequate; 3 were double blind	Consistent	Direct for short versus long course antibiotics. Direct for elderly people for outcomes and time periods reported. Indirect for other populations. Type of antibiotic in each RCT arm a possible confounder in RCT that vary antibiotic type between trial arms.	Large samples wide CI	Most evidence is based on lower-quality RCTs	Moderate recommendation for short- or long-course treatment over single dose for elderly people
Children								
Cranberry products	Griffiths 2003	Systematic overview	Randomized RCT mostly low quality (unclear allocation concealment, most not blinded)	Consistent	Direct comparisons for cranberry products (juice, capsules) versus none. Indirect evidence for children.	No data could be synthesized	High number of dropouts; reporting bias may be evident	No recommendation for cranberry products for children

	Jepson 2008	Cochrane review	1 RCT used adequate concealment, 1 used unclear methods, 1 was double blind; 1 was single blind	Consistent	Direct for cranberry products (juice, capsules) versus none. Indirect evidence for children.	Data for children could not be analyzed separately	Considerable variation in drop out rate; some dropped out because of cranberry product intolerance	—
Prophylactic antibiotics	Williams 2006	Cochrane review	Of the 4 RCTs contributing data, 2 had adequate allocation concealment, 1 implied randomization, and 1 used inadequate methods; 1 was double blind	Inconsistent: heterogeneity partly explained by different antibiotics	Direct for children. Direct for antibiotic versus other. Indirect for different types of antibiotics and for different duration.	Large samples, wide CI	Results not significant when subgroup analysis included only high-quality studies	Low recommendation for prophylactic antibiotics for children
Antibiotic class	Hodson 2007	Cochrane review	All 3 RCTs contributing data to the meta-analysis had unclear reporting of methods	Consistent	Direct for children with acute pyelonephritis. Direct for third-generation cephalosporins versus either amoxicillin or trimethoprim/ sulphasoxazole.	Small RCT	—	No recommendation for any class of antibiotic of any other class for children

(continued on next page)

Table 4
(continued)

Intervention	Study	Design	Quality	Consistency	Directness	Precision	Other	Overall
Antibiotic duration	Hodson 2007	Cochrane review	Both RCTs contributing data had unclear or inadequate methods	Consistent	Direct for children with acute pyelonephritis. Direct for single or short versus longer treatment; differing durations and antibiotics were used.	Small to moderate-size RCT	—	Moderate recommendation for longer-course antibiotic compared with single dose for children
	Keren 2002	Review: abstract only	16 RCTs: quality details of RCTs not specified; mentions only that quality was assessed	Unclear	Direct for children who have acute, symptomatic UTI. Direct for single, short, or longer treatment. Indirect for different durations and antibiotics used.	Unclear	Meta-regression showed results did not differ when quality was used as a covariate	—
	Michael 2003	Cochrane review	2 of 10 RCTs had adequate allocation concealment; 8 had implied randomization	Consistent	Direct for children with lower-tract UTI. Direct for short (2–4 days) versus standard duration (7–14 days).	Large samples	—	—

	Tran 2001	Children ≤ 18 years	22 RCTs that stated they were randomized, no details of allocation concealment; 1 study was double blind, and 12 used ITT analysis	Inconsistent: some heterogeneity partly explained by drug type	Direct for children with asymptomatic UTI. Direct for short (2–4 days) versus standard duration (7–14 days).	Large samples	—
Route of administration	Hodson 2007 Cochrane review		Of the 10 RCTs contributing data, 5 reported adequate randomization and allocation concealment, no mention of blinding. The remainder had unclear or inadequate methods	Consistent	Direct for children with acute pyelonephritis. Direct for oral versus IV, differing duration, combinations of oral + IV, and different antibiotics.	Large samples	No recommendation for route of administration for children

a Summarized using the Grading of Recommendations Assessment, Development and Evaluation Working Group (GRADE) system (http://www.gradeworkinggroup.org/).

prophylactic antibiotics in children is weak, with unexplained heterogeneity among RCTs, indirect comparisons within RCTs, and imprecision of results.

Treatment of Urinary Tract Infections

Among nonpregnant women who have symptomatic and asymptomatic uncomplicated UTI, long-course antibiotic regimens are better than 3-day or single-dose courses for achieving bacteriologic cure. For patients who have acute pyelonephritis, IV or IM administration routes are better than oral administration for improving the rate of bacteriologic cure. Recommendations are less certain for pregnant women, because no difference was seen for any outcomes in meta-analyses comparing class, duration, or route of antibiotic administration. For elderly patients who have uncomplicated UTI, both short- and long-course antibiotics seem to be significantly more effective than a single dose in reducing symptomatic UTI for up to 2 weeks posttreatment, but not after 2 weeks posttreatment, although it is expected that the risk of late recurrence is the result of predisposing causes for recurrent UTI and is not related to acute treatment. For children who have asymptomatic or symptomatic UTI, evidence supports the use of longer-course rather than short-course or single-dose treatment, although these findings were not consistent across all meta-analyses. The route of administration does not seem to alter cure, re-infection, or relapse rates in children or to affect the side-effect profile significantly.

FUTURE DIRECTIONS IN RESEARCH

Although the authors were able to summarize meta-analyses in the prophylaxis and treatment of UTI in several populations, it is evident that there are evidence gaps for particular subgroups of people. Cranberry products remain untested in pregnant women, the elderly, and among children, and the optimum daily dose of cranberry product for preventing UTI in women has not been established. In general, when considering prophylactic measures, longer-term outcomes would increase knowledge of post-prophylaxis events.

For the active treatment of UTI, unconfounded comparisons across RCT arms would help guide therapy, and direct head-to-head comparisons of antibiotic classes would be informative in specific population subgroups. RCTs comparing the same antibiotic administered by the same route but for differing lengths of time and RCTs using the same antibiotic for the same duration of treatment but with differing routes of administration would provide evidence that is not confounded by antibiotic class, route of administration, or duration effect. Consistent and complete reporting of the methodologic quality of RCT design would increase confidence in the evidence that does exist, because much of the evidence in meta-analyses was qualified by concern about the lack of detail describing methods in the RCTs that contributed data. Furthermore, important outcomes were missing from the evidence, such as development of bacterial resistance, the rate of hospitalization, cost-effectiveness, and adherence to therapy.

REFERENCES

1. Jepson RG, Craig JC. Cranberries for preventing urinary tract infections. [update of Cochrane Database Syst Rev. 2004;(2):CD001321; PMID: 15106157]. Cochrane Database Syst Rev 2008;(1):CD001321.
2. Albert X, Huertas I, Pereiro II, et al. Antibiotics for preventing recurrent urinary tract infection in non-pregnant women. Cochrane Database Syst Rev 2004;(3): CD001209.

3. Milo G, Katchman EA, Paul M, et al. Duration of antibacterial treatment for uncomplicated urinary tract infection in women. Cochrane Database Syst Rev 2005;(2): CD004682.
4. Pohl A. Modes of administration of antibiotics for symptomatic severe urinary tract infections. Cochrane Database Syst Rev 2007;(4):CD003237.
5. Smaill F, Vazquez JC. Antibiotics for asymptomatic bacteriuria in pregnancy. [update of Cochrane Database Syst Rev. 2001;(2):CD000490; PMID: 11405965]. Cochrane Database Syst Rev 2007;(2):CD000490.
6. Vazquez JC, Villar J. Treatments for symptomatic urinary tract infections during pregnancy. [update of Cochrane Database Syst Rev. 2000;(3):CD002256; PMID: 10908537]. Cochrane Database Syst Rev 2003;(4):CD002256.
7. Villar J, Lydon-Rochelle MT, Gulmezoglu AM, et al. Duration of treatment for asymptomatic bacteriuria during pregnancy. Cochrane Database Syst Rev 2000;(2):CD000491.
8. Regal RE, Pham CQ, Bostwick TR. Urinary tract infections in extended care facilities: preventive management strategies. Consult Pharm 2006;21(5):400–9.
9. Lutters M, Vogt N. Antibiotic duration for treating uncomplicated, symptomatic lower urinary tract infections in elderly women. Cochrane Database Syst Rev 2002;(3):CD001535.
10. Williams GJ, Wei L, Lee A, et al. Long-term antibiotics for preventing recurrent urinary tract infection in children. [update of Cochrane Database Syst Rev. 2001;(4):CD001534; PMID: 11687116]. Cochrane Database Syst Rev 2006;3: CD001534.
11. Hodson EM, Willis NS, Craig JC. Antibiotics for acute pyelonephritis in children. [update of Cochrane Database Syst Rev. 2005;(1):CD003772; PMID: 15674914]. Cochrane Database Syst Rev 2007;(4):CD003772.
12. Keren R, Chan E. A meta-analysis of randomized, controlled trials comparing short- and long-course antibiotic therapy for urinary tract infections in children. [see comment]. Pediatrics 2002;109(5):E70.
13. Michael M, Hodson EM, Craig JC, et al. Short versus standard duration oral antibiotic therapy for acute urinary tract infection in children. Cochrane Database Syst Rev 2003;(1):CD003966.
14. Tran D, Muchant DG, Aronoff SC. Short-course versus conventional length antimicrobial therapy for uncomplicated lower urinary tract infections in children: a meta-analysis of 1279 patients. J Pediatr 2001;139(1):93–9.

Systematic Reviews in Malaria: Global Policies Need Global Reviews

Paul Garner, MB, BS, MD, FFPHM[a],*, Hellen Gelband, MHS[b],
Patricia Graves, MSPH, PhD[c], Katharine Jones, MBChB, MRCGP, DTM&H[a],
Harriet MacLehose, BSc, PhD, MA[a], Piero Olliaro, MD, PhD[d], on behalf of the
Editorial Board, Cochrane Infectious Diseases Group

KEYWORDS

- Malaria • Systematic review • Policy • Meta-analysis
- Research synthesis

An estimated 247 million cases of malaria occur every year, resulting in about 1 million deaths, mostly of children aged less than 5 years.[1] Families, endemic country governments, and donors spend considerable amounts in treating and preventing the disease. Indeed, in the last 5 years, a large amount of money has gone into malaria control from governments, aid agencies, and international organizations, so it is critical that it is spent wisely. Basing policies on the best available evidence will help ensure maximum impact in terms of reducing death and illness globally, and, with such a high disease burden globally, this has to be a priority in international health.

Randomized controlled trials evaluating comparative benefits and harms of new drugs to treat malaria, or the effect of public health policies such as using mosquito nets treated with insecticide, help delineate best policies within regions. But over the last 15 years, the number of published trials in malaria has increased, from 56 in 1980 to 1984 to 540 in 2000 to 2004 (**Fig. 1**). For policy makers, interpreting and keeping up to date with this emerging literature are difficult, if not impossible. In parasitic diseases, as in other areas of health care, expert opinion is not enough. There is a clear need to summarize knowledge using formal, accepted methods of research synthesis in the form of systematic reviews (**Box 1**). Yet early on, infectious and parasitic diseases largely had escaped the net of research synthesis; the techniques were

[a] International Health Group, Liverpool School of Tropical Medicine, Liverpool, L3 5QA, UK
[b] Resources for the Future, 1616 P Street NW, Washington, DC 20036, USA
[c] Epidemiologist, Health Programs, The Carter Center, 1 Copenhill, 453 Freedom Parkway, Atlanta, GA 30307, USA
[d] United Nations Children's Fund/the United Nations Development Programme/World Bank/ World Health Organization Special Programme for Research & Training in Tropical Diseases (TDR), World Health Organization, Geneva, Switzerland
* Corresponding author.
E-mail address: pgarner@liverpool.ac.uk (P. Garner).

Infect Dis Clin N Am 23 (2009) 387–404
doi:10.1016/j.idc.2009.01.007
0891-5520/09/$ – see front matter Crown Copyright © 2009 Published by Elsevier Inc. All rights reserved.
id.theclinics.com

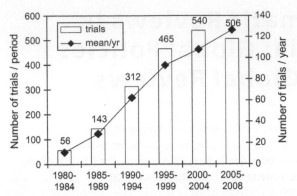

Fig. 1. Malaria trials indexed in PubMed. Search terms: malaria and clinical trial and randomized controlled trial.

honed and applied by researchers in wealthy countries, and the health conditions they addressed were important there. If they also affected the poor in developing countries, that was serendipity.

Applying the methods of research synthesis to an infectious disease like malaria is not straightforward. Countries vary substantially in the epidemiology of malaria, available resources, capacity of their health systems, and in their ability to mount effective prevention programs. Indeed, the outcomes of research in appropriate interventions often have been seen to be locally relevant but difficult to generalize and apply globally, as factors around host immunity, patterns of transmission, and types of parasite tend to be country- or region-specific. For these reasons, the application of research synthesis to malaria initially was regarded with skepticism. Up to the 1990s it had been

---

Box 1
Clarification of terms

Systematic review

A review that "attempts to collate all empiric evidence that fits prespecified eligibility criteria to answer a specific research question"[28]

Key characteristics of a systematic review

A clearly stated set of objectives with predefined eligibility criteria for studies

An explicit, reproducible methodology

A systematic search that attempts to identify all studies that would meet the eligibility criteria

An assessment of the validity of the findings of the included studies (eg, through the assessment of risk of bias)

A systematic presentation and synthesis of the characteristics and findings of the included studies[28]

Meta-analysis

A systematic review may include a meta-analysis, which is a statistical approach to combining data from two or more studies

Cochrane review

A systematic review prepared with the support of a Cochrane Review Group (which is part of The Cochrane Collaboration) and is published in the *Cochrane Database of Systematic Reviews* (part of *The Cochrane Library*)

consensus groups, drawing on expert opinion alone, which decided on the best global policies. Over the last 15 years, however, the World Health Organization (WHO) has shown considerable leadership in malaria research, in particular ensuring the application of research synthesis to this field. It has developed partnerships between key researchers and specialists in research synthesis, particularly with The Cochrane Collaboration, to prepare and regularly update systematic reviews about the benefits and harms of new and emerging interventions to prevent and treat malaria. The WHO now formally endorses systematic reviews as integral parts of its guideline development process.[2]

This article highlights some of these systematic reviews and what has been learned about applying methods of research synthesis in this particular infectious disease over the last 15 years. The authors' objectives in writing this article are to (1) illustrate how systematic reviews have been used to guide policy, (2) show what has been learned about synthesizing research in this area, and (3) reflect on how best to maximize their uptake in policy and practice.

COCHRANE INFECTIOUS DISEASES GROUP

The Cochrane Infectious Diseases Group was formed in 1994, one of the original review groups of The Cochrane Collaboration, an international nonprofit organization dedicated to preparing and keeping up-to-date reliable reviews about the effects of health care interventions.

In the early 1990s, systematic review and meta-analytic methods rarely were applied to parasitic diseases; early systematic reviews were of interventions for pregnancy and childbirth.[3] Iain Chalmers (now Sir Iain), founder of The Cochrane Collaboration, persuaded the authors to summarize all randomized controlled trials evaluating malaria chemoprophylaxis during pregnancy on substantive outcomes, including perinatal mortality. The authors were staggered how thin the evidence was for prophylaxis, yet it was WHO policy at the time.[4] This systematic review was performed at the epicenter of a tidal force emanating from the United Kingdom that was intent on summarizing research in a way that minimized bias.[5] This led the authors to explore how to establish a process to prepare and update systematic reviews in parasitic and other infections relevant to the tropics. In the process, the authors would carry out meta-analysis—the statistical combination of the results—where appropriate. What was to become the Cochrane Infectious Diseases Group started as a meeting of malaria specialists hosted by Professor Chitr Sitthiamorn at Chulalongkorn University in Thailand. The concept, developed as part of the wider Cochrane Collaboration, was to establish a network of authors who would offer their time to carry out and update systematic reviews of interventions and policies in malaria, to help make decisions more evidence-informed, and to guide priorities in research. The group was registered with The Cochrane Collaboration in 1994 under Professor Paul Garner's leadership and, following the guidelines of The Cochrane Collaboration as a whole, it is committed to conducting reviews that minimize bias, ensuring quality, and keeping reviews up to date. This is done in various ways:

    Protocols for Cochrane Reviews are mandatory and are published. These outline
        the materials and methods of the systematic review, including inclusion criteria,
        search strategy, and the analytical plan. No data are contained in them. Proto-
        cols are refereed by specialists in statistics, research synthesis, malaria, and
        health policy, and then published.
    Experienced information retrieval specialists carry out searches across multiple
        databases. In some cases, before literature indexing had improved, the

Cochrane Infectious Diseases Group employed people to search specialist journals by hand to identify relevant trials.

Protocols and Reviews are prepared using standard methods and software developed by The Cochrane Collaboration.

Extensive development by The Cochrane Collaboration and its associates to improve general methods and special methods in meta-analysis (eg, for cluster randomized trials that often are used in the trials of interest to Cochrane Infectious Diseases Group authors).

Central coordination of topics for reviews to avoid duplication, and to encourage academic groups to work together rather than compete.

Inclusiveness, enabling participation of authors whatever their background or experience, with more experienced volunteers providing training and mentorship in research synthesis.

The Cochrane Infectious Diseases Group always has focused on diseases of importance in low-income tropical countries and not all infectious diseases. Part of its mission has been to help develop expertise in systematic reviews in these countries. The group's editorial team is a mixture of grant- and university-supported staff and a volunteer editorial board (**Box 2**), which has involved technical staff from the WHO from the outset. There is now a group of over 200 authors (**Fig. 2**) who are committed to preparing and updating systematic reviews in relevant areas of parasitic and infectious diseases in the tropics. To date, the authors have prepared 35 reviews in malaria, 16 in tuberculosis, 13 in diarrhea, and 25 in other neglected tropical diseases and health problems relevant to middle- and low-income countries. The only reason this endeavor is possible is through the substantial amount of time that editors and authors donate as volunteers. On top of this, some support staff and funds for larger reviews come through the Department for International Development, which is part of the UK government, for the benefit of people living in developing countries, and commissioned projects through the WHO, in particular the WHO's Special Programme for Research & Training in Tropical Diseases (TDR).

Overall, there has been a shift toward using these systematic reviews in policy. The Technical Expert Group for the World Health Organization Malaria Treatment Guidelines drew on research evidence in systematic reviews in the first edition in 2006,[6] categorizing decisions and recommendations using the standard approach (highest based on systematic reviews, and lowest based on expert opinion). In 2008, the WHO had decided that all guideline development needed to follow an explicit, transparent process where systematic reviews were used,[2] and then the evidence formally assessed using one particular system called GRADE, which stands for Grading of Recommendations Assessment, Development, and Evaluation.[7] These GRADE profiles then are considered by the consensus panel in forming recommendations and provide a measure of the strength of evidence behind a recommendation, and will appear in the next edition of the Global Malaria Treatment Guidelines.[6,8]

The article now turn to topics in malaria prevention and treatment, and the systematic reviews conducted through the Cochrane Infectious Diseases Group to discuss how they came about, and what has been learned from them.

PREVENTING MALARIA

Drugs to Prevent Malaria in Pregnancy: A Place to Start

The most vulnerable members of the population in malarial areas are infants, children, and pregnant women. For reasons that are partially understood, women—especially low-parity women—lose some of their acquired immunity to malaria

---

Box 2
The Cochrane Collaboration: a global organization[29]

The Cochrane Collaboration is dedicated to improving health care decision making globally, through systematic reviews of the effects of health care interventions, published in the *Cochrane Database of Systematic Reviews*, part of *The Cochrane Library.*

The Cochrane Collaboration is a global network of dedicated volunteers and researchers. It relies on grants and donations, and does not accept conflicted funding. There are about 11,500 volunteers in more than 90 countries. The Cochrane Collaboration has 10 principles:

1. Collaboration

2. Building on the enthusiasm of individuals

3. Avoiding duplication

4. Minimizing bias

5. Keeping up to date

6. Striving for relevance

7. Promoting access

8. Ensuring quality

9. Continuity

10. Enabling wide participation

Production is coordinated through 52 Cochrane Review Groups. Methods groups help develop and advise on best methods, and Cochrane Centers coordinate activities within region.

Cochrane Infectious Diseases Group

Scope

> The scope covers health care interventions for communicable diseases. The focus is mainly, but not exclusively, on diseases that affect people in low-income and middle-income countries. These diseases include malaria, acute diarrhea, tuberculosis, helminth infections, scabies and head lice, and other protozoan, bacterial, and viral infections that are found predominantly but not exclusively in tropical and subtropical regions of the world.

Editorial team

> The editorial base is located in the Liverpool School of Tropical Medicine, United Kingdom. Thirteen editors, based around the world, provide support for individual reviews and editorial policies and decisions. The Group Web site is http://www.cidg.cochrane.org.

---

when pregnant. In the early 1990s, spreading resistance to 4-aminoquinolines (eg, chloroquine and amodiaquine) meant the options for prophylaxis were limited, and this reopened the debate: if prophylaxis or intermittent preventive treatment or malaria prevention is worth doing, then one really needs to know if it is of benefit to women and their infants. Although some authors had noted a positive influence of prophylaxis on birth weight, there was a debate as to whether this might do more harm than good.[9]

The first systematic review on the topic was published in the *Bulletin of the WHO.*[4] At this time, the authors pointed out that, although policies encouraging prophylaxis and intermittent preventive treatment looked promising, the impact of various approaches was not evident for pregnant women of all parity groups together, and impacts on substantive outcomes, including anemia in the mother and perinatal mortality in the fetus, were not sufficient to be sure the intervention was effective. In

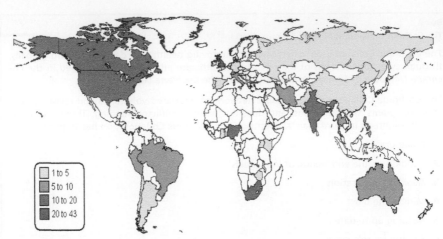

☐	1 to 5
☐	5 to 10
☐	10 to 20
☐	20 to 43

Fig. 2. Global spread of Cochrane Infectious Diseases Group authors.

particular, none of the trials reported on the effect of the intervention in preventing anemia.

This first systematic review provided insight to preparing systematic reviews in malaria, and the first lesson was the degree to which researchers are willing to help with additional data analysis. One of the concerns raised by referees and literature at the time was whether malaria prophylaxis shifted the whole birth weight curve and caused an increase in high birth weight infants.[9] Authors of the original trials were cooperative in providing unpublished data that helped answer this question, and there did not appear to be an increased number of high birth weight infants in the intervention group. Professor Brian Greenwood and colleagues in The Gambia provided unpublished data (1991) on perinatal mortality, and Dr. François Nosten and colleagues in Thailand reanalyzed their birth weight data to examine for differences between prophylaxis and control groups in relation to the number of high birth weight infants. More than just reviewing the published literature, then, this systematic review helped reframe the questions relevant to the policy being tested, and then allowed the authors of the systematic review to obtain these data from the researchers who conducted the original studies.

In addition to summarizing existing evidence, systematic reviews aim to help identify research priorities. The first systematic review pointed out that none of the trials looked at point prevalence of anemia in the mothers, and it was recommended this be included in future studies. The first subsequent study, by Shulman and colleagues,[10] identified severe anemia in the mother as the primary outcome, and actually showed a significant effect of intermittent preventive treatment with sulfadoxine–pyrimethamine on this outcome. This finding was an important impetus in this intervention being recommended by the WHO, and it was adopted and promoted as national policy in countries.

Over time, the effects on perinatal mortality have accumulated, and the current reading is suggestive of a protective effect of drugs taken to prevent the effects of malaria in pregnancy (relative risk [RR] 0.73, 95% CI, 0.53 to 0.99; 1986 participants, three trials, **Fig. 3**).[11] This demonstrates how a systematic review can highlight the gaps in the knowledge and provide pointers for research, and how the accumulation of global knowledge can be captured by updating the systematic review over time.

First edition: 1994

Latest edition: 2001

Trials included: 19

Current status: Update in progress

Learning points

- Trialists can be very helpful in providing outcomes not published in the trials

- The review highlighted important outcomes to be measured in future trials

- Meta-analysis of uncommon but important outcomes (in this case perinatal mortality) helps generate new knowledge

---

Comparison: Any drug for preventing malaria given to women in first or second pregnancy vs placebo or no drug

Outcome: Perinatal death

Summary statistic: Risk ratio 0.73, 95% confidence interval 0.53 to 0.99

Finding: Antimalarial drugs in pregnancy reduce the number of perinatal deaths

Study or Subgroup	Antimalarial drug Events	Total	No drug Events	Total	Weight	Risk Ratio M-H, Fixed, 95% CI	Risk Ratio M-H, Fixed, 95% CI
4.1.1 Prophylaxis							
Greenwood 1909	23	193	34	190	39.9%	0.67 [0.41, 1.09]	
Ndyomugyenyi 2000	1	186	2	180	2.4%	0.48 [0.04, 5.29]	
Subtotal (95% CI)		379		370	42.3%	0.66 [0.41, 1.06]	
Total events	24		36				
Heterogeneity: Chi² = 0.07, df = 1 (P = 0.80); I² = 0%							
Test for overall effect: Z = 1.72 (P = 0.08)							
4.1.2 Intermittent preventive treatment							
Shulman 1999	39	626	49	611	57.7%	0.78 [0.52, 1.17]	
Subtotal (95% CI)		626		611	57.7%	0.78 [0.52, 1.17]	
Total events	39		49				
Heterogeneity: Not applicable							
Test for overall effect: Z = 1.22 (P = 0.22)							
Total (95% CI)		1005		981	100.0%	0.73 [0.53, 0.99]	
Total events	63		85				
Heterogeneity: Chi² = 0.34, df = 2 (P = 0.84); I² = 0%							
Test for overall effect: Z = 2.03 (P = 0.04)							

0.01   0.1   1   10   100
Favours antimalarial   Favours no drug

Fig. 3. Malaria prophylaxis in pregnancy. (*From* Garner P, Gülmezoglu AM. Drugs for preventing malaria in pregnant women. Cochrane Database Syst Rev 2006;2; with permission.)

Insecticide-Treated Nets for Malaria: Public Health Interventions to the Test

Preventing malaria by sleeping under mosquito nets treated with insecticide was a new technology in the 1970s. It was clear that the intervention was potentially powerful, a substantive technology that could have impacts similar in magnitude to insecticide spraying, but bringing it to scale would require considerable global investment. But before making the investment, further research was needed to evaluate this intervention. Major funders began embarking on cluster randomized trials comparing insecticide-treated nets to untreated nets or no nets with mortality in children as an outcome, and the WHO along with academic groups sought to ensure a systematic review was performed.

The trend in the trials in terms of lower mortality was encouraging, but when taken together in a meta-analysis,[12] with careful adjustment for design effects related to clustering, the effect was consistent, clear, and statistically significant in favor of the insecticide-treated nets (**Fig. 4**). This particular analysis provides graphic and

First edition: 1998

Latest edition: 2004

Trials included: 14 cluster randomized controlled trials and 8 randomized controlled trials of individuals

Current status: Monitoring for new trials

Learning points

- Trials and meta-analysis of potentially powerful, community-based interventions in poor areas is possible

- Statistical adjustment for clustering is required for all cluster randomized designs

---

Comparison: Insecticide-treated nets vs untreated nets or no nets

Outcome: All-cause child mortality

Summary statistic: Relative rate 0.82, 95% confidence interval 0.76 to 0.89

Finding: Insecticide-treated nets reduce mortality in children living in endemic areas

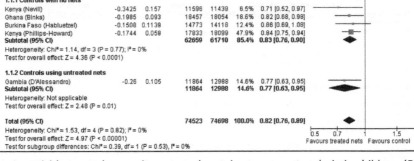

Study or Subgroup	log[Relative rate]	SE	Treated nets Total	Control Total	Weight	Relative rate IV, Fixed, 95% CI	Relative rate IV, Fixed, 95% CI
1.1.1 Controls with no nets							
Kenya (Nevill)	-0.3425	0.157	11598	11439	6.5%	0.71 [0.52, 0.97]	
Ghana (Binka)	-0.1985	0.093	18457	18054	18.6%	0.82 [0.68, 0.98]	
Burkina Faso (Habluetzel)	-0.1508	0.1139	14773	14118	12.4%	0.86 [0.69, 1.08]	
Kenya (Phillips-Howard)	-0.1744	0.058	17833	18099	47.9%	0.84 [0.75, 0.94]	
Subtotal (95% CI)			62659	61710	85.4%	0.83 [0.76, 0.90]	
Heterogeneity: Chi² = 1.14, df = 3 (P = 0.77); I² = 0%							
Test for overall effect: Z = 4.36 (P < 0.0001)							
1.1.2 Controls using untreated nets							
Gambia (D'Alessandro)	-0.26	0.105	11864	12988	14.6%	0.77 [0.63, 0.95]	
Subtotal (95% CI)			11864	12988	14.6%	0.77 [0.63, 0.95]	
Heterogeneity: Not applicable							
Test for overall effect: Z = 2.48 (P = 0.01)							
Total (95% CI)			74523	74698	100.0%	0.82 [0.76, 0.89]	
Heterogeneity: Chi² = 1.53, df = 4 (P = 0.82); I² = 0%							
Test for overall effect: Z = 4.97 (P < 0.00001)							
Test for subgroup differences: Chi² = 0.39, df = 1 (P = 0.53), I² = 0%							

0.5　0.7　1　1.5
Favours treated nets　Favours control

Fig. 4. Insecticide-treated mosquito nets and curtains to prevent malaria in children. (*From* Lengeler C. Insecticide-treated bed nets and curtains for preventing malaria. Cochrane Database Syst Rev 2004;2; with permission.)

statistically robust evidence that this intervention reduces child deaths. This evidence has been tremendously important in establishing the effectiveness of insecticide-treated nets, and ensuring further development of the technology. When the concept first was tested, it relied on cloth nets that had to be treated by hand and renewed every few months. Several generations later, the insecticide is integrated into the fabric itself and lasts as long as the net, providing long-lasting protection.

Insecticide-Treated Nets in Pregnancy: Meta-analysis Helps Consumers Understand

Once it was clear that malaria prophylaxis or intermittent preventive treatment using drugs was effective during pregnancy in preventing severe anemia, increasing mean birth weight, and possibly lowering the risk of perinatal mortality,[11] the question remained as to whether insecticide-treated nets also would be beneficial for pregnant women. Several large trials were set up to address this question. It became particularly important as emerging drug resistance meant the options for malaria prophylaxis or intermittent preventive treatment were becoming more limited; expensive drugs with toxic effects (eg, mefloquine) were being tested.[13]

Policy makers in the WHO wanted a systematic review to help guide their policies in relation to insecticide-treated nets in pregnancy. The Cochrane Review[14] showed a clear effect in women of low parity on parasitemia and anemia. When data were extracted carefully on fetal loss, an interesting trend emerged, which in meta-analysis demonstrated statistical significance (**Fig. 5**). This was a powerful message—that insecticide-treated nets reduced fetal loss—useful in communicating to pregnant women the true value of nets in terms of outcomes that have meaning to them.

Malaria Vaccines: Focusing on Disease Outcomes and Improving Trial Design

The world has been waiting a long time for a malaria vaccine; the cycle of promise and disappointment has been constant since the 1960s. By the mid-1990s, a good deal of early phase malaria vaccine research had been performed, much of it leading to dead ends for particular antigens. When starting to synthesize the evidence on this topic, trials with only immunologic (mainly antibody titers) endpoints were eliminated from consideration, and reviews were focused on trials that tested the efficacy of vaccines in preventing or mitigating disease (either in laboratory or natural challenge). Data on

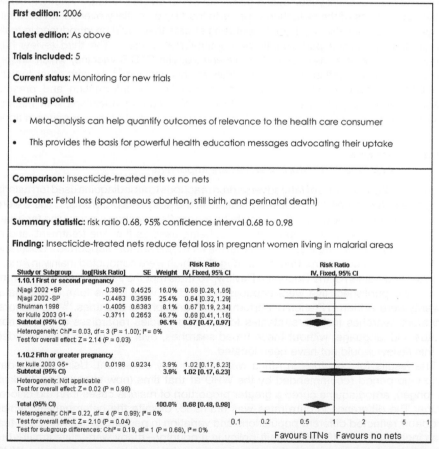

First edition: 2006

Latest edition: As above

Trials included: 5

Current status: Monitoring for new trials

Learning points

- Meta-analysis can help quantify outcomes of relevance to the health care consumer

- This provides the basis for powerful health education messages advocating their uptake

Comparison: Insecticide-treated nets vs no nets

Outcome: Fetal loss (spontaneous abortion, still birth, and perinatal death)

Summary statistic: risk ratio 0.68, 95% confidence interval 0.68 to 0.98

Finding: Insecticide-treated nets reduce fetal loss in pregnant women living in malarial areas

Fig. 5. Insecticide-treated mosquito nets in pregnancy. (*From* Gamble C, Ekwaru JP, ter Kuile FO. Insecticide-treated nets for preventing malaria in pregnancy. Cochrane Database Syst Rev 2006;2; with permission.)

adverse effects were extracted from immunologic trials for those vaccines that also had challenge endpoints in other trials.

Careful attention was paid to the stage of parasites used in a vaccine, the length of follow-up, the intensity of local transmission, and the effect of booster doses. A particular issue was how malaria cases were detected (active or passive), which can bias results, but were reported poorly in early trials. The authors believe that highlighting this in Cochrane Reviews has, resulted in standardized and improved collection methodology and reporting of outcomes in vaccine trials.

As trials of malaria vaccines have accumulated, what was originally a single Cochrane Review has been reorganized into three:

1. A systematic review that captures the history of SPf66 (**Fig. 6**)
2. One for pre-erythrocytic vaccines (intended to protect against or delay malaria infection)
3. One for blood-stage vaccines (intended to prevent invasion of red blood cells or diminish the severity of malaria)[15–17]

Together, they have helped to confirm a lack of effectiveness in Africa of SPf66, one early and controversial vaccine, and its limited effect outside Africa.[17] Another review raised awareness of the reduction in parasite load by potentially overlooked asexual-stage vaccines but also highlighted confusing effects that could be introduced in trials by predosing vaccine participants with antimalarial drugs.[15] The third review has summarized the effectiveness of the pre-erythrocytic RTS,S vaccine, which underlined the need for further multicountry trials of this vaccine.[16] As with other topics, the updating process allows authors to reorganize the information and present research questions and assembled data to reflect current questions with malaria vaccines — and here highlight the most promising vaccines at particular points in time.

TREATING MALARIA
Amodiaquine: Broad Literature Searches are Important

In the mid-1980s, reports of fatal adverse drug reactions to amodiaquine used for malaria prophylaxis led the WHO to stop recommending the drug in its programs.[18] There were some suggestions, however, that it might be more effective than chloroquine for treatment. In some countries, amodiaquine was being used as first-line treatment, and in others it was banned entirely. Working with the WHO, the authors supported a Cochrane Review of amodiaquine treatment trials (**Fig. 7**), which were conducted mainly in Africa.

In the first edition of the Cochrane Review, 40 trials met the inclusion criteria. Seventeen were published; five were unpublished, and 18 were in the form of raw data. Twenty were written in French or performed in Francophone countries.[19] The authors' literature searches include strategies for locating studies regardless of publication status and language; without these broad searches, over half of the trials included in this review would not have been located.

The results for countries in Africa were remarkably consistent. Using the 14-day follow-up period recommended by the WHO at that time (now changed to 28 days or longer), amodiaquine cured a greater proportion of malaria cases than did chloroquine. The difference in cure rates was dramatic, despite the heterogeneity, which probably reflected different populations and variation in parasite sensitivity. Each trial was individually insufficient to shift policy in a country — many were quite small — but overall the picture was clear. As a consequence of this systematic review, the WHO listed amodiaquine again as an option for treating malaria,[20] and the drug was made more widely available again in Africa.

First edition: 1997

Latest edition: 2006

Trials included: 10

Current status: Monitoring for new trials

Learning points

- It is helpful sometimes to stratify results of trials by region

- In deciding on the balance between benefits and harms, summaries of adverse events are important

- Defining outcomes clearly as clinical malaria or infection

- Helps define implications for research

Comparison: SPf66 vaccine vs placebo

Outcome: New malaria episode (*Plasmodium falciparum*)

Summary statistic for Africa: risk ratio 098, 95% confidence interval 0.90 to 1.07

Summary statistic for South America: risk ratio 0.72, 95% confidence interval 0.63 to 0.82

Finding: No evidence of protection in Africa

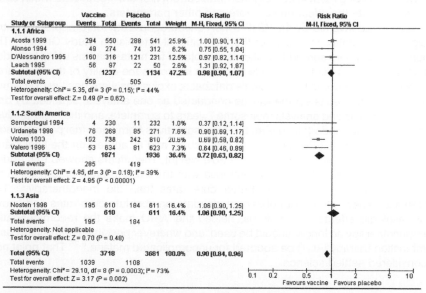

Fig. 6. SPf66 malaria vaccine. (*From* Graves P, Gelband H. Vaccines for preventing malaria (SPf66). Cochrane Database Syst Rev 2006;2; with permission.)

Artemisinin Combinations: Individual Patient Data Meta-analysis

Reviews of artemisinin derivatives[21,22] have evaluated 41 trials of various different artemisinin monotherapy and combination treatments, in various regimens and doses. In 1998, the systematic review then current was used by the WHO in considering next priorities in research in a meeting convened by the WHO in Annecy, France.[23]

Study or subgroup	Amodiaquine n/N	Chloroquine n/N	Peto Odds Ratio Peto,Fixed,95% CI	Weight	Peto Odds Ratio Peto,Fixed,95% CI
2 Day 14					
Burkina Faso 1998	44/46	30/46		5.3%	6.77 [2.43, 18.87]
Cameroon 1998	17/17	8/15		2.0%	14.09 [2.70, 73.58]
Colombia-Antioquia98	15/15	3/29		3.5%	37.51 [10.71, 131.35]
Equatorial Guinea 91	33/42	14/43		7.7%	6.29 [2.69, 14.73]
Gabon 1997-8	13/13	4/9		1.4%	20.48 [2.82, 148.57]
Gabon-Libreville 98	13/15	3/16		2.9%	13.90 [3.47, 55.61]
Kenya 1989	59/68	7/71		12.6%	21.37 [11.00, 41.49]
Kenya-Kilifi 1993	30/40	11/43		7.6%	7.05 [3.00, 16.60]
Kenya-Malindi 1984	58/60	53/69		5.6%	5.16 [1.91, 13.95]
Kenya-Turiani 1992	48/51	28/42		5.0%	6.16 [2.15, 17.62]
Madagascar 1983-4	54/56	42/59		5.8%	6.14 [2.30, 16.36]
Madagascar 1985-6	54/62	43/60		7.2%	2.56 [1.07, 6.14]
Nigeria-Ibadan 1990	52/52	39/46		2.4%	9.69 [2.09, 44.86]
Nigeria-Ibadan 2000	102/104	84/102		6.6%	5.96 [2.37, 14.96]
Philippines 1984-5	2/13	13/14		2.5%	0.05 [0.01, 0.22]
Senegal-Dakar 1996-8	32/33	16/27		3.5%	10.15 [2.88, 35.82]
Senegal-Mlomp 1996-8	17/28	8/33		5.4%	4.41 [1.60, 12.17]
Sénégal-Diohine 1996	73/87	47/84		13.0%	3.77 [1.96, 7.25]
Subtotal (95% CI)	802	808		100.0%	6.44 [5.09, 8.15]

Total events: 716 (Amodiaquine), 453 (Chloroquine)
Heterogeneity: Chi² = 73.16, df = 17 (P<0.00001); I² =77%
Test for overall effect: Z = 15.49 (P < 0.00001)

0.0010 0.1 1.0 10.0 1000.0
Chloroquine   Amodiaquine

Fig. 7. Amodiaquine for *Plasmodium falciparum* malaria. (*From* Graves P, Gelband H. Vaccines for preventing malaria (SPf66). Cochrane Database Syst Rev 2006;2; with permission.)

Researchers recommended a more strategic approach to evaluating these compounds, giving them in combination with current first-line treatments within countries, to evaluate the effect on cure rate and other parameters.

A taskforce convened by the WHO's TDR encouraged a standard approach to trial design and facilitated formation of the International Artemisinin Study Group.[24] This group of researchers agreed to a standard protocol for meta-analysis using individual patient data across continents. This approach improves the quality of the meta-analysis. All trials were compiled in a single database; exclusions were dealt with in similar fashion, and the results synthesis was conducted as one analysis, stratified by drug and site. The trials and analysis took some 7 years to complete, and the meta-analysis was a substantive undertaking (**Fig. 8**). Representatives from each trial participated in a meeting to discuss the analysis and the results, and all agreed on the final manuscript, which gave the findings considerable weight. The effects showed that adding artemisinin derivatives for 3 days combined with the existing base drug used in the country resulted in substantially better cure rates than did monotherapy.[24] This systematic review, along with observational data on absolute cure rates and known pharmacologic effects of the drugs, helped the WHO make the recommendation that monotherapy no longer should be used, and wherever possible artemisinin-based combination therapy (ACT) be adopted for uncomplicated malaria.[6,25] That point now is considered settled science.

Head-to-Head Comparisons of Artemisinin-Based Combination Therapies: Adopting Grading of Recommendations Assessment, Development, and Evaluation Summaries

Once ACTs were established as the recommended first-line treatment for uncomplicated malaria, consideration of the best option needed evaluation, particularly as new combinations emerged, and resistance patterns varied around the world. A veritable explosion of trials obscured the overall picture. It is important, however, for the WHO to make timely decisions in this area.

Published in *The Lancet*: 2004

Trials included: 16

Learning points

- Individual patient data meta-analysis is a powerful methodological and political approach.
- Global questions can be answered despite varying drug resistance.
- Once the question is answered, updating is not required.

Comparison: Artesunate for 3 days plus base drug vs base drug. Base drugs either chloroquine (CQ), amodiaquine (AQ), sulfadoxine-pyrimethamine (SP), or mefloquine (MQ)

Outcome: Parasite failure at day 28 (not adjusted to exclude new infections)

Summary statistic: Risk ratio 0.30, 95% confidence interval 0.26 to 0.35

Finding: Adding artesunate substantially reduces parasitological failure by day 28 of follow up

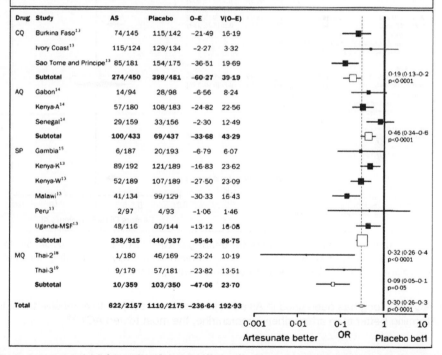

Fig. 8. Artesunate combinations for treatment of malaria: meta-analysis. (*From* Adjuik M, Babiker A, Garner P, et al. Artesunate combinations for treatment of malaria: meta-analysis. Lancet 2004;363:9; with permission.)

Over the last 2 years, an increasing number of head-to-head comparison trials have been performed. These trials, when put into meta-analysis, are beginning to show there are probably clinically significant differences in cure rate between different ACTs. Some are local, but others are applicable globally. This means that keeping systematic reviews up to date is important to inform decision making. A Cochrane Review of ACTs is in progress (**Fig. 9**); it demonstrates that dihydroartemisinin–piperaquine,

First edition: For publication in 2008

Trials included: 46

Learning points

• Despite variations in drug resistance, systematic reviews by continent are valid and helpful

• Systematic reviews are helpful when differences between alternative drug regimens may be more modest

Comparison: Dihydroartemisinin-piperaquine (DHAP) vs artemether-lumefantrine

Outcome: Total failure (P. falciparum) by day 42, adjusted to exclude new infections

Summary statistic: Risk ratio 0.42, 95% confidence interval 0.26 to 0.67

Finding: In the trials to date, DHAP is more effective than artemether-lumefantrine

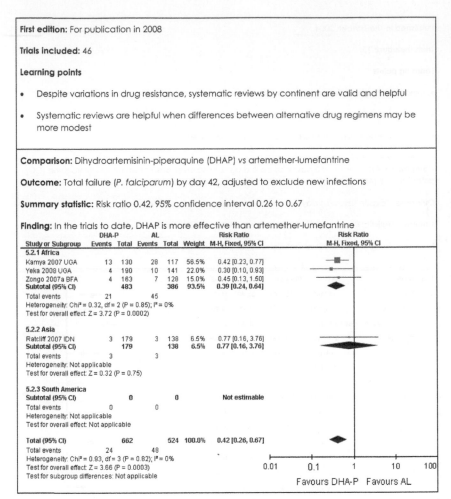

Fig. 9. Artemisinin combination therapy for treating uncomplicated malaria. (From Sinclair D, Zani B, Bukirwa H, et al. Artemisinin-based combination therapy for treating uncomplicated malaria. Cochrane Database Syst Rev 2008;4; with permission.)

an ACT that long has been used in Asia but has not been subject to extensive trials, is performing better than artemether–lumefantrine, the most tested ACT.[26]

Primaquine for Plasmodium Vivax: Policy Influence in India and Sri Lanka

For some years, the WHO has recommended a 14-day regimen of primaquine to prevent relapses of Plasmodium vivax, but in Sri Lanka and India, policy was for a 5-day regimen. A senior policy maker from Sri Lanka on study leave in Liverpool, United Kingdom, performed a Cochrane Review[27] of primaquine for preventing relapses of P vivax malaria with support from colleagues in India. As shown in Fig. 10, the included trials demonstrated lower relapse rates for P vivax with the 14-day regimen and no effect of the 5-day regimen. This evidence opened discussion about standard treatment both in Sri Lanka and India; Ministries of Health in both countries approved of a shift from the 5-day to 14-day regimen in the national guidelines.

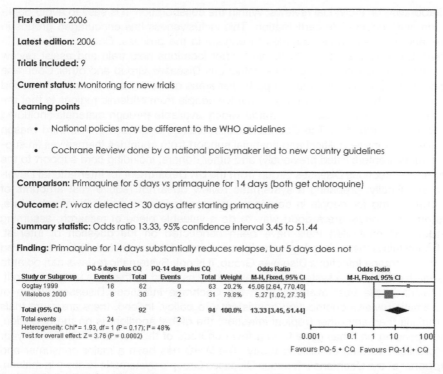

Fig. 10. Primaquine for *Plasmodium vivax*: changing regional policies. (*From* Galappaththy GN, Omari AA, Tharyan P. Primaquine for preventing relapses in people with *Plasmodium vivax* malaria. Cochrane Database Syst Rev 2007;1:CD004389; with permission.)

This illustrates that there is often a gap between global policies set by the WHO and national guidelines. In this instance, a systematic review that involved policy staff from the relevant countries facilitated a rapid change in national guidelines in line with the available evidence, and consistent with the WHO guidelines.

REFLECTIONS ON THE PROCESS

Malaria is a parasitic disease of massive global importance, with varying sensitivity to drugs related to time, place, host immunity, and the resistance profile of local parasites. Despite this variation, carefully conducted systematic reviews (some with meta-analysis) can provide substantive guidance to global policy. The collaboration between the WHO and the Cochrane Infectious Diseases Group has been constructive in providing solid evidence for policy change.

Although much of the developed world moved fast with systematic reviews and meta-analysis underpinning the treatment of chronic diseases, tropical diseases have not moved quite as quickly. Malaria, however, has been an important flagship to show it can be done for problems in low- and middle-income countries, involving researchers from endemic areas in gathering and evaluating the evidence. In malaria, the first author on over half of the Cochrane Reviews is from endemic regions. In such a rapidly growing organization, this is remarkable and has been possible for several reasons.

The first is the structure of The Cochrane Collaboration itself. It is international, and from the outset determined to have a global community contributing to it and collaborating on individual reviews. Within the collaboration, it is easy to avoid duplication and enable wide participation. This inclusiveness has encouraged groups in low- and middle-income countries to engage in the process. Cochrane Centers in Brazil, South Africa, India, China, and other locations help train and assist review authors working with the Cochrane Infectious Diseases Group and other Cochrane Review Groups reviewing trials in particular areas of medicine and health. A second reason it has been relatively easy to involve people from endemic regions is that the methods are clear, explicit, and made widely available through materials (including software developed by The Cochrane Collaboration) and training. The third reason has been extensive political and financial support from countries themselves (in supporting the centers listed previously) and other donors, including core support to the Cochrane Infectious Diseases Group from the UK Department for International Development. Finally, preparing a systematic review does not require vast amounts of resources, and for people in countries with constraints on research infrastructure, systematic reviews are a good way to do a valuable piece of research, assuming randomized controlled trials have been conducted on the question of interest. Although this is the case today for malaria, in some of the neglected diseases covered by the Cochrane Infectious Diseases Group, it is not. Systematic reviews can point to research needs, but a systematic review is only as good as the trials underpinning it.

Malaria is the best example from the Cochrane Infectious Diseases Group of systematic reviews contributing consistently to policy. Indeed, there are more trials in malaria than any other tropical infection; the global spotlight is on the condition, and spending on it has gone from a few hundreds of thousands of dollars per year before 2000 to tens of millions today. The WHO has been a major consumer and supporter of the Cochrane Infectious Diseases Group's systematic reviews in malaria, particularly in understanding new preventive interventions (such as insecticide-treated mosquito nets) and treatment with ACTs—both of which have large, beneficial effects. The reviews have helped reinforce the optimism around these developments by quantifying the beneficial effect more precisely than is possible in individual trials. Also, in summary, three main factors appear to have helped make this an effective process:

The structure and principles of The Cochrane Collaboration, avoiding duplication, encouraging a collective effort, and enabling wide participation.

Commitment of technical scientists working at policy level and involvement of key malaria researchers, inside and outside endemic countries, in the systematic review preparation process.

The editorial process is independent, although the WHO and the key researchers have been involved in critiquing and refereeing reviews during the development process.

Cochrane Reviews aim to be timely, good quality, accurate, and independent. In malaria, there is a true partnership between those synthesizing the research, those producing it, and those responsible for global policy. This helps ensure that reviews are timed to inform current policy decisions.

REFERENCES

1. World Health Organization. World malaria report 2008. Geneva (Switzerland): World Health Organization; 2008.
2. World Health Organization In: World Health Organization manual, September 2008, Part VIII, Section 1, Annex B. Geneva (Switzerland): World Health Organization; 2008.

3. Starr M, Chalmers I. The evolution of he Cochrane Library, 1988–2003. Available at: www.update-software.com/history/clibhist.htm. Accessed November 20, 2008.

4. Garner P, Brabin B. A review of randomized controlled trials of routine antimalarial drug prophylaxis during pregnancy in endemic malarious areas. Bull World Health Organ 1994;72:89–99.

5. Chalmers I, Dickersin K, Chalmers TC. Getting to grips with Archie Cochrane's agenda. BMJ 1992;305:786–8.

6. World Health Organization. Roll Back Malaria Department: guidelines for the treatment of malaria. Geneva (Switzerland): World Health Organization; 2006.

7. GRADE working group. Available at: http://www.gradeworkinggroup.org/. Accessed November 20, 2008.

8. Guyatt GH, Oxman AD, Vist GE, et al. GRADE: an emerging consensus on rating quality of evidence and strength of recommendations. BMJ 2008;336:924–6.

9. Garner P, Kramer MS, Chalmers I. Might efforts to increase birthweight in undernourished women do more harm than good? Lancet 1992;340:1021–3.

10. Shulman CE, Dorman EK, Cutts F, et al. Intermittent sulphadoxine–pyrimethamine to prevent severe anaemia secondary to malaria in pregnancy: a randomised placebo-controlled trial. Lancet 1999;353:632–6.

11. Garner P, Gülmezoglu AM. Drugs for preventing malaria in pregnant women. Cochrane Database Syst Rev 2006;4:CD000169.

12. Lengeler C. Insecticide-treated bed nets and curtains for preventing malaria. Cochrane Database Syst Rev 2004;2:CD000363.

13. Steketee RW, Wirima JJ, Slutsker L, et al. Malaria treatment and prevention in pregnancy: indications for use and adverse events associated with use of chloroquine or mefloquine. Am J Trop Med Hyg 1996;55:50–6.

14. Gamble C, Ekwaru JP, ter Kuile FO. Insecticide-treated nets for preventing malaria in pregnancy. Cochrane Database Syst Rev 2006;2:CD003755.

15. Graves P, Gelband H. Vaccines for preventing malaria (blood-stage). Cochrane Database Syst Rev 2006;4:CD006199.

16. Graves P, Gelband H. Vaccines for preventing malaria (pre-erythrocytic). Cochrane Database Syst Rev 2006;4:CD006198.

17. Graves P, Gelband H. Vaccines for preventing malaria (SPf66). Cochrane Database Syst Rev 2006;2:CD005966.

18. World Health Organization In: Practical chemotherapy of malaria. WHO Technical Report Series; 1990. p. 805.

19. Olliaro P, Mussano P. Amodiaquine for treating malaria. Cochrane Database Syst Rev 2000;2:CD000016.

20. World Health Organization. Management of uncomplicated malaria and the use of antimalarial drugs for the protection of travellers: report of an informal consultation, Geneva, 18–21 September 1995. Geneva (Switzerland): World Health Organization; 1997.

21. McIntosh HM, Olliaro P. Artemisinin derivatives for treating severe malaria. Cochrane Database Syst Rev 2000;2:CD000527.

22. McIntosh HM, Olliaro P. Artemisinin derivatives for treating uncomplicated malaria. Cochrane Database Syst Rev 2000;2:CD000256.

23. McIntosh HM, Olliaro P. Cochrane systematic reviews of published and unpublished randomized controlled trials in uncomplicated and complicated malaria. In Annex to the working papers of the Rational Use of Quinghaosu and its Derivatives conference: 1998 April 19–22; Annecy, France. Rhone-Polulenc (France): International Laveran Assocation, Marcel Merieux Foundation; 1998.

24. Adjuik M, Babiker A, Garner P, et al. Artesunate combinations for treatment of malaria: meta-analysis. Lancet 2004;363:9–17.
25. Arrow KJ, Panosian CB, Gelband H, editors. Saving lives, buying time. Economics of malaria drugs in an age of resistance. Washington, DC: The National Academies Press; 2004.
26. Sinclair D, Zani B, Bukirwa H, et al. Artemisinin-based combination therapy for treating uncomplicated malaria. Cochrane Database Syst Rev, in press.
27. Galappaththy GN, Omari AA, Tharyan P. Primaquine for preventing relapses in people with Plasmodium vivax malaria. Cochrane Database Syst Rev 2007;1: CD004389.
28. Higgins PT, Green S, editors. Cochrane handbook for systematic reviews of interventions. Chichester (UK): Wiley-Blackwell; 2008.
29. The Cochrane Collaboration. Available at: www.cochrane.org. Accessed November 5, 2008.

Meta-analysis on Surgical Infections

Dimitrios K. Matthaiou, MD[a,b], George Peppas, MD, PhD[a,c],
Matthew E. Falagas, MD, MSc, DSc[a,d,e],*

KEYWORDS

- Intra-abdominal infections • Prophylaxis • Mortality
- Wound infections • Surgical site infections
- Appendicitis • Pancreatitis

Surgical infections are a set of different infections that are roughly divided into two major groups: surgical site infections (SSIs) and other infections that require surgical intervention to resolve along with antibiotic treatment. SSIs are further divided into superficial incisional, deep incisional, and organ/space infections.[1]

Surgical infections are an important clinical entity, as almost 3% of the operations performed in the United States are complicated by SSIs.[2] Patients in whom SSIs develop are more likely to be admitted to an intensive care unit, return to the hospital after discharge, or even die than patients who do not.[3] Specific types of surgical infections, such as intra-abdominal infections or bone and joint infections, may further contribute to mortality and morbidity.

Meta-analysis is a statistical approach that was first used during the late 1980s in the field of psychology and social sciences[4] and soon found its place in medical research. It combines the findings of similar studies regarding the outcomes of various treatments in certain populations and settings using quantitative methods. In this regard, the pooling of data included in different studies confers a larger sample size and consequently a more accurate estimate of the outcomes of different interventions. Thus, an adequately powered quantitative conclusion is frequently derived, which may be used in the formation of guidelines and the promotion of medical practice.

Under this perspective, we sought to conduct a review focusing on the application of this analytical tool and its potential contribution to the field of surgical infections.

[a] Alfa Institute of Biomedical Sciences (AIBS), 9 Neapoleos Street, 151 23 Marousi, Athens, Greece
[b] Department of Medicine, "G. Gennimatas" General Hospital, 41 Ethnikis Amynis Street, 546 35 Thessaloniki, Greece
[c] Department of Surgery, Henry Dunant Hospital, 107 Mesogeion Avenue, 115 26 Athens, Greece
[d] Department of Medicine, Tufts University School of Medicine, Boston, MA 02111, USA
[e] Department of Medicine, Henry Dunant Hospital, 107 Mesogeion Avenue, 115 26 Athens, Greece
* Corresponding author.
E-mail address: m.falagas@aibs.gr (M.E. Falagas).

Infect Dis Clin N Am 23 (2009) 405–430
doi:10.1016/j.idc.2009.01.012
0891-5520/09/$ – see front matter © 2009 Elsevier Inc. All rights reserved.

id.theclinics.com

LITERATURE SEARCH

The literature was systematically reviewed to identify meta-analyses focusing on surgical infections. One reviewer (DKM) performed the literature search in PubMed until 30/09/2008 using the search terms "meta-analysis AND (appendicitis OR peritonitis OR diverticulitis OR intra-abdominal infection OR intra-abdominal infections OR cholecystitis OR necrotizing pancreatitis OR surgical infection OR surgical infections OR surgical site infection OR surgical site infections OR abscess OR empyema)."

STUDY SELECTION AND EXTRACTION

An article was considered eligible to be included in this review if it was a meta-analysis including randomized controlled trials with a focus on surgical infections and (1) it compared different surgical procedures for the treatment of diseases requiring surgical intervention and reported data on SSIs and other surgical complications, (2) it evaluated antimicrobial prophylaxis for different surgical procedures and reported outcomes of SSIs, (3) it compared different antimicrobial regimens used for the treatment of patients with surgical infections and reported data on effectiveness, and/or (4) it compared different preventive procedures and reporting data on SSIs and other surgical complications. Additionally, the outcomes of interest should have been considered as primary outcomes and consistent with the outcomes of interest of this review. Meta-analyses that included patients with mixed infections reporting separate outcomes on surgical infections were also included. Consecutive updates of the same meta-analysis (except for the most recent version), meta-analyses including less than 100 patients in total, duplicate publications, as well as conference abstracts were excluded. There was no language limitation for an article to be included in this review.

Data extracted and tabulated from each meta-analysis were: author name, year of publication, intervention studied (focus of the meta-analysis), number of included studies, number of included patients, and effect on primary outcomes.

The total number of the retrieved articles was 693, of which, 518 were excluded at first screening of title and abstract. After excluding 85 for other various reasons, 90 meta-analyses were considered eligible to be included in the review and are presented in **Tables 1** and **2** .

META-ANALYSES FOCUSING ON ANTIBIOTIC PROPHYLAXIS FOR SURGICAL INFECTIONS

Table 1 summarizes 45 meta-analyses with a focus on antibiotic prophylaxis for surgical infections.[5–49] Specifically, 19 of these 45 (42.2%)[5–23] focused on antibiotic prophylaxis in abdominal surgery, 6 (13.3%)[36,37,40,42,45,49] on perioperative prophylaxis in surgery, 5 (11.19%)[27–31] on antibiotic prophylaxis in thoracic and vascular surgery, 4 (8.9%)[35,44,46,47] on prophylaxis in neurosurgery, 3 (6.7%)[38,39,48] on prophylaxis in breast surgery, 3 (6.7%)[32–34] on obstetrics and gynecology, 3 (6.7%)[24–26] on antibiotic prophylaxis in orthopedics, and 2 (4.4%)[41,43] on other topics.

Meta-analyses Focusing on Antibiotic Prophylaxis in Abdominal Surgery

Seven of 19 abdominal surgery meta-analyses (36.8%)[5,7,8,14–16,19] focused on acute pancreatitis requiring surgery (six on necrotizing pancreatitis [31.6%][5,7,8,14,15,19] and one nonnecrotizing [5.3%][16]). Five of these seven meta-analyses (26.3%)[5,14–16,19] found no advantage in the use of prophylaxis, whereas two (10.5%)[7,8] found antibiotic prophylaxis to be superior regarding pancreatic infection rates. In terms of mortality, four meta-analyses (21.1%)[5,7,14,16] found no advantage in the use of prophylaxis, whereas three (15.8%)[8,15,19] found prophylaxis to be superior.

Four of 19 abdominal meta-analyses (21.1%)[6,10–12] focused on hernia surgery, three of which (15.8%)[6,10,11] found antibiotic prophylaxis to be superior regarding wound infection rates. The remaining meta-analysis[12] found no difference between the protocols. Two of these meta-analyses[10,12] included studies focusing on mesh hernia repair, whereas the remaining ones[6,11] included both studies using prosthetic material or not. No data were provided regarding the types of meshes used.

Three of 19 meta-analyses (15.8%)[9,13,20] studied the use of antibiotic prophylaxis in percutaneous endoscopic gastrostomy. All of them (15.8%) found antibiotic prophylaxis to be superior regarding wound infection rates.

Two of 19 meta-analyses (10.5%)[18,23] focused on biliary surgery. The more recent meta-analysis (5.3%)[18] found no benefit in the use of antibiotic prophylaxis, whereas the other (5.3%)[23] found prophylaxis to be superior regarding wound infection rates.

Of the remaining three meta-analyses (15.8%), one (5.3%)[22] focused on colorectal surgery, one (5.3%)[17] on antimicrobial prophylaxis after appendicectomy, and one (5.3%)[21] on prophylaxis for the prevention of infections in cirrhotic patients with gastrointestinal bleeding. All of them found antibiotic prophylaxis to be superior regarding wound infection rates.

Meta-analyses Focusing on Antibiotic Prophylaxis in Thoracic and Vascular Surgery

Four of 5 (80%)[28–31] meta-analyses concerning thoracic and vascular surgery focused on thoracic surgery. Two of them (40%)[28,31] examined the effect of antibiotic prophylaxis in isolated chest trauma and in tube thoracostomy for trauma, both of which favored the use of antibiotic prophylaxis. Two of them (40%)[29,30] focused on cardiothoracic surgery, one on the comparison of glycopeptides with b-lactams as prophylaxis against wound infection after cardiac surgery,[29] and the other on the use of prophylaxis for permanent pacemaker implantation.[30] The remaining meta-analysis (20%)[27] focused on the use of antimicrobial prophylaxis in arterial reconstruction.

Meta-analyses Focusing on Antibiotic Prophylaxis in Peri-Operative Prophylaxis in Surgery

Three of six meta-analyses (50%)[42,45,49] focusing on perioperative prophylaxis in surgery compared ceftriaxone with other drugs,[42] ceftriaxone with other cephalosporins,[45] and amoxicillin-clavulanate with other drugs,[49] respectively. Two of six meta-analyses (33.3%)[36,40] examined the prophylactic effect of mupirocin in developing wound infections after surgery, of which, one found mupirocin to be superior regarding postoperative *Staphylococcus aureus* infection rates,[36] whereas the other was consistent with the former only regarding wound infection rates in nongeneral surgery.[40] The remaining study examined the prophylactic effect of antiseptic bathing with chlorhexidine gluconate, in which no difference was found between antiseptic bathing and other methods for prevention of SSIs.[37]

Meta-analyses Focusing on Antibiotic Prophylaxis in Neurosurgery, Obstetrics and Gynecology, and Breast Surgery

All four meta-analyses (100%)[35,44,46,47] focusing on antimicrobial prophylaxis in neurosurgical procedures found prophylaxis to be superior regarding wound infection rates. All three meta-analyses (100%)[32–34] focusing on antimicrobial prophylaxis in obstetrics and gynecology, of which, two (66.7%)[32,34] concerned cesarean delivery and one (33.3%)[33] abdominal hysterectomy, found antimicrobial prophylaxis to be superior regarding wound infection. All three meta-analyses (100%)[38,39,48] focusing

Table 1
Meta-analyses focusing on antibiotic prophylaxis

Study	Intervention Studied (Focus of the Meta-analysis)	Studies Included	Patients Included	Effect on Primary Outcomes
Intra-abdominal				
Bai et al, 2008[5]	Prophylactic antibiotics in acute necrotizing pancreatitis (antibiotics versus placebo/no treatment)	7	467	Infected pancreatic necrosis rates: RR = 0.81 (0.54–1.22) Mortality: RR = 0.70 (0.42–1.17)
Gravante et al, 2008[6]	Single-dose antibiotic prophylaxis versus placebo in open inguinal repair	10	4336	Wound infection: OR = 0.67 (0.48–0.93)
Xu and Cai, 2008[7]	Prophylactic antibiotic treatment in acute necrotizing pancreatitis	8	540	Pancreatic or peripancreatic infection: RR = 0.69 (0.50–0.95) Mortality: RR = 0.76 (0.50–1.18) Non-pancreatic infection: RR = 0.66 (0.48–0.91) Surgical intervention: RR = 0.90 (0.66–1.23)
Dambrauskas et al, 2007[8]	Prophylactic antibiotics in acute necrotizing pancreatitis	10	1079	Infected necrosis: RR = 0.57 (0.42–0.78) Mortality: RR = 0.76 (0.59–0.98)
Jafri et al, 2007[9]	Antibiotic prophylaxis to prevent peristomal infection after percutaneous endoscopic gastrostomy (antibiotics versus placebo/no intervention)	10	1059	Wound infection: RR = 0.36 (0.26–0.50)
Sanabria et al, 2007[10]	Prophylactic antibiotics for mesh inguinal hernioplasty antibiotics versus placebo/no treatment)	6	2507	Surgical site infection: OR = 0.48 (0.27–0.85)
Sanchez-Manuel et al, 2007[11]	Antibiotic prophylaxis for hernia repair	12	6705	Wound infection: OR = 0.64 (0.48–0.85)

Aufenacker et al, 2006[12]	8	2861	Antibiotic prophylaxis in prevention of wound infection after mesh repair of abdominal wall hernia (antibiotics versus placebo) — Wound infection (inguinal hernia): OR = 0.54 (0.24–1.21) Deep wound infection (inguinal hernia): OR = 0.50 (0.12–2.09)
Lipp and Lusardi, 2006[13]	10	1100	Systemic antimicrobial prophylaxis for percutaneous endoscopic gastrostomy (prophylaxis versus no prophylaxis) — Peristomal infection: OR = 0.31 (0.22–0.44)
Mazaki et al, 2006[14]	6	329	Prophylactic antibiotic use in acute necrotizing pancreatitis — Infected necrosis: RR = 0.77 (0.54–1.12) Mortality: RR = 0.78 (0.44–1.39)
Villatoro et al, 2006[15]	5	294	Antibiotic therapy for prophylaxis against infection of pancreatic necrosis in acute pancreatitis — Mortality: OR = 0.37 (0.17–0.83) Infected pancreatic necrosis: OR = 0.62 (0.35–1.09)
Xiong et al, 2006[16]	6	338	Prophylactic antibiotic administration in severe acute pancreatitis (antibiotics versus placebo) — Pancreatic infection: RR = 0.77 (0.48–1.24) Surgical intervention: RR = 0.84 (0.40–1.74) Extra-pancreatic infection: RR = 0.52 (0.31–0.88) Mortality: RR = 0.54 (0.28–1.04)
Andersen et al, 2005[17]	71	8812	Antibiotics versus placebo for prevention of postoperative infection after appendicectomy — Wound infection: OR = 0.33 (0.29–0.38) Postoperative intra-abdominal abscess: OR = 0.43 (0.25–0.73)
Catarci et al, 2004[18]	6	974	Antibiotic prophylaxis in elective laparoscopic cholecystectomy — Perioperative infection: OR = 0.69 (0.34–1.43) Surgical site infection: OR = 0.82 (0.36–1.86) Other site infection: OR = 0.82 (0.18–1.90)
Sharma and Howden, 2001[19]	3	160	Antibiotic prophylaxis in acute necrotizing pancreatitis (prophylaxis versus no prophylaxis) — Pancreatic infection: ARR = 12% (-2.4%–26.4%) Sepsis: ARR = 21.1% (6.5%–35.6%) Mortality: ARR = 12.3% (2.7%–22%)

(continued on next page)

Table 1
(continued)

Study	Intervention Studied (Focus of the Meta-analysis)	Studies Included	Patients Included	Effect on Primary Outcomes
Sharma and Howden, 2000[20]	Antibiotic prophylaxis before percutaneous endoscopic gastrostomy (antibiotics versus placebo/no treatment)	7	777	Wound infection: ARR = 17.5% (12.5%–22.5%)
Bernard et al, 1999[21]	Antibiotic prophylaxis for the prevention of bacterial infections in cirrhotic patients with gastrointestinal bleeding (prophylaxis versus no prophylaxis)	5	534	Infection: Improvement rate = 32% (22%–42%) Bacteremia and/or SBP: Improvement rate = 19% (11%–26%) SBP: Improvement rate = 7% (2.1%–12.6%) Survival: Improvement rate = 9.1% (2.9%–15.3%)
Glenny and Song, 1999[22]	Antimicrobial prophylaxis in colorectal surgery (antibiotics versus no antibiotics)	4	293	Surgical wound infection: OR = 0.24 (0.13–0.43)
Meijer et al, 1990[23]	Antibiotic prophylaxis in biliary tract surgery (antibiotics versus no antibiotics)	42	4129	Wound infection: OR = 0.30 (0.23–0.38)
Orthopedic				
Albuhairan et al, 2008[24]	Antibiotic prophylaxis for wound infections in total joint arthroplasty (prophylaxis versus no prophylaxis)	7	3065	Wound infection Absolute risk reduction by 8% and relative risk reduction by 81% (P<.00001)
Slobogean et al, 2008[25]	Single- versus multiple-dose antibiotic prophylaxis in the surgical treatment of closed fractures	7	3808	Surgical wound infection: RR = 1.24 (0.60–2.60)

Southwell-Keely et al, 2004[26]	Antibiotic prophylaxis in hip fracture surgery	10	2417	Surgical wound infection (antibiotics at any dose or duration versus placebo): OR = 0.55 (0.35–0.85)
Thoracic surgery/vascular				
Stewart et al, 2007[27]	Prevention of infection in peripheral arterial reconstruction (antibiotics versus placebo)	10	1297	Wound infection: RR = 0.25 (0.17–0.38); Early graft infection: RR = 0.31 (0.11–0.85)
Sanabria et al, 2006[28]	Prophylactic antibiotics in isolated chest trauma (antibiotics versus placebo)	5	614	Empyema: RR = 0.19 (0.07–0.5); Pneumonia: RR = 0.44 (0.27–0.73)
Bolon et al, 2004[29]	Glycopeptides versus b-lactams for prevention of surgical site infection after cardiac surgery	7	5761	Surgical site infection at 30 days: RR = 1.14 (0.91–1.42)
Da Costa et al, 1998[30]	Antibiotic prophylaxis for permanent pacemaker implantation (prophylaxis versus no prophylaxis)	7	2023	Protective effect of antibiotic pretreatment: OR = 0.26 (0.10–0.66)
Fallon and Wears, 1992[31]	Antibiotic prophylaxis in tube thoracostomy for trauma	6	507	Empyema: RR = 5.27 (1.82–15.32); All infectious complications: RR = 4.30 (2.20–8.41)
Obstetric				
Martins and Krauss-Silva, 2006[32]	Antibiotic prophylaxis in cesarean sections (antibiotics versus placebo)	27	4470	Endometritis: RR = 0,33 (0.27–0.39); Surgical wound infection: RR = 0,32 (0.24–0.43)
Costa and Krauss-Silva, 2004[33]	Antibiotic prophylaxis in abdominal hysterectomy (antibiotics versus placebo)	20	2456	Surgical site infection: RR = 0.49 (0.41–0.59)

(continued on next page)

Table 1
(continued)

Study	Intervention Studied (Focus of the Meta-analysis)	Studies Included	Patients Included	Effect on Primary Outcomes
Chelmow et al, 2001[34]	Prophylactic use of antibiotics for nonlaboring patients undergoing cesarean delivery with intact membranes (antibiotics versus placebo)	7	446	Postoperative fever: RR = 0.25 (0.14–0.44); Endometritis: RR 0.05 (0.01–0.38); Wound infection: RR = 0.59 (0.24–1.45)
Other				
Ratilal et al, 2008[35]	Antibiotic prophylaxis for surgical introduction of intracranial ventricular shunts (antibiotics versus placebo/no antibiotics)	17	2134	Shunt infection: OR = 0.51 (0.36–0.73)
van Rijen et al, 2008[36]	Prevention of S aureus infections in nasal S aureus carriers after surgery (nasal mupirocin versus placebo/no treatment)	4	1372	Postoperative S aureus infection rate: RR = 0.55 (0.34–0.89)
Webster and Osborne, 2007[37]	Preoperative antiseptic bathing for prevention of surgical site infection (chlorhexidine gluconate versus placebo/bar soap/no washing)	6	10,007	Surgical site infection Antiseptic versus placebo: RR = 0.91 (0.80–1.04); Antiseptic versus soap: RR = 1.02 (0.57–1.84)
Cunningham et al, 2006[38]	Antibiotic prophylaxis after breast cancer surgery	6	—	Surgical site infection: RR = 0.66 (0.48–0.89)
Tejirian et al, 2006[39]	Antibiotic prophylaxis after breast surgery (antibiotics versus placebo)	5	1307	Wound infection: RR = 0.60 (0.45–0.81)
Kallen et al, 2005[40]	Perioperative intranasal mupirocin versus no mupirocin for the prevention of surgical site infections	7	11,088	Surgical site infection General surgery: RR = 1.04 (0.81–1.33); Nongeneral surgery: RR = 0.80 (0.58–1.10)

Study	Description	RCTs	Patients	Outcome
Vardakas et al, 2005[41]	Perioperative teicoplanin compared with cephalosporins in orthopedic and vascular surgery involving prosthetic material	6	2886	Surgical site infection: OR = 1.32 (0.45–3.84)
Esposito et al, 2004[42]	Ceftriaxone versus other antibiotics for surgical prophylaxis	48	17,565	Surgical site infection: log OR = −0.30 (−0.50 to −0.13)
Strippoli et al, 2004[43]	Antimicrobial agents for preventing peritonitis in peritoneal dialysis patients	19	1949	Early peritonitis: RR = 0.35 (0.15–0.80) Exit site and tunnel infection: RR = 0.32 (0.02–4.81)
Barker, 2002[44]	Prophylactic antibiotic therapy in spinal surgery (antibiotics versus placebo/no intervention)	6	843	Wound infection: OR = 0.37 (0.17–0.78)
Dietrich et al, 2002[45]	Ceftriaxone versus other cephalosporins for perioperative antibiotic prophylaxis	43	13,482	Surgical wound infection: RR = 0.7 (98.3% confidence interval 0.55–0.89)
Barker, 1994[46]	Prophylactic antibiotics for craniotomy (antibiotics versus placebo)	8	2075	Infection: Antibiotics arm 2% and placebo arm 8% ($P < 10^{-8}$)
Langley et al, 1993[47]	Antimicrobial prophylaxis in placement of cerebrospinal fluid shunts (prophylaxis versus no prophylaxis)	12	1359	cerebrospinal fluid shunt infection: Weighted RR = 0.52 (0.37–0.73)
Platt et al, 1993[48]	Perioperative antibiotic prophylaxis in breast surgery	—	2587	Wound infection: OR = 0.62 (0.40–0.95)
Wilson et al, 1992[49]	Amoxicillin-clavulanate in surgical prophylaxis	21	4905	Wound infection: OR = 0.84 (0.68–1.03)

Abbreviations: RCTs, Randomized clinical trials; RR, Risk ratio; OR, Odds ratio; ARR, Absolute risk reduction.

on antimicrobial prophylaxis in breast surgery found prophylaxis to be superior regarding wound infection rates.

Meta-analyses Focusing on Antibiotic Prophylaxis in Orthopedics

Two of three meta-analyses (66.7%)[25,26] focusing on orthopedics examined the use of prophylaxis in fracture surgery, of which, one (33.3%)[26] compared prophylaxis with no prophylaxis, and one (33.3%)[25] compared single- with multiple-dose antibiotic prophylaxis. In the former study, an absolute risk reduction by 8% and relative risk reduction by 81% for wound infection was found, whereas in the latter, no difference was found between single- and multiple-dose prophylaxis. In the remaining meta-analysis (33.3%)[24] comparing prophylaxis with no prophylaxis in total joint arthroplasty, prophylaxis was found to be superior regarding wound infection rates.

Meta-analyses Focusing on Antibiotic Prophylaxis in Other Patient Settings

The remaining two meta-analyses examined the use of prophylaxis in peritoneal dialysis patients[43] and the comparison of teicoplanin with cephalosporins in orthopedic and vascular surgery involving prosthetic material,[41] respectively. In both meta-analyses, no difference was found between the two antibiotic regimens regarding SSI rates.

META-ANALYSES FOCUSING ON TOPICS OTHER THAN ANTIBIOTIC PROPHYLAXIS

Table 2 summarizes 44 meta-analyses[50–93] (one was not reported in the table because of the large number of outcomes of interest)[94] that focused on other aspects of surgical infections apart from antibiotic prophylaxis—mostly comparisons of different surgical techniques and procedures, as well as comparisons of the efficacy of different antibiotics for the treatment of surgical infections. Thirty-one of them (68.9%)[50–79,94] regarded techniques and procedures used in abdominal surgery, four (8.9%)[80–83] concerned cardiothoracic and vascular surgery, three (6.7%)[85–87] focused on orthopedics, two (4.4%)[84,85] regarded obstetrics and gynecology, and five (11.1%)[89–93] dealt with various other topics.

Meta-analyses Focusing on Abdominal Surgery

Nine of the 31 (29%)[61,64,67,70,74–78] abdominal surgery meta-analyses focused on appendicitis, nine (29%)[52–54,56,63,66,69,71,72] on colorectal surgery, five (16.1%) on biliary surgery, five (16.1%)[50,55,65,73,79] on comparing different antibiotic regimens for the treatment of intra-abdominal infections, one (3.2%)[68] on gastrointestinal surgery, and one (3.2%)[60] on the use of drainage for uncomplicated liver resection, respectively. The meta-analysis not reported in the table because of the large number of primary analyses[94] focused on the comparison of 16 different antibiotic regimens for the treatment of secondary peritonitis of gastrointestinal origin in adults. None of the comparisons favored any of the compared regimens in terms of clinical success or mortality.

Six of nine meta-analyses (66.7%)[61,70,74,76–78] concerning appendicitis compared laparoscopic with conventional techniques for appendectomy, four (44.4%)[70,74,76,77] of which found laparoscopic techniques to be superior regarding wound infection rates, whereas one[61] found no difference between the techniques. All meta-analyses reporting relevant data found no difference between the techniques regarding the rate of intra-abdominal abscesses. Three of 9 (33.3%)[64,67,75] meta-analyses compared different wound closure methods during appendectomy.

Three of 9 (33.3%)[66,69,72] meta-analyses concerning colorectal surgery compared mechanical bowel preparation with no preparation. In two of these[69,72] anastomotic leakage was less in mechanical bowel preparation, whereas in the remaining one,[66] no difference was found regarding the anastomotic leakage rate. In two of three meta-analyses[69,72] in which wound infection and intra-abdominal abscess rates were reported, no difference between the two methods was found. The remaining six meta-analyses (66.7%) compared (1) laparoscopic with open surgery for resection of colorectal cancer,[52] in which laparoscopic techniques were associated with fewer wound infections; (2) different methods for ileocolic anastomoses,[53] in which anastomotic leaks were significantly fewer with stapled method; (3) supplemental perioperative oxygen versus no oxygen in colorectal surgery patients,[54] in which no difference was found between the protocols; (4) ileostomy with colostomy for colorectal anastomotic decompression,[56] in which no difference was found in terms of wound infection or mortality; (5) drainage with no drainage in elective colorectal surgery,[63] in which no advantage was found in the use of drainage; and (6) primary repair versus fecal diversion for penetrating colon injuries,[71] in which primary repair was associated with fewer complications in general, but not with less mortality of infectious complications.

Three of five meta-analyses (60%)[57–59] concerning biliary surgery compared the use of different types of drainage in various types of cholecystectomy with mixed results. The remaining meta-analyses (40%)[51,62] compared early with delayed laparoscopic cholecystectomy, in which no difference was found between the two techniques regarding complication rates.

The five meta-analyses studying different antibiotic regimens for the treatment of intra-abdominal infections compared ertapenem with other antibiotic regimens,[50] clindamycin/aminoglycoside with b-lactam monotherapy,[55] ciprofloxacin/metronidazole with b-lactam based regimens,[65] aminoglycosides with other antibiotic regimens,[73] and meropenem with other antimicrobials.[79] Ertapenem was found to be as effective as other antimicrobials for the treatment of complicated intra-abdominal infections. Ciprofloxacin/metronidazole[65] and aminoglycosides[73] were found to be more effective, whereas clindamycin/aminoglycoside was less effective than comparators for the treatment of intra-abdominal infections. No difference regarding the response rates was found between meropenem and other antibiotic regimens. The meta-analysis focusing on the treatment of secondary peritonitis of gastrointestinal origin in adults[94] compared virtually each available antibiotic class with all the other for various outcomes, of which the primary outcomes were clinical success and mortality.

Of the remaining two meta-analyses concerning abdominal surgery, one focused on the use of drainage for uncomplicated liver resection,[60] and 1 on the comparison of different techniques for the treatment of perforated peptic ulcer.[68]

Meta-analyses Focusing on Cardiothoracic and Vascular Surgery

Three of 4 meta-analyses (75%)[80,81,83] concerning cardiothoracic and vascular surgery focused on vascular surgery. Two of them (50%)[81,83] compared minimally invasive with conventional vein harvesting, in which minimally invasive vein harvesting was superior regarding wound infection rates. The remaining one (25%)[80] compared closed suction drainage with no drainage in lower limb arterial surgery, in which no difference was found between the two techniques regarding various outcomes. One meta-analysis (25%)[82] focused on the comparison of off-pump surgery with traditional coronary artery bypass grafting, in which off-pump surgery was superior.

Table 2
Meta-analyses focusing on the effect of various interventions (other than antimicrobial prophylaxis) on surgical infections

Study	Intervention Studied (Focus of the Meta-analysis)	Studies Included	Patients Included	Effect on Primary Outcomes
Intra-abdominal				
Falagas et al, 2008[50]	Ertapenem versus other antimicrobial regimens for complicated intra-abdominal infections	6	2691	Clinical success: OR = 1.11 (0.89–1.39)
Siddiqui et al, 2008[51]	Early versus delayed laparoscopic cholecystectomy for acute cholecystitis	4	375	Complications: OR = 1.07 (0.60–1.92); Conversion rate: OR = 0.92 (0.57–1.48)
Yamamoto et al, 2008[52]	Laparoscopic versus open surgery for resection of colorectal cancer	10	3821	Wound infection: RR = 0.70 (0.51–0.95)
Choy et al, 2007[53]	Stapled versus handsewn methods for ileocolic anastomoses	6	955	Anastomotic leaks: OR 0.34 (0.14–0.82)
Chura et al, 2007[54]	Supplemental perioperative oxygen versus no oxygen in colorectal surgery patients	4	943	Surgical site infection: RR = 0.73 (0.42–1.28)
Falagas et al, 2007[55]	Treatment of intra-abdominal infections (clindamycin/aminoglycoside versus b-lactam monotherapy)	28	4518	Clinical success: OR = 0.67 (0.55–0.81)
Güenaga et al, 2007[56]	Ileostomy versus colostomy for temporary decompression of colorectal anastomosis	5	334	Mortality: RD = 0.02 (-0.02 - 0.05); Wound infection: RR = 0.57 (0.31–1.07); Reoperation: RD = 0.01 (−0.06–0.09); Colorectal anastomotic dehiscence: RR = 0.72 (0.36–1.47)
Gurusamy and Samraj, 2007[57]	Primary closure versus T-tube drainage after open common bile duct exploration	5	324	Positive bile culture: OR = 0.22 (0.10–0.45); Wound infection: OR = 0.29 (0.15–0.56)
Gurusamy et al, 2007[58]	Routine abdominal drainage versus no drainage for uncomplicated laparoscopic cholecystectomy	6	741	Wound infection: OR = 5.86 (1.05–32.70)
Gurusamy and Samraj, 2007[59]	Routine abdominal drainage versus no drainage for uncomplicated open cholecystectomy	28	3659	Mortality: OR = 0.79 (0.21–2.97); Bile peritonitis: OR = 1.33 (0.22–8.01)

Study	Trials	Patients	Comparison	Results
Gurusamy et al, 2007[60]	5	465	Routine abdominal drainage versus no drainage for uncomplicated liver resection	Mortality at maximal follow-up: OR = 1.17 (0.37–3.70); Reoperation for any reason: OR = 1.35 (0.44–4.11); Reoperation for intra-abdominal collection: OR = 1.86 (0.50–6.96)
Aziz et al, 2006[61]	7	1237	Laparoscopic versus open appendectomy in children	Wound infection: OR = 0.47 (0.16–1.35); Intra-abdominal abscess: OR = 1.7 (1–2.87); Postoperative ileus: OR = 0.48 (0.21–1.1)
Gurusamy and Samraj, 2006[62]	5	451	Early versus delayed laparoscopic cholecystectomy for acute cholecystitis	Bile duct injury: OR = 0.63 (0.15–2.70); Bile leak requiring ERCP: OR = 5.78 (1.00–33.29); Intra-abdominal collections requiring drainage: OR = 1.86 (0.56–6.18); Superficial infection: OR = 1.39 (0.56–3.44); Deep infection: OR = 0.43 (0.09–1.98)
Karliczek et al, 2006[63]	6	1140	Drainage versus nondrainage in elective colorectal anastomosis	Mortality: OR = 0.71 (0.39–1.31); Anastomotic leakage: OR = 1.55 (0.61–3.95)
Kazemier et al, 2006[64]	4	427	Endoscopic linear stapling versus loop ligatures of the stump during laparoscopic appendectomy for acute appendicitis	Superficial wound infections: OR = 0.21 (0.06–0.71); Postoperative ileus: OR = 0.36 (0.14–0.89); Intra-abdominal abscesses: OR = 0.62 (0.20–1.94)
Matthaiou et al, 2006[65]	5	1431	Treatment of intra-abdominal infections (ciprofloxacin/metronidazole versus b-lactam–based antibiotics)	Clinical success: OR = 1.69 (1.20–2.39)
Güenaga et al, 2005[66]	9	1592	Mechanical bowel preparation versus no preparation for elective colorectal surgery	Anastomotic leakage; Low anterior resection: Peto OR = 1.45 (0.57–3.67); Colonic surgery: Peto OR = 1.80 (0.68–4.75); Overall anastomotic leakage: Peto OR = 2.03 (1.28–3.26)
Henry and Moss, 2005[57]	6	347	Primary versus delayed wound closure in complicated appendicitis	Wound infection: RR = 0.64 (0.46–0.91)

(continued on next page)

Table 2
(continued)

Study	Intervention Studied (Focus of the Meta-analysis)	Studies Included	Patients Included	Effect on Primary Outcomes
Sanabria et al, 2005[68]	Laparoscopic versus open surgical treatment in patients with perforated peptic ulcer	2	214	Intra-abdominal abscess: OR = 4.82 (0.55–42.00) Anastomotic leakage: OR = 0.93 (0.13–6.71) Surgical site infection: OR = 0.33 (0.08–1.26)
Bucher et al, 2004[69]	Mechanical bowel preparation versus nonmechanical bowel preparation for elective colorectal surgery	7	1297	Anastomotic dehiscence: OR = 1.85 (1.06–3.22) Intra-abdominal infection: OR = 1.69 (0.76–3.75) Wound infection: OR = 1.38 (0.89–2.15) Reoperation rate: OR = 1.72 (0.81–3.65) General complications: OR = 1.15 (0.79–1.70) Mortality: OR = 1.42 (0.37–5.45)
Sauerland et al, 2004[70]	Laparoscopic versus open surgery for suspected appendicitis	45	5366	Laparoscopic versus conventional appendectomy in adults Wound infections: OR = 0.45 (0.35–0.58) Intra-abdominal abscesses: OR = 2.48 (1.45–4.21) Laparoscopic versus conventional appendectomy in children Wound infections: OR = 0.20 (0.08–0.54) Intra-abdominal abscesses: OR = 1.97 (0.20–19.14) Diagnostic laparoscopy (and open appendectomy if necessary) versus immediate open appendectomy Wound infections: OR = 7.54 (0.47–122.29) Intra-abdominal abscesses: OR = 0.14 (0.01–2.16)

Study			Results
Nelson and Singer, 2003[71]	Primary repair versus fecal diversion for penetrating colon injuries	6	705	Mortality: Peto OR = 1.22 (0.40–3.74) Complications: Peto OR = 0.54 (0.39–0.76) Total infectious complications: Peto OR = 0.44 (0.17–1.1) Abdominal infections including dehiscence: Peto OR = 0.67 (0.35–1.3) Abdominal infections excluding dehiscence: Peto OR = 0.69 (0.34–1.39) Wound complications including dehiscence: Peto OR = 0.73 (0.38–1.39) Wound complications excluding dehiscence: Peto OR = 0.67 (0.32–1.39)
Wille-Jorgensen et al, 2003[72]	Mechanical bowel preparation versus no preparation in patients undergoing elective colorectal surgery	6	1204	Anastomotic leakage Rectal resection: OR = 1.17 (0.35–3.96) Colonic surgery: OR = 1.75 (0.18–17.02) Overall: OR = 1.94 (1.09–3.43) Peritonitis: OR = 1.90 (0.78–4.64) Wound infection: OR = 1.34 (0.85–2.13)
Bailey et al, 2002[73]	Aminoglycosides versus other antibiotics in intra-abdominal infections	47	7772	Efficacy: OR = 1.19 (1.01–1.40)
Eypasch et al, 2002[74]	Laparoscopic versus open surgery for suspected appendicitis	45	>4000	Wound infection: Peto OR = 0.47 (0.36–0.62) Intra-abdominal abscesses: Peto OR = 2.77 (1.61–4.77)
Rucinski et al, 2000[75]	Primary versus delayed closure for gangrenous or perforated acute appendicitis	27	2532	Wound infection rates Primary closure: 4.7% (3.7%–5.7%) Delayed closure: 4.6% (3.2%–5.9%)
Meynaud-Kraemer et al, 1999[76]	Laparoscopic versus open appendectomy	8	907	Wound infection: OR = 0.33 (0.18–0.61)
Temple et al, 1999[77]	Laparoscopic versus open appendectomy in suspected acute appendicitis	12	1383	Wound infections: OR = 0.40 (0.24–0.69) Intra-abdominal abscesses: OR = 1.94 (0.68–5.58)
Sauerland et al, 1998[78]	Laparoscopic versus conventional appendectomy	28	2877	Operating time: +15.7 min (+11.9–+19.6) Total complications: RD = −1.3% (−4.2 to +1.5) Wound infections: RD = −4.2% (−6.1 to 2.3) Deep abscesses: RD = +0.9% (−0.4 to 2.3)

(continued on next page)

Table 2
(continued)

Study	Intervention Studied (Focus of the Meta-analysis)	Studies Included	Patients Included	Effect on Primary Outcomes
Chang and Wilson, 1997[79]	Meropenem monotherapy versus other antimicrobial regimens in intra-abdominal infections	10	1227	Overall difference in response rate: −1.6% (−5.7% to 2.5%) Overall response ratio: 0.99 (0.90–10.9)
Thoracic surgery/vascular				
Karthikesalingam et al, 2008[80]	Closed suction drainage versus no drainage in lower limb arterial surgery	4	429	Wound infection: OR = 1.56 (0.56–1.91) Seroma/lymphocele formation: OR = 2.01 (0.42–9.93) Hematoma formation: OR = 0.62 (0.37–1.04)
Reed, 2008[81]	Leg infections after great saphenous vein harvesting (minimally invasive versus conventional)	17	5215	Wound infection: OR = 0.19 (0.14–0.28) Wound healing disturbances: OR = 0.26 (0.20–0.34)
Sedrakyan et al, 2006[82]	Off-pump surgery versus traditional coronary artery bypass grafting	41	3996	Stroke: RR =0.5 (0.07–0.73) Atrial fibrillation: RR = 0.7 (0.16–0.43) Wound infection: RR = 0.52 (0.26–0.63)
Athanasiou et al 2003[83]	Leg wound infection after coronary artery bypass grafting (minimally invasive versus conventional vein harvesting)	14	1527	Wound infection: OR = 0.22 (0.14–0.34)
Obstetric				
Hellums et al, 2007[84]	Prophylactic drainage for prevention of wound complications after cesarean delivery (subcutaneous drainage versussubcutaneous suture alone/no intervention)	6	1066	Wound disruption: OR = 0.74 (0.39–1.42) Wound infection: OR = 1.15 (0.70–1.90) Wound hematoma: OR = 1.05 (0.33–3.30) Wound seroma: OR = 0.44 (0.14–1.43)
Gates and Anderson, 2005[85]	Wound drain versus no drain for cesarean section	7	1993	Wound infection: RR = 0.91 (0.58–1.43) Wound complication (seroma ± hematoma ± dehiscence): RR = 0.87 (0.41–1.84) Febrile morbidity: RR = 0.89 (0.66–1.20)

Orthopedic

Parker and Gurusamy, 2006[86]	Internal fixation versus arthroplasty for intracapsular proximal femoral fractures in adults	36	5464	All wound infection: RR = 0.84 (0.61–1.15); Deep wound infection: RR = 0.70 (0.29–1.68)
Parker et al, 2004[87]	Closed suction drainage versus no drainage for hip and knee arthroplasty	18	3495	Wound infection: RR = 0.73 (0.47–1.14); Wound hematoma: RR = 1.73 (0.74–4.07); Reoperations for wound complications: RR = 0.52 (0.13–1.99)
Parker and Pryor, 1996[88]	DHS versus Gamma nailing for extracapsular femoral fractures	10	1794	Percentage increase for the DHS; Wound infection: 1.7 (−0.9 to 4.2); Mortality: 0.4 (−3.5 to 4.3)

Other

McCallum et al, 2008[89]	Healing by primary closure versus open healing after surgery for pilonidal sinus	18	1573	Surgical site infection: RR = 1.20 (0.55–2.63); Recurrence rate: RR = 0.42 (0.26–0.66)
Rabindranath et al, 2007[90]	Continuous ambulatory peritoneal dialysis versus automated peritoneal dialysis for end-stage renal disease	3	139	Mortality: RR = 1.49 (0.51–4.37); Peritonitis: RR = 0.75 (0.50–1.11)
Webster and Alghamdi, 2007[91]	Plastic adhesive drapes (iodine-impregnated or not) versus no drape during surgery	7	4195	Surgical site infection; Adhesive drape versus no drape: RR = 1.23 (1.02–1.48); Iodine-impregnated adhesive drape versus no drape: RR = 1.03 (0.064–1.66)
Delaney et al, 2006[92]	Percutaneous dilatational tracheostomy versus surgical tracheostomy in critically ill patients	17	1212	Wound infection: OR = 0.28 (0.16–0.49); Bleeding: OR = 0.80 (0.45–1.41); Mortality: OR = 0.79 (0.59–1.07)
Tanner et al, 2006[93]	Preoperative hair removal to reduce surgical site infection	11	4501	Wound infection – existence of pus; Shaving versus no hair removal: RR = 1.59 (0.77–3.27); Cream versus no hair removal: RR = 1.02 (0.45–2.31)

Abbreviations: RCTs, Randomized controlled trials; OR, Odds ratio; RR, Risk ratio; RD, Risk difference.

Meta-analyses Focusing on Orthopedics

Two of 3 meta-analyses (66.7%)[86,88] concerning orthopedics compared different procedures for the treatment of femoral fractures; none of the compared techniques was found to be superior in terms of wound infection rates or mortality. The remaining meta-analysis (33.3%)[87] focused on the use of closed suction drainage versus no drainage for hip and knee arthroplasty, in which no difference was found between the two techniques for the examined outcomes.

Meta-analyses Focusing on Obstetrics

Both meta-analyses (100%)[84,85] concerning obstetrics focused on the use of drainage versus no drainage for cesarean section. No difference was found between the compared techniques regarding the various outcomes.

Meta-analyses Focusing on Other Topics

Of the remaining meta-analyses (20% each), one focused on the comparison of different techniques for the treatment of pilonidal sinus,[89] in which primary closure was associated with lower recurrence rates; one on the comparison of continuous ambulatory dialysis with automated peritoneal dialysis for end-stage renal diseases,[90] in which no difference was found between the types of dialysis in terms of mortality or peritonitis; one on the use of plastic adhesive drapes versus no drape during surgery,[91] in which no advantage was found in the use of drapes regarding the surgical site infection rates; one on the comparison of different techniques of tracheostomy,[92] in which percutaneous dilatational tracheostomy was superior to surgical tracheostomy in terms of wound infections rates; and one on the comparison of different hair removal techniques to reduce SSIs,[93] in which no advantage was found in preoperative hair removal of any type.

DISCUSSION

Meta-analysis is a useful statistical approach, which offers quantitative measures of studied outcomes and can be applied in virtually any field of science. As such, it has also been used in the study of surgical infections. According to our findings, meta-analyses regarding surgical infections may be divided in studies focusing on the use of antimicrobial prophylaxis, and in studies focusing on the comparison of different techniques and procedures or therapeutic regimens for the treatment of surgical infections.

Administration of antibiotics may have an impact on the postoperative course regarding the wound infection rates. This depends on the type of surgery or infection for which they are used. Thus, in acute necrotizing pancreatitis, it is not clear if antibiotic prophylaxis has a role in the reduction of pancreatic necrosis or mortality. Although the majority of meta-analyses focusing on the subject show no benefit from the administration of prophylaxis regarding the infected necrosis rates, the most recent studies suggest that prophylaxis may be superior. Safe conclusions regarding mortality are even more difficult to be drawn, as merely half of the meta-analyses found prophylaxis to be superior. The same results may be observed in meta-analyses regarding SSI rates in biliary surgery. However, all meta-analyses that have been conducted in other patient settings, such as percutaneous endoscopic gastrostomy, thoracic surgery, neurosurgery, obstetrics and gynecology, and breast surgery, as well as the majority of meta-analysis regarding hernia surgery, suggest an advantage in the use of antibiotic prophylaxis.

The natural history of each type of surgical infection as well as the degree of contamination during surgery are important determinants of outcomes. In patients with acute necrotizing pancreatitis, for example, the extent of necrosis varies. It is a process on which antibiotics have no direct effect and may have a serious impact on patients' courses. Pancreatic necrosis, tissue debris, and surrounding inflammation may decompensate antibiotic effectiveness when intestinal bacteria infect necrotic tissues. Similarly, in contaminated surgery, as in nonelective gastrointestinal surgery or perforation of hollow organs, tissue destruction and bacterial contamination is greater, resulting in more severe disease manifestations.

Furthermore, new procedures have been introduced in surgery to improve outcomes. Such methods include laparoscopy and postoperative use of wound drainage. All but one meta-analysis comparing laparoscopic with conventional surgery found an advantage of laparoscopy regarding wound infection rates. However, no difference was found in the rate of intra-abdominal abscesses. It should be noted that most of these meta-analyses included patients with appendicitis. Furthermore, meta-analyses comparing minimally invasive with conventional vein harvesting techniques found minimally invasive techniques to be superior regarding wound infection rates. On the contrary, no advantage was found regarding SSI rates or mortality in the use of drainage in any of the meta-analyses reporting relevant data.

Tissue destruction caused by conventional, more invasive methods, has a capital role in the postoperative course. The maneuvers used in conventional procedures may cause ischemia and subsequent reduced flow of drugs and nutrients, which delay healing and facilitate bacterial growth.

It should be noted that apart from the usage of prosthetic materials during surgery itself, the properties of these materials may have a role in the perioperative course as well as in the rates of SSIs, eg, meshes used in hernia repair. According to their pore size, they are divided into microporous (PTFE) and macroporous (Dacron). The pore diameter of the former group is smaller than that of leucocytes, thus preventing them from penetrating the mesh and reaching the site of a potential infection, whereas the pores of the latter group are large enough to allow the passage of leucocytes, resulting in lower mesh infection rates. Although such mesh properties are not specifically reported in the relevant meta-analyses, all of them suggest the use of antibiotic prophylaxis when mesh hernia repair is performed.

There is a debate of increasing interest regarding whether surgical infections such as diverticulitis or appendicitis should receive nonsurgical treatment. No meta-analysis has been performed comparing conservative with surgical treatment for diverticulitis, whereas one systematic review focuses on conservative treatment of appendiceal abscess or phlegmon.[95] Although virtually all of the included studies are retrospective, the authors perform "meta-analytical" analyses and support that patients with appendiceal abscess or phlegmon should receive nonsurgical treatment without appendectomy. Furthermore, opinions are gaining ground that support the shortening of antimicrobial treatment in septicemic surgical patients. However, no meta-analysis has been performed on the subject as well.

The advent of different antimicrobial classes has led to several comparisons between different antibiotics in terms of effectiveness in various types of infections, including surgical infections. However, almost half of the included meta-analyses (2 of 5, 40%) that compared different antimicrobial regimens for the treatment of surgical infections found no difference in terms of effectiveness. The design of the included randomized controlled trials, which are noninferiority studies, as well as the type of statistical tests that are used, may lead to such results. However, there are many factors that may influence randomized controlled trial outcomes, especially in intra-abdominal infections.[96] General factors, which are independently associated with clinical failure, are the isolation of an organism resistant to the treatment regimen, including *Pseudomonas* spp, being on antibiotic therapy at the time of admission, and diagnosis of a complicated intra-abdominal infection.[97]

Given the size of the field of surgical infections, one would expect meta-analysis to have been used in the study of virtually every type of surgical infection. However, the topics that have been studied are limited. More than half of the included meta-analyses focused on surgical infections in abdominal surgery (50 of 90, 55.6%). Furthermore, many meta-analyses with similar topics include practically the same studies. This is expected to some extent, because the conduction of a randomized controlled trial is a costly and time-consuming process. Thus, in the short interval between two meta-analyses on the same topic, few new randomized trials may have been published to substantially alter the former meta-analyses' outcomes.

It should be noted that, although the topic of two meta-analyses may be the same and the included studies are similar, the outcome estimates are different. Apart from the additional inclusion of a small number of more recent, if any, studies, there are other factors that may also influence the outcome estimates. Such factors may be the analytical methodology that has been used, and the variability in the number of patients of each evaluable trial that are included in the analyses. Although discrepancies among the point estimates of meta-analyses on the same topic may be expected to some extent, scores calculating the overall quality of each meta-analysis should be developed, as for other types of studies. Thus, quality of meta-analyses may be quantified to help in the evaluation of findings and correct application of conclusions.

It is interesting that the retrieved meta-analyses focusing exclusively on surgical infections most often concern antibiotic prophylaxis or the comparison of specific techniques and procedures but not comparisons of different antibiotic regimens for the treatment of surgical infections. Antibiotics as therapeutic regimens are more easily evaluated in patients with various infections. Prospective studies are designed to include patients from broad settings, because the applicability and extrapolation of the findings are greater, whereas the cost of the study and the time needed to find the appropriate participants are smaller.

Furthermore, few meta-analyses (15 of 90, 16.7%) report data on mortality as primary outcomes. All but four (11 of 15, 73.3%) were meta-analyses focusing on surgical infections in abdominal surgery. One would expect this outcome to be reported more often, because mortality is a crucial determinant in the evaluation of different treatments, as it encompasses both efficacy and safety.

According to the definition by the Centers for Disease Control, surgical infections are very common, but also diverse clinical entities and cannot be considered as a whole. Data regarding wound infections, among other numerous outcomes, were reported in a large number of meta-analyses, which included studies evaluating or comparing various types of interventions, but they were not considered primary outcomes, resulting in their exclusion. However, practically any surgical procedure may have an SSI as a possible complication. Although this may be a methodologic limitation of the review, presenting all these diverse data would make a meaningful interpretation difficult.

SUMMARY

Meta-analysis on surgical infections may be a useful tool that can provide more accurate outcome estimates than other conventional types of studies. Published meta-analyses in surgical infections tend to focus mainly on the use of antimicrobial prophylaxis and on the comparison of different procedures or techniques for the treatment of surgical infections. The majority concern surgical infections in abdominal surgery. However, mortality is reported as primary outcome in few meta-analyses. Meta-analyses focusing exclusively on surgical infections, reporting data on mortality as a primary outcome, and comparing different antibiotic regimens for the treatment of surgical infections should be conducted.

REFERENCES

1. Horan TC, Gaynes RP. Surveillance of nosocomial infections. In: Mayhall CG, editor. Hospital epidemiology and infection control. 3rd edition. Philadelphia: Lippincott Williams & Wilkins; 2004. p. 1659–702.
2. Gaynes RP, Culver DH, Horan TC, et al. Surgical site infection (SSI) rates in the united states, 1992–1998: the national nosocomial infections surveillance system basic SSI risk index. Clin Infect Dis 2001;33(Suppl 2):69–77.
3. Bratzler DW, Houck PM. Antimicrobial prophylaxis for surgery: an advisory statement from the national surgical infection prevention project. Clin Infect Dis 2004; 38(12):1706–15.
4. Kazrin A, Durac J, Agteros T. Meta-meta analysis: a new method for evaluating therapy outcome. Behav Res Ther 1979;17(4):397–9.
5. Bai Y, Gao J, Zou D-W, et al. Prophylactic antibiotics cannot reduce infected pancreatic necrosis and mortality in acute necrotizing pancreatitis: evidence from a meta-analysis of randomized controlled trials. Am J Gastroenterol 2008; 103(1):104–10.
6. Gravante G, Venditti D, Filingeri V. The role of single-shot antibiotic prophylaxis in inguinal hernia repair: a meta-analysis approach of 4336 patients. Ann Surg 2008; 248(3):496–7.
7. Xu T, Cai Q. Prophylactic antibiotic treatment in acute necrotizing pancreatitis: results from a meta-analysis. Scand J Gastroenterol 2008;43(10): 1249–58.
8. Dambrauskas Z, Gulbinas A, Pundzius J, et al. Meta-analysis of prophylactic parenteral antibiotic use in acute necrotizing pancreatitis. Medicina (Kaunas) 2007;43(4):291–300.
9. Jafri NS, Mahid SS, Minor KS, et al. Meta-analysis: antibiotic prophylaxis to prevent peristomal infection following percutaneous endoscopic gastrostomy. Aliment Pharmacol Ther 2007;25(6):647–56.
10. Sanabria A, Dominguez LC, Valdivieso E, et al. Prophylactic antibiotics for mesh inguinal hernioplasty: a meta-analysis. Ann Surg 2007;245(3):392–6.
11. Sanchez-Manuel FJ, Lozano-Garcia J, Seco-Gil JL. Antibiotic prophylaxis for hernia repair. Cochrane Database Syst Rev 2007.
12. Aufenacker TJ, Koelemay MJW, Gouma DJ, et al. Systematic review and meta-analysis of the effectiveness of antibiotic prophylaxis in prevention of wound infection after mesh repair of abdominal wall hernia. Br J Surg 2006;93(1):5–10.
13. Lipp A, Lusardi G. Systemic antimicrobial prophylaxis for percutaneous endoscopic gastrostomy. Cochrane Database Syst Rev 2006.
14. Mazaki T, Ishii Y, Takayama T. Meta-analysis of prophylactic antibiotic use in acute necrotizing pancreatitis. Br J Surg 2006;93(6):674–84.
15. Villatoro E, Bassi C, Larvin M. Antibiotic therapy for prophylaxis against infection of pancreatic necrosis in acute pancreatitis. Cochrane Database Syst Rev 2006.

16. Xiong G-S, Wu S-M, Wang Z-H. Role of prophylactic antibiotic administration in severe acute pancreatitis: a meta-analysis. Med Princ Pract 2006;15(2):106–10.

17. Andersen BR, Kallehave FL, Andersen HK. Antibiotics versus placebo for prevention of postoperative infection after appendicectomy. Cochrane Database Syst Rev 2005.

18. Catarci M, Mancini S, Gentileschi P, et al. Antibiotic prophylaxis in elective laparoscopic cholecystectomy. Lack of need or lack of evidence? Surg Endosc 2004; 18(4):638–41.

19. Sharma VK, Howden CW. Prophylactic antibiotic administration reduces sepsis and mortality in acute necrotizing pancreatitis: a meta-analysis. Pancreas 2001; 22(1):28–31.

20. Sharma VK, Howden CW. Meta-analysis of randomized, controlled trials of antibiotic prophylaxis before percutaneous endoscopic gastrostomy. Am J Gastroenterol 2000;95(11):3133–6.

21. Bernard B, Grange JD, Khac EN, et al. Antibiotic prophylaxis for the prevention of bacterial infections in cirrhotic patients with gastrointestinal bleeding: a meta-analysis. Hepatology 1999;29(6):1655–61.

22. Glenny AM, Song F. Antimicrobial prophylaxis in colorectal surgery. Qual Health Care 1999;8(2):132–6.

23. Meijer WS, Schmitz PI, Jeekel J. Meta-analysis of randomized, controlled clinical trials of antibiotic prophylaxis in biliary tract surgery. Br J Surg 1990;77(3): 283–90.

24. AlBuhairan B, Hind D, Hutchinson A. Antibiotic prophylaxis for wound infections in total joint arthroplasty: a systematic review. J Bone Joint Surg Br 2008;90(7): 915–9.

25. Slobogean GP, Kennedy SA, Davidson D, et al. Single- versus multiple-dose antibiotic prophylaxis in the surgical treatment of closed fractures: a meta-analysis. J Orthop Trauma 2008;22(4):264–9.

26. Southwell-Keely JP, Russo RR, March L, et al. Antibiotic prophylaxis in hip fracture surgery: a metaanalysis. Clin Orthop Relat Res 2004;(419):179–84.

27. Stewart AH, Eyers PS, Earnshaw JJ. Prevention of infection in peripheral arterial reconstruction: a systematic review and meta-analysis. J Vasc Surg 2007;46(1): 148–55.

28. Sanabria A, Valdivieso E, Gomez G, et al. Prophylactic antibiotics in chest trauma: a meta-analysis of high-quality studies. World J Surg 2006;30(10):1843–7.

29. Bolon MK, Morlote M, Weber SG, et al. Glycopeptides are no more effective than beta-lactam agents for prevention of surgical site infection after cardiac surgery: a meta-analysis. Clin Infect Dis 2004;38(10):1357–63.

30. Da Costa A, Kirkorian G, Cucherat M, et al. Antibiotic prophylaxis for permanent pacemaker implantation: a meta-analysis. Circulation 1998;97(18):1796–801.

31. Fallon WF, Wears RL. Prophylactic antibiotics for the prevention of infectious complications including empyema following tube thoracostomy for trauma: results of meta-analysis. J Trauma 1992;33(1):110–6.

32. Martins AC, Krauss-Silva L. [Systematic reviews of antibiotic prophylaxis in cesareans]. Cad Saude Publica 2006;22(12):2513–26 [in Portugese].

33. Costa RJ, Krauss-Silva L. [Systematic review and meta-analysis of antibiotic prophylaxis in abdominal hysterectomy]. Cad Saude Publica 2004;20(Suppl 2): 175–89 [in Portugese].

34. Chelmow D, Ruehli MS, Huang E. Prophylactic use of antibiotics for nonlaboring patients undergoing cesarean delivery with intact membranes: a meta-analysis. Am J Obstet Gynecol 2001;184(4):656–61.

35. Ratilal B, Costa J, Sampaio C. Antibiotic prophylaxis for surgical introduction of intracranial ventricular shunts: a systematic review. J Neurosurg Pediatrics 2008;1(1):48–56.
36. van Rijen MML, Bonten M, Wenzel RP, et al. Intranasal mupirocin for reduction of *Staphylococcus aureus* infections in surgical patients with nasal carriage: a systematic review. J Antimicrob Chemother 2008;61(2):254–61.
37. Webster J, Osborne S. Preoperative bathing or showering with skin antiseptics to prevent surgical site infection. Cochrane Database Syst Rev 2007.
38. Cunningham M, Bunn F, Handscomb K. Prophylactic antibiotics to prevent surgical site infection after breast cancer surgery. Cochrane Database Syst Rev 2006.
39. Tejirian T, DiFronzo LA, Haigh PI. Antibiotic prophylaxis for preventing wound infection after breast surgery: a systematic review and metaanalysis. J Am Coll Surg 2006;203(5):729–34.
40. Kallen AJ, Wilson CT, Larson RJ. Perioperative intranasal mupirocin for the prevention of surgical-site infections: systematic review of the literature and meta-analysis. Infect Control Hosp Epidemiol 2005;26(12):916–22.
41. Vardakas KZ, Soteriades ES, Chrysanthopoulou SA, et al. Perioperative anti-infective prophylaxis with teicoplanin compared to cephalosporins in orthopaedic and vascular surgery involving prosthetic material. Clin Microbiol Infect 2005; 11(10):775–7.
42. Esposito S, Noviello S, Vanasia A, et al. Ceftriaxone versus other antibiotics for surgical prophylaxis: a meta-analysis. Clin Drug Investig 2004;24(1):29–39.
43. Strippoli GFM, Tong A, Johnson D, et al. Antimicrobial agents for preventing peritonitis in peritoneal dialysis patients. Cochrane Database Syst Rev 2004.
44. Barker FG. Efficacy of prophylactic antibiotic therapy in spinal surgery: a meta-analysis. Neurosurgery 2002;51(2):391–400.
45. Dietrich ES, Bieser U, Frank U, et al. Ceftriaxone versus other cephalosporins for perioperative antibiotic prophylaxis: a meta-analysis of 43 randomized controlled trials. Chemotherapy 2002;48(1):49–56.
46. Barker FG. Efficacy of prophylactic antibiotics for craniotomy: a meta-analysis. Neurosurgery 1994;35(3):484–90.
47. Langley JM, LeBlanc JC, Drake J, et al. Efficacy of antimicrobial prophylaxis in placement of cerebrospinal fluid shunts: meta-analysis. Clin Infect Dis 1993; 17(1):98–103.
48. Platt R, Zucker JR, Zaleznik DF, et al. Perioperative antibiotic prophylaxis and wound infection following breast surgery. J Antimicrob Chemother 1993;31(Suppl B):43–8.
49. Wilson AP, Shrimpton S, Jaderberg M. A meta-analysis of the use of amoxycillin-clavulanic acid in surgical prophylaxis. J Hosp Infect 1992;22(Suppl A):9–21.
50. Falagas ME, Peppas G, Makris GC, et al. Meta-analysis: ertapenem for complicated intra-abdominal infections. Aliment Pharmacol Ther 2008;27(10):919–31.
51. Siddiqui T, MacDonald A, Chong PS, et al. Early versus delayed laparoscopic cholecystectomy for acute cholecystitis: a meta-analysis of randomized clinical trials. Am J Surg 2008;195(1):40–7.
52. Yamamoto S, Fujita S, Ishiguro S, Akasu T, Moriya Y. Wound infection after a laparoscopic resection for colorectal cancer. Surg Today 2008;38(7):618–22.
53. Choy PYG, Bissett IP, Docherty JG, et al. Stapled versus handsewn methods for ileocolic anastomoses. Cochrane Database Syst Rev 2007.
54. Chura JC, Boyd A, Argenta PA. Surgical site infections and supplemental perioperative oxygen in colorectal surgery patients: a systematic review. Surg Infect (Larchmt) 2007;8(4):455–61.

55. Falagas ME, Matthaiou DK, Karveli EA, et al. Meta-analysis: randomized controlled trials of clindamycin/aminoglycoside vs. beta-lactam monotherapy for the treatment of intra-abdominal infections. Aliment Pharmacol Ther 2007; 25(5):537–56.
56. Guenaga KF, Lustosa SAS, Saad SS, et al. Ileostomy or colostomy for temporary decompression of colorectal anastomosis. Cochrane Database Syst Rev 2007.
57. Gurusamy KS, Samraj K. Primary closure versus t-tube drainage after open common bile duct exploration. Cochrane Database Syst Rev 2007.
58. Gurusamy KS, Samraj K, Mullerat P, et al. Routine abdominal drainage for uncomplicated laparoscopic cholecystectomy. Cochrane Database Syst Rev 2007.
59. Gurusamy KS, Samraj K. Routine abdominal drainage for uncomplicated open cholecystectomy. Cochrane Database Syst Rev 2007.
60. Gurusamy KS, Samraj K, Davidson BR. Routine abdominal drainage for uncomplicated liver resection. Cochrane Database Syst Rev 2007.
61. Aziz O, Athanasiou T, Tekkis PP, et al. Laparoscopic versus open appendectomy in children: a meta-analysis. Ann Surg 2006;243(1):17–27.
62. Gurusamy KS, Samraj K. Early versus delayed laparoscopic cholecystectomy for acute cholecystitis. Cochrane Database Syst Rev 2006.
63. Karliczek A, Jesus EC, Matos D, et al. Drainage or nondrainage in elective colorectal anastomosis: a systematic review and meta-analysis. Colorectal Dis 2006; 8(4):259–65.
64. Kazemier G, in't Hof KH, Saad S, et al. Securing the appendiceal stump in laparoscopic appendectomy: evidence for routine stapling? Surg Endosc 2006;20(9): 1473–6.
65. Matthaiou DK, Peppas G, Bliziotis IA, et al. Ciprofloxacin/metronidazole versus beta-lactam-based treatment of intra-abdominal infections: a meta-analysis of comparative trials. Int J Antimicrob Agents 2006;28(3):159–65.
66. Guenaga KF, Matos D, Castro AA, et al. Mechanical bowel preparation for elective colorectal surgery. Cochrane Database Syst Rev 2005.
67. Henry MCW, Moss RL. Primary versus delayed wound closure in complicated appendicitis: an international systematic review and meta-analysis. Pediatr Surg Int 2005;21(8):625–30.
68. Sanabria AE, Morales CH, Villegas MI. Laparoscopic repair for perforated peptic ulcer disease. Cochrane Database Syst Rev 2005.
69. Bucher P, Mermillod B, Gervaz P, et al. Mechanical bowel preparation for elective colorectal surgery: a meta-analysis. Arch Surg 2004;139(12):1359–64.
70. Sauerland S, Lefering R, Neugebauer EAM. Laparoscopic versus open surgery for suspected appendicitis. Cochrane Database Syst Rev 2004.
71. Nelson R, Singer M. Primary repair for penetrating colon injuries. Cochrane Database Syst Rev 2003.
72. Wille-Jorgensen P, Guenaga KF, Castro AA, et al. Clinical value of preoperative mechanical bowel cleansing in elective colorectal surgery: a systematic review. Dis Colon Rectum 2003;46(8):1013–20.
73. Bailey JA, Virgo KS, DiPiro JT, et al. Aminoglycosides for intra-abdominal infection: equal to the challenge? Surg Infect (Larchmt) 2002;3(4):315–35.
74. Eypasch E, Sauerland S, Lefering R, et al. Laparoscopic versus open appendectomy: between evidence and common sense. Dig Surg 2002;19(6): 518–22.
75. Rucinski J, Fabian T, Panagopoulos G, et al. Gangrenous and perforated appendicitis: a meta-analytic study of 2532 patients indicates that the incision should be closed primarily. Surgery 2000;127(2):136–41.

76. Meynaud-Kraemer L, Colin C, Vergnon P, et al. Wound infection in open versus laparoscopic appendectomy. a meta-analysis. Int J Technol Assess Health Care 1999;15(2):380–91.
77. Temple LK, Litwin DE, McLeod RS. A meta-analysis of laparoscopic versus open appendectomy in patients suspected of having acute appendicitis. Can J Surg 1999;42(5):377–83.
78. Sauerland S, Lefering R, Holthausen U, et al. Laparoscopic vs conventional appendectomy–a meta-analysis of randomised controlled trials. Langenbecks Arch Surg 1998;383(3–4):289–95.
79. Chang DC, Wilson SE. Meta-analysis of the clinical outcome of carbapenem monotherapy in the adjunctive treatment of intra-abdominal infections. Am J Surg 1997;174(3):284–90.
80. Karthikesalingam A, Walsh SR, Sadat U, et al. Efficacy of closed suction drainage in lower limb arterial surgery: a meta-analysis of published clinical trials. Vasc Endovascular Surg 2008;42(3):243–8.
81. Reed JF. Leg wound infections following greater saphenous vein harvesting: minimally invasive vein harvesting versus conventional vein harvesting. Int J Low Extrem Wounds 2008;7(4):210–9.
82. Sedrakyan A, Vaccarino V, Elefteriades JA, et al. Health related quality of life after mitral valve repairs and replacements. Qual Life Res 2006;15(7): 1153–60.
83. Athanasiou T, Aziz O, Skapinakis P, et al. Leg wound infection after coronary artery bypass grafting: a meta-analysis comparing minimally invasive versus conventional vein harvesting. Ann Thorac Surg 2003;76(6):2141–6.
84. Hellums EK, Lin MG, Ramsey PS. Prophylactic subcutaneous drainage for prevention of wound complications after cesarean delivery–a metaanalysis. Am J Obstet Gynecol 2007;197(3):229–35.
85. Gates S, Anderson ER. Wound drainage for caesarean section. Cochrane Database Syst Rev 2005.
86. Parker MJ, Gurusamy K. Internal fixation versus arthroplasty for intracapsular proximal femoral fractures in adults. Cochrane Database Syst Rev 2006.
87. Parker MJ, Roberts CP, Hay D. Closed suction drainage for hip and knee arthroplasty. A meta-analysis. J Bone Joint Surg Am 2004;86-A(6):1146–52.
88. Parker MJ, Pryor GA. Gamma versus DHS nailing for extracapsular femoral fractures. Meta-analysis of ten randomised trials. Int Orthop 1996;20(3): 163–8.
89. McCallum IJD, King PM, Bruce J. Healing by primary closure versus open healing after surgery for pilonidal sinus: Systematic review and meta-analysis. BMJ 2008;336(7649):868–71.
90. Rabindranath KS, Adams J, Ali TZ, et al. Continuous ambulatory peritoneal dialysis versus automated peritoneal dialysis for end-stage renal disease. Cochrane Database Syst Rev 2007.
91. Webster J, Alghamdi AA. Use of plastic adhesive drapes during surgery for preventing surgical site infection. Cochrane Database Syst Rev 2007.
92. Delaney A, Bagshaw SM, Nalos M. Percutaneous dilatational tracheostomy versus surgical tracheostomy in critically ill patients: a systematic review and meta-analysis. Crit Care 2006;10(2).
93. Tanner J, Woodings D, Moncaster K. Preoperative hair removal to reduce surgical site infection. Cochrane Database Syst Rev 2006.
94. Wong PF, Gilliam AD, Kumar S, et al. Antibiotic regimens for secondary peritonitis of gastrointestinal origin in adults. Cochrane Database Syst Rev 2005.

95. Andersson RE, Petzold MG. Nonsurgical treatment of appendiceal abscess or phlegmon: a systematic review and meta-analysis. Ann Surg 2007;246(5): 741–8.
96. Solomkin JS, Meakins JL, Allo MD, et al. Antibiotic trials in intra-abdominal infections. A critical evaluation of study design and outcome reporting. Ann Surg 1984;200(1):29–39.
97. Falagas ME, Barefoot L, Griffith J, et al. Risk factors leading to clinical failure in the treatment of intra-abdominal or skin/soft tissue infections. Eur J Clin Microbiol Infect Dis 1996;15(12):913–21.

Meta-analyses on Pediatric Infections and Vaccines

Alexandros P. Grammatikos, MD, MSc[a,b], Elpis Mantadakis, MD, PhD[c],
Matthew E. Falagas, MD, MSc, DSc[a,d,e],*

KEYWORDS

- Children • Infections • Meta-analyses • Vaccines
- Acute gastroenteritis • Bronchiolitis • Influenza vaccines
- Pneumococcal vaccines

Meta-analysis, the statistical analysis of a large collection of results from individual studies for the purpose of integrating their findings, is a useful tool for solving controversial medical issues.

Two of the scientific fields where meta-analyses have contributed substantially are those of pediatric infections and vaccines. Serious infections are less common in children than in adults and, moreover, children are also generally more difficult to recruit into clinical trials. As a result, isolated trials on pediatric infections are usually small, making them less useful than larger trials for drawing conclusions. Meta-analyses solve this problem by combining the results of different studies, and thus enabling clinicians to draw firmer conclusions.

Meta-analyses played a role in making vaccines so successful. Over the last century, meta-analyses were often used to measure the success and failure of vaccines and to gauge such factors as immunogenicity, clinical efficiency, and toxicity. Conclusions drawn from metaanalyses helped researchers refine and improve vaccines. A recent report from the Centers for Disease Control and Prevention ranked vaccines first on the list of the most important public health advances of the twentieth century.[1] Meta-analyses summarizing the current evidence on various aspects of vaccine use, including immunogenicity, clinical efficiency, and toxicity, have helped achieve this goal.

[a] Alfa Institute of Biomedical Sciences (AIBS), 9 Neapoleos Street, 15123 Marousi, Athens, Greece
[b] Department of Medicine, "G. Gennimatas" Hospital, Thessaloniki, Greece
[c] Department of Pediatrics, University District Hospital of Alexandroupolis and Democritus University of Thrace, Alexandroupolis, Thrace, Greece
[d] Department of Medicine, Tufts University School of Medicine, Boston, MA, USA
[e] Department of Medicine, Henry Dunant Hospital, Athens, Greece
* Corresponding author.
E-mail address: m.falagas@aibs.gr (M.E. Falagas).

Infect Dis Clin N Am 23 (2009) 431–457
doi:10.1016/j.idc.2009.01.008
0891-5520/09/$ – see front matter © 2009 Elsevier Inc. All rights reserved.

id.theclinics.com

In preparing an overview of the contribution of meta-analyses into these two important scientific fields—pediatric infections and vaccinology—we searched various electronic databases for relevant articles. Our search produced more than 200 related meta-analyses. Below we summarize our findings into those areas of vaccines and pediatric infections where meta-analyses seem to have focused the most (eg, where the topic was covered in four or more reviews). For the purposes of this review, neonatal and adult meta-analyses on infectious diseases were excluded,[2] whereas mixed-population studies were included only if they presented relevant data and if the majority of their observations were derived from children.

META-ANALYSES ON PEDIATRIC INFECTIONS
Acute Gastroenteritis and Diarrhea

A substantial number of studies have been performed in recent years on acute gastroenteritis (AGE) and diarrhea. Even though morbidity of AGE has fallen sharply in recent years, it still afflicts a substantial proportion of children globally, particularly in the developing world, accounting for a large number of pediatric deaths. Although other causes are also implicated in the development of AGE and diarrhea, infections account for the majority of the cases.

Oral rehydration therapy (ORT) is considered to be one of the most important advances in the treatment of AGE in recent years, and many investigators attribute to ORT the recent decline in AGE-related mortality worldwide. Three previous meta-analyses have focused on evaluating ORT in comparison to intravenous rehydration treatments, and all confirmed that the former is equally effective in children with diarrhea.[3–5] Regarding the best type of ORT, two solutions have been tested in clinical trials: reduced osmolarity solutions and rice-based oral rehydration solutions.[6,7] Reduced osmolarity solutions, which contain less sodium and glucose than standard solutions, fare better and, indeed, have become the current standard.[7,8] Meanwhile, rice-based solutions were effective only in children with cholera.[7] According to another meta-analysis, nonhuman, nonhydrolyzed milk can also be administered with safety to children with diarrhea.[9]

Other studies have focused on the supplementation of minerals and vitamins to children with AGE because malnutrition is known to be one of the most important adverse prognostic indicators in this disease, particularly in developing countries. Based on the findings of three meta-analyses, zinc supplementation offers relief to children suffering from AGE.[10–12] By contrast, vitamin A has no consistent protective effect on the incidence of diarrhea, as shown by nine randomized controlled trials (RCTs).[13]

Another promising treatment option for pediatric AGE is probiotics. At least nine meta-analyses have attempted to summarize the evidence available on probiotics in children. Although some evidence exists on the value of probiotics in treating AGE, this evidence is generally inconclusive and further trials are clearly necessary to elucidate the potential of these agents.[14–22] Three of these reviews evaluated the use of Lactobacillus and Saccharomyces, and concluded that both bacterial genera have a moderate potential to prevent acute diarrhea in children.[19–21] Although the use of probiotics has also been advocated to prevent antibiotic-associated diarrhea in children, current evidence seems to be controversial.[15,18,22]

Regarding the use of certain antidiarrheal agents (smectite) and antiemetics (ondansetron and metoclopramide) in children with AGE, their benefit is rather minimal and their use entails some dangers.[23–26] Finally, one meta-analysis on the efficacy of homeopathy in the treatment of acute diarrhea in children found that this modality can significantly decrease the duration of a diarrheal episode by 0.66 days.[27]

However, although statistically significant, this result has rather minimal clinical significance.

Regarding prevention of AGE, two vaccines against rotaviruses, the most common infectious cause of diarrhea worldwide, are commercially available. The first vaccine against rotaviruses was first licensed in 1998, but it was withdrawn the next year because of its possible association with intussusception. Since then, two large phase III clinical trials with more than 70,000 infants showed that the currently available vaccines are both safe and effective in preventing diarrhea in children.[28]

Bronchiolitis and Pneumonia

Bronchiolitis, a virally induced lower respiratory tract infection (LRTI) most frequently caused by respiratory syncytial virus, is a common infection in children. According to current recommendations, clinical treatment of children with bronchiolitis should be supportive and limited to administration of oxygen in cases of hypoxia. Indeed, several recent meta-analyses have shown that bronchodilator therapy is associated with modest or no benefit at all in children with bronchiolitis (**Table 1**).[29-33] Likewise, antibiotics do not seem to confer any significant advantage to children with bronchiolitis, as one would expect considering the viral nature of the disease.[34] The use of surfactant, although a promising therapy, is not yet supported by adequate evidence and, moreover, is applicable only for the most severely affected infants.[35] Ribavirin treatment seems to be beneficial for some infants with severe bronchiolitis due to respiratory syncytial virus.[36] Although one previous meta-analysis found some evidence to support the use of systemic corticosteroids for bronchiolitis in infants,[37] two more recent studies concluded that corticosteroids are not associated with any significant benefits.[38,39] In accordance with these studies, a recent meta-analysis evaluating the strength of evidence in support of the various treatments for bronchiolitis in critically ill infants did not come up with any clear beneficial effects.[40] Finally, chest physiotherapy does not offer much benefit to infants with acute bronchiolitis.[41]

In contrast to bronchiolitis, pneumonia in children is frequently of bacterial etiology. Although various risk factors have been associated with the development of pneumonia in children, a recent meta-analysis suggests that indoor air pollution from unprocessed solid fuels may represent a major risk factor by increasing the risk 1.8-fold (**Table 2**).[42] However, indoor air pollution can hardly explain the majority of cases of pneumonia in children.

The diagnosis of pneumonia relies mainly on the identification of certain clinical signs and symptoms along with a positive chest radiograph. Although C-reactive protein measurements have been used to differentiate bacterial from viral pneumonias, current evidence suggests that C-reactive protein may only weakly predict a bacterial cause.[43] The World Health Organization case-management approach appears to be more successful in identifying those cases of pneumonia most likely to be of a bacterial origin in children. This approach relies on the use of a simple algorithm based on the child's respiratory rate. A recent meta-analysis showed that the use of this approach has had a substantial effect in reducing the neonatal, infant, and childhood mortality due to pneumonia worldwide.[44]

Several trials have compared different antibiotics in the treatment of pediatric pneumonia. A recent meta-analysis summarized their findings and concluded that amoxicillin is better than trimethoprim-sulfamethoxazole (TMP-SMX), while there is no difference between azithromycin and erythromycin or between cefpodoxime and amoxicillin-clavulanic acid in ambulatory children.[45] For hospitalized children, procaine penicillin seems superior to TMP-SMX, the combination of penicillin plus gentamicin is better than chloramphenicol alone, and intravenous penicillin and oral

Table 1
Meta-analyses on acute bronchiolitis in children

Author, Year	Intervention/ Parameter Studied	Outcomes/ Conclusions	Number of Trials, Population Analyzed
Spurling et al, 2007[34,a]	Antibiotics for bronchiolitis	No benefit	1 trial, 52 infants
Ventre et al, 2007[36,a]	Ribavirin for respiratory syncytial virus LRTI	May reduce the duration of mechanical ventilation and length of stay	12 trials, 227 infants <6 mo old
Blom et al, 2007[38,a]	Inhaled corticosteroids for bronchiolitis	No benefit	5 trials, 374 infants <2 y old
Patel et al, 2004[39,a]	Systemic corticosteroids for bronchiolitis	No benefit	13 trials, 1198 infants <30 mo old
Garrison et al, 2000[37]	Systemic corticosteroids for bronchiolitis	Improvement in symptoms, length of stay, and duration of symptoms	6 trials, 347 hospitalized infants <2 y old
Smucny et al, 2006[32,a]	B_2-agonists for bronchitis	No benefit	2 trials, 109 children >2 y old
Gadomski et al, 2006[29,a]	Bronchodilators for bronchiolitis	Small, short-term benefit	22 trials, 1428 infants <2 y old
Hartling et al, 2004[31,a]	Epinephrine for bronchiolitis	Possible benefit (outpatients)	14 trials, 916 infants <2 y old
Flores et al, 1997[33]	B_2-agonists for bronchiolitis	No benefit (outpatients)	8 trials, 333 infants <2 y old
Kellner et al, 1996[30]	Bronchodilators for bronchiolitis	Modest, short-term benefit	15 trials, children with first-time wheezing
Ventre et al, 2006[35,a]	Surfactant therapy for bronchiolitis	Insufficient data	3 trials, 79 mechanically ventilated children <60 mo old
Davison et al, 2004[40]	Efficacy of interventions for bronchiolitis	Surfactant therapy: promising; corticosteroids/ ribavirin: may be beneficial	16 trials, 523 critically ill infants
Perrotta et al, 2007[41,a]	Chest physiotherapy for bronchiolitis	No benefit	3 trials, hospitalized infants <2 y old

[a] Cochrane systematic review.

amoxicillin have similar efficacy rates.[45] Shorter courses of therapy (3 days) are adequate for cases of community-acquired pneumonia that are not severe.[46] For more severe cases, hospitalization is generally recommended. However, even in these cases, oral treatment, instead of intravenous treatment, can be administered with safety, at least to those children who can tolerate oral antibiotics.[47] The use of antibiotic therapy for LRTIs with *Mycoplasma pneumoniae* in children is still under debate

Table 2
Meta-analyses on pneumonia in children

Author, Year	Intervention/Parameter Studied	Outcomes/Conclusions	Number of Trials, Population Analyzed
Dherani et al, 2008[42]	Indoor air pollution from unprocessed solid fuel on risk of pneumonia	Risk of pneumonia increased	24 trials, children <5 y old
Flood et al, 2008[43]	Serum C-reactive protein as a predictor of bacterial pneumonia	C-reactive protein >40–60 mg/dL weakly predicts a bacterial etiology	8 trials, 1230 children 1 mo–18 y old
Sazawal et al, 2003[44]	Mortality impact of case-management approach for pneumonia	Substantial effect on reducing mortality	9 trials, children <4 y old
Haider et al, 2008[46,a]	Short vs long courses of antibiotics for nonsevere community-acquired pneumonia	Short courses (3 d) are effective	3 trials, 5763 children 2 mo–5 y old
Kabra et al, 2006[45,a]	Antibiotics for community-acquired pneumonia	Amoxicillin/procaine penicillin better than trimethoprim-sulfamethoxazole; penicillin plus gentamicin better than chloramphenicol	20 trials, 8110 hospitalized and ambulatory children <18 y old
Rojas et al, 2006[47,a]	Oral vs parenteral antibiotics for severe pneumonia	Oral therapy is effective and safe	3 trials, 172 hospitalized children 2 mo–5 y old
Gavranich et al, 2005[48,a]	Antibiotics for LRTIs with *Mycoplasma pneumoniae*	Insufficient evidence	6 trials, 1352 children <18 y old
Chen et al, 2008[49,a]	Vitamin A for LRTIs	Only benefits children with retinol deficiency or poor nutritional status	9 trials, 33,179 children <7 y old
Ni et al, 2005[50,a]	Vitamin A for nonmeasles pneumonia	No benefit	5 trials, 1453 children <15 y old
Grotto et al, 2003[13]	Vitamin A for respiratory infections	Slightly increases the incidence of respiratory tract infections	9 trials, children 6 mo–7 y old
Aggarwal et al, 2007[12]	Zinc for respiratory illness	Reduced the frequency and severity of LRTIs	17 trials, children <5 y old
Smith et al, 2008[51,a]	Over-the-counter medications for acute cough	Insufficient evidence	8 trials, 616 ambulatory children <18 y old
Marchant et al, 2005[52,a]	Antibiotics for prolonged moist cough	Probably beneficial	2 trials, 140 children <7 y old

[a] Cochrane systematic review.

and a recent meta-analysis was unable to reach any firm conclusions regarding its value.[48]

Except for antibiotics, vitamin A supplementation has also been proposed as an adjunct for the treatment of LRTIs in children. However, current evidence does not support its use, at least in children with a normal nutritional status.[13,49,50] Meanwhile, a recent meta-analysis shows zinc supplementation to be potentially useful to children, irrespective of their nutritional status.[12]

Acute cough, one of the commonest symptoms in everyday clinical practice, is quite frequently treated in children with nonprescription over-the-counter medications, such as decongestants, expectorants, and antihistamines. A recent review summarizing evidence from eight RCTs did not conclude for or against their use.[51] However, antibiotic treatment seems to be beneficial for children with prolonged (>10 days), moist cough.[52]

Otitis Media

Acute otitis media (AOM) is extremely common in children, particularly those aged 3 months to 3 years. Currently published guidelines support a "watchful waiting" approach for the treatment of children with AOM. This means delaying the administration of antibiotics for at least 72 hours, especially for children 6 months old or older.[53,54] This recommendation is based on the observation that spontaneous remission can occur in a substantial number of children, presumably those suffering from viral infections. Indeed, six different meta-analyses confirm that antibiotics provide only a modest benefit to children with AOM.[55–60]

Antibiotic therapy is important in children under 2 years of age with bilateral AOM,[56] in children with AOM and otorrhoea,[56] and in children at higher risk for mastoiditis.[57] When a decision to prescribe antibiotics is taken, 5 days of therapy is usually adequate for most cases of uncomplicated AOM.[61,62] Long prophylactic courses of antibiotics (>6 months) can be used to reduce the probability of recurrent AOM in children who had three or more episodes of AOM within the last 6 months or four episodes within the last year.[63]

Neither decongestants nor antihistamines offer any additional benefit to the treatment of children with AOM.[64] Moreover, although otic preparations with analgesic agents (excluding antibiotics) are frequently prescribed in children with AOM, their use is not supported by solid scientific evidence.[65]

Another inflammatory condition frequently encountered in pediatric patients is otitis media with effusion (OME). Although OME is not directly attributed to infectious agents, it can be a precursor of AOM or follow its resolution.[66] OME is the most common cause of acquired hearing loss in childhood and has been associated with both delayed language development and behavioral problems. However, a recent meta-analysis on the effect of OME in later language development failed to show a substantial negative impact.[67] Moreover, the use of screening programs for OME in the general population, as a means to prevent these problems, does not seem to have any positive effects.[68]

OME has a high percentage of spontaneous resolution and current research shows that adjunctive treatment with antihistamines or decongestants is unnecessary.[69] Intranasal and oral corticosteroids offer a marginal benefit to the treatment of these patients, albeit only in the short term.[70,71] Tympanostomy tubes do not seem to offer significant benefits to children with OME, and are associated with some complications.[72,73] Finally, autoinflation (ie, placing air into the middle ear cavity though a nasal balloon), although a promising low-cost and safe technique, lacks sufficient evidence to recommend its use.[74]

Tonsillitis and Croup

Laryngotracheitis or croup is a virally induced infection of the trachea below the level of the vocal cords that affects almost exclusively children under 6 years of age. Two of the most widely used agents against this disease are epinephrine and corticosteroids. Although no meta-analysis has been published regarding the effects of epinephrine against croup, two recent [75,76] and one older[77] meta-analyses confirm that corticosteroids are effective in relieving the symptoms and reducing the length of hospital stay for children with croup. Although treatment with humidified air has also been widely used against croup, recent reports shed doubts over the value of this practice.[78]

Tonsillitis, an infection of the tonsils and pharynx, is a common infection in children of all ages. Although most cases are of viral origin, a substantial number of cases (5%–20%) are due to group A beta-hemolytic streptococci (GABS).

Although penicillin has for decades been considered as the treatment of choice for GABS tonsillitis, several reports of treatment failure associated with its use have been published over the years. Cephalosporins represent an alternative antibiotic in this setting because of their good overall antimicrobial spectrum and excellent safety profile. Four meta-analyses concluded that in comparison to penicillin, cephalosporins are indeed associated with better treatment outcomes (clinical and especially bacteriologic cure rates) in children with GABS tonsillitis.[79–82] Moreover, all available cephalosporin formulations seem to work equally well, with no major efficacy differences among agents of different generations.[82]

Regarding penicillin, one previous meta-analysis compared twice-a-day versus four-times-a-day dosing and concluded that the former regimen was superior.[83] Ten days of penicillin are a reasonable treatment option for GABS tonsillitis, since shorter treatment courses are associated with inferior bacteriologic outcomes (ie, lower GABS eradication rates).[84] To promote patient adherence to the prescribed medications, various behavioral and educational interventions have been proposed and their use in combination seems to work best.[85] Although some clinicians advocate the use of antibiotics to prevent posttonsillectomy complications (ie, postoperative bacterial infections of the tonsillar fossa and the associated pain), this practice is not supported by sufficient data.[86]

One meta-analysis evaluated the practice of administering antibiotics for sore throat and found some evidence to support their use as a means of preventing serious complications, albeit this is only applicable to developing countries, where rheumatic fever continues to be common.[87]

Urinary Tract Infections

Urinary tract infections (UTIs) are common in children of all ages and a recent meta-analysis reported an overall prevalence of 7% among febrile infants (**Table 3**).[88] Although girls are more commonly affected, boys predominate in infants under 1 year of age, and the highest incidence occurs in uncircumcised boys under 3 months old.[88]

Because urine cultures are not available for at least 24 hours, more rapid techniques are commonly used in everyday clinical practice to make a presumptive diagnosis of UTI. Two meta-analyses reviewed the available literature to identify the best laboratory test available to rapidly diagnose UTIs. The older meta-analysis concluded that the use of (1) Gram stain to identify bacteria on uncentrifuged urine and (2) dipstick analysis for nitrite and leukocyte esterase can perform equally well in detecting UTIs in children.[89] A more recent review by Huicho and colleagues[90] suggested that the presence of concurrent pyuria and bacteriuria was best suited for assessing the risk of UTIs in children.

Table 3
Meta-analyses on UTIs in children

Author, Year	Intervention/ Parameter Studied	Outcomes/Conclusions	Number of Trials, Population Analyzed
Shaikh et al, 2008[88]	Prevalence of UTIs in children	Infants presenting with fever: 7%; febrile uncircumcised boys <3 mo old: 20.1%	18 trials, 22,919 children <19 y old
Huicho et al, 2002[90]	Urine screening tests for UTIs	Presence of pyuria (≥10 high-power field) and bacteriuria (any) are best suited	48 trials, children <18 y old
Gorelick et al, 1999[89]	Urine screening tests for UTIs	Gram stain for bacteria or dipstick analysis for nitrite and leukocyte esterase are best suited	26 trials, children <12 y old
Michael et al, 2003[93,a]	Short- vs long-course oral antibiotics for lower UTIs	Short (2–4 days) duration was as effective as longer duration	10 trials, 652 children 3 mo–18 y old
Keren et al, 2002[92]	Short- vs long-course oral antibiotics for UTIs	Long-course therapy: fewer treatment failures	16 trials, children <18 y old
Tran et al, 2001[94]	Short- vs long-course antibiotics for uncomplicated lower UTIs	3 days of trimethoprim-sulfamethoxazole therapy was equally effective with longer-duration regimens	22 trials, 1279 children <18 y old
Hodson et al, 2007[91,a]	Antibiotics for acute pyelonephritis	Oral and combinations of oral with short intravenous antibiotic courses are as effective as exclusive intravenous antibiotic courses	23 trials, 3295 children <18 y old
Williams et al, 2006[95,a]	Long-term antibiotics for recurrent UTIs	Insufficient evidence	8 trials, 618 children <18 y old

[a] Cochrane systematic review.

Antibiotic therapy is the mainstay of treatment for UTIs, particularly for acute pyelonephritis, a UTI with renal parenchymal involvement. A Cochrane review assessed the efficacy of different antibiotic regimens in children with acute pyelonephritis and concluded that both (1) oral regimens and (2) sequential short-oral (for 2 to 4 days) and intravenous regimens are as effective as standard intravenous-only therapies.[91] For cases where intravenous treatment is chosen, current evidence supports single- over multiple-dose aminoglycoside regimens.[91]

Antibiotic therapy is also frequently used for lower UTIs, like cystitis and urethritis, and shorter treatment regimens seem to be adequate for these infections. Three different meta-analyses examined the efficacy of short antibiotic regimens for lower UTIs in children, and each reached a different conclusion by either refuting[92] or confirming their value for all[93] or for specific (TMP-SMX) antibiotics alone.[94] Finally, the administration of long-term prophylactic antibiotics to prevent recurrent UTIs in children with reflux or other predisposing conditions, a very common practice, awaits further evidence to support its use.[95]

Bacterial Meningitis

Bacterial meningitis is a life-threatening infection that is quite common in children, particularly those under 5 years old. Some physicians advocate the use of preadmission antibiotics to all children with suspected meningitis to prevent the critical delay associated with seeking bacterial confirmation before antibiotic administration. No RCTs have been performed to test the value of this approach, and such a study is unlikely to ever be completed.[96]

Most current guidelines recommend the use of a third-generation cephalosporin to treat bacterial meningitis, although conventional antibiotic therapy with either chloramphenicol or ampicillin-chloramphenicol combinations seems to perform equally well.[96,97] Such treatment regimens have the additional advantage of being much more affordable in comparison to third-generation cephalosporins and are still widely used in poor countries. Although the use of intraventricular antibiotics has been proposed as a means of achieving higher cerebrospinal fluid antibiotic concentrations, a recent meta-analysis recommended against their use.[98] For individuals in close contact with a meningitis patient and for populations with a high carriage rate of *Neisseria meningitis*, prophylactic antibiotics are recommended and, in this setting, both ciprofloxacin and ceftriaxone are equally effective.[99]

Three meta-analyses have evaluated the evidence on the efficacy of antibiotics for preventing serious sequelae in children with bacteremia. Although an older review found that antibiotic therapy can indeed help prevent incidents of bacterial meningitis,[100] two more recent ones discovered only a minor benefit associated with their use.[101,102] In this regard, oral antibiotic therapy seems to be as effective as intravenous therapy.[103] However, it has been estimated that a study with more than 7500 bacteremic children or more than 300,000 febrile children would be needed to have an 80% power to prove that intravenous antibiotics are superior to oral ones in preventing serious bacterial infections, such as meningitis.[103]

Corticosteroids are also frequently used in children with bacterial meningitis to inhibit the inflammatory process and thus avert the development of adverse neurologic outcomes. A recent meta-analysis confirmed the value of this practice, when applied to children from rich countries, in reducing the incidence of severe hearing loss and short-term neurologic sequelae.[104] The reasons why their efficacy is suboptimal in children from poor countries are not yet clear, although methodological differences among trials are the most plausible explanation. Four older studies confirm the above findings, and support the use of short (2 days) corticosteroid regimens in cases of bacterial meningitis.[105–108]

Regarding supportive treatment, many physicians advocate restricting the amount of intravenous fluids to children with bacterial meningitis to avoid the development of inappropriate antidiuretic hormone secretion. However, this practice has not been thoroughly evaluated, and a recent Cochrane review concluded that it might be better to maintain fluids than to restrict them, at least for those cases associated with high mortality or late hospital admission.[109]

Cystic Fibrosis

Thirteen meta-analyses, all performed by the Cochrane group, have examined the infectious complications of patients with cystic fibrosis, focusing mainly on the treatment of LRTIs.

Antimicrobial susceptibility tests are frequently used in these patients to choose the best antibiotic therapy. For resistant microorganisms, combination antimicrobial testing has been proposed to identify the most synergistic antibiotic combinations. However, a recent meta-analysis was unable to come up with enough data to support the use of in vitro combination antimicrobial testing over simple antimicrobial susceptibility testing.[110]

For treating cystic fibrosis patients with an LRTI, physicians traditionally apply several antibiotic agents, such as b-lactams, macrolides, and aminoglycosides. Treatment with azithromycin, a macrolide antibiotic, confers a small, albeit significant, improvement to the respiratory function of these patients.[111] Aminoglycoside–b-lactam combinations are also widely used in cystic fibrosis patients, even though the comparative value of these combinations against monotherapies is still uncertain.[112] Regarding the best dosing schemes for aminoglycosides for the treatment of pulmonary exacerbations in these patients, once-a-day treatment regimens seem to be equally effective and more convenient than three-times-a-day regimens.[113]

Although cystic fibrosis patients are traditionally treated in a hospital environment using intravenous therapy, a recent meta-analysis concluded that home intravenous antibiotic treatment is equally effective.[114] Current evidence is still insufficient to support the use of oral antibiotics for these patients.[115] Most physicians use 14 days of intravenous treatment for pulmonary exacerbations in cystic fibrosis patients, although no trials have been performed on this issue to date.[116] Nebulized antibiotic therapy represents an alternative for the treatment of pulmonary exacerbations in patients with cystic fibrosis, although more research is still necessary to establish the efficacy of this practice.[117]

A number of studies have examined when antimicrobial therapy should best be administered in patients with cystic fibrosis. A proposed strategy is to use intravenous antipseudomonal antibiotics at regular intervals, irrespective of symptoms. However, this practice is not adequately supported.[118] Other researchers recommend the early use of antibiotics in the course of an infection to prevent long-term colonization with *Pseudomonas aeruginosa*. Although short-term eradication is achievable with this policy, concrete, long-term clinical benefits are yet to be proven.[119]

Most of the trials performed to date on the treatment of chest exacerbations in cystic fibrosis patients have focused on *P aeruginosa* and *Staphylococcus aureus*. A recent meta-analysis summarized the evidence currently available on the use of antistaphylococcal antibiotics and concluded that these agents can reduce the rates of colonization with *S aureus* when commenced early in infancy and continued up to 6 years of age.[120]

Various vaccines have been tested in cystic fibrosis patients to prevent respiratory tract infections and the relentless deterioration of the lung function. Two meta-analyses summarized the current evidence available for vaccines against influenza and *P aeruginosa* and concluded that there is insufficient evidence to recommend their use.[121,122]

META-ANALYSES ON VACCINES

Influenza Vaccines

Influenza (the flu), a highly contagious respiratory illness due to influenza viruses, continues to represent a significant cause of morbidity and mortality worldwide. Some rich countries have incorporated vaccines against influenza in their vaccination programs for children aged 6 to 59 months, for the elderly, and for certain high-risk groups.

Currently, two types of influenza vaccines are licensed. These are (1) conventional, trivalent, inactivated vaccines, administered intramuscularly, and (2) live-attenuated vaccines (LAVs) for intranasal administration. Both of these vaccines are effective in preventing culture-positive influenza illness (**Table 4**).[123] Among the inactivated vaccines, the whole-virus, subunit, and split-virus vaccines seem to be equally immunogenic.[124] Few adverse events have been reported for both inactivated vaccines and LAVs. However, due to its route of administration, the inactivated vaccine seems to produce more local reactions.[125]

Three previous meta-analyses studied the role of influenza vaccines on healthy children and concluded that they reduce laboratory-confirmed cases of influenza (efficacy), albeit being less successful against influenzalike illnesses (effectiveness).[126–128] Although both inactivated vaccines and LAVs exhibit very good efficacy rates in children, a recent Cochrane review suggested that LAVs might perform even better in these ages.[126] Contrary to current recommendations, this last review found enough evidence on the efficacy of these vaccines only for children over 2 years of age.

Most national guidelines do not recommend influenza vaccines for healthy adults. However, influenza vaccines are as efficacious in adults as they are in children, even though their ability to reduce cases of influenzalike illnesses is much lower than their ability to reduce confirmed cases of influenza.[129,130]

Influenza vaccines are generally recommended for persons suffering from chronic diseases. Indeed, several RCTs show that the administration of inactivated influenza vaccines to persons suffering from chronic obstructive pulmonary disease can significantly reduce their pulmonary exacerbations.[131] However, several trials carried on in other groups, including patients with asthma, coronary heart disease, AIDS, and bronchiectasis, were unable to gather enough evidence to strongly support anti-influenza vaccination in any of these conditions.[132–136]

A proposed strategy currently adopted by some developed countries is to vaccinate all persons over 65 years old, as elderly people are more prone to influenza infections and their complications. Indeed, four different meta-analyses give credit to this practice by concluding that influenza vaccinations can reduce influenza complications, particularly for those elderly residing in long-term care facilities.[137–140] Another strategy is to vaccinate health care workers to protect those under their care, although a recent review did not find this approach to be particularly effective.[141]

Pneumococcal Vaccines

Streptococcus pneumoniae is a major cause of morbidity and mortality in children and adults, and is responsible for a heterogeneous array of infections, both invasive (eg, meningitis, pneumonia, bacteremia) and noninvasive (eg, AOM, sinusitis). Increasing antibiotic resistance of *S pneumoniae* strains in recent years has made the search for an effective vaccine much more compelling.

Currently, two different types of pneumococcal vaccines are available: the 23-valent pneumococcal polysaccharide vaccine (PPV) and the 7-valent pneumococcal conjugate vaccine (PCV). The latter was more recently developed as a solution to the problem of low immunogenicity exhibited by PPV in children under 2 years old. In contrast to PPV, PCV can induce sufficient immune responses and can adequately protect children under 2 years old against invasive pneumococcal infections.[142] Based on these observations, the PCV vaccine is recommended for all children aged 2 to 23 months and for those children aged 24 to 59 months who are at increased risk for pneumococcal infections.

Despite the good efficacy of PCV against invasive pneumococcal diseases, its ability to prevent noninvasive pneumococcal infections has yet to be proven.[143] Furthermore,

Table 4
Meta-analyses on influenza vaccines

Author, Year	Intervention/Parameter Studied	Outcomes/Conclusions	Number of Trials, Population Analyzed
Beyer et al, 2002[123]	LAV vs inactivated influenza vaccines	Similar efficacy	18 RCTs, 5000 subjects of all ages
Beyer et al, 1998[124]	Subunit vs whole-virus vs split-virus influenza vaccines	Similar efficacy; subunit vaccines are safer	22 RCTs, 5416 subjects of all ages
Beyer et al, 1996[125]	Gender differences in reported adverse events to inactivated influenza vaccine	Females reported more local reactions than males	14 trials, 1800 subjects of all ages
Jefferson et al, 2008[126,a]	Influenza vaccines (inactivated vaccines and LAVs) for healthy children	Both inactivated vaccines and LAVs efficacious in children >2 y old (LAVs more efficacious than inactivated vaccines)	51 trials, 294,159 children <16 y old
Manzoli et al, 2007[127]	Influenza vaccines for healthy children	Efficacious	19 RCTs, 247,517 children <18 y old
Negri et al, 2005[128]	Influenza vaccines (inactivated vaccines and LAVs) for healthy children	Both efficacious (LAVs and inactivated vaccines equally efficacious)	13 RCTs, children <18 y old
Jefferson et al, 2007[129,a]	Influenza vaccines for healthy adults	Efficacious	48 trials, 66,248 healthy adults 16–65 y old
Villari et al, 2004[130]	Influenza vaccines for healthy adults	Efficacious	26 trials, healthy adults 15–65 years old
Thomas et al, 2006[141,a]	Influenza vaccines for health care workers who work with the elderly	Do not reduce complications in those in workers' care	3 trials, health care workers <60 y old
Rivetti et al, 2006[137,a]	Influenza vaccines for the elderly	Effective in long-term care facilities; modest effect in the community	64 trials, elderly >65 y old

Vu et al, 2002[138]	Influenza vaccines for the elderly living in the community	Effective	15 trials, elderly >65 y old
Gross et al, 1995[139]	Influenza vaccines for the elderly	Effective	26 trials, elderly >65 y old
Puig-Barbera et al, 1995[140]	Influenza vaccines for the elderly living in the community	Effective	8 trials, elderly >65 y old
Chang et al, 2007[135,a]	Influenza vaccines for bronchiectasis patients	Insufficient evidence	No trials
Poole et al, 2006[131,a]	Influenza vaccines for chronic obstructive pulmonary disease patients	Inactivated vaccine is effective	6 RCTs, 2469 chronic obstructive pulmonary disease patients
Cates et al, 2008[134,a]	Influenza vaccines for asthma patients	Insufficient evidence	15 RCTs, adults and children >2 y old with asthma
Keller et al, 2008[133,a]	Influenza vaccines to prevent coronary heart disease	Insufficient evidence	2 RCTs, 778 coronary heart disease and non-coronary heart disease patients
Anema et al, 2008[136]	Influenza vaccines for HIV-positive patients	Insufficient evidence	4 trials, 1346 HIV-positive patients
Atashili et al, 2006[132]	Influenza vaccines for HIV-positive patients	Moderately effective	4 trials, 646 HIV-positive patients

[a] Cochrane systematic review.

PCV cannot confer protection to infants under 3 months old, even when administered at birth. A proposed strategy to protect this high-risk group is to immunize their mothers during pregnancy, although current evidence cannot support this policy.[144]

Other groups at high risk for pneumococcal infections include the elderly, patients with chronic diseases (eg, sickle cell anemia and chronic lung diseases), and patients who are immunocompromised. Recommendations on the efficacy of pneumococcal vaccines in these populations are contradictory. In a recent Cochrane review, PPV was found to prevent invasive pneumococcal disease in healthy adults, but was not effective in adults with chronic illnesses.[145] Another meta-analysis found that, although PPV can prevent the development of pneumococcal pneumonia in adults, it doesn't do so in those over 55 years old.[146] A third meta-analysis found that PPV can reduce the risk of pneumonia in immunocompetent but not in immunocompromised adults.[147] An older review also concluded that pneumococcal vaccination cannot prevent pneumonia and bronchitis in high-risk patients.[148] However, two other meta-analyses conclude that the PPV vaccine is indeed protective in the elderly and in those with chronic diseases.[149,150]

Three different meta-analyses limited to particular groups of high-risk individuals confuse matters even more. Pneumococcal vaccines were unable to prevent acute exacerbations in patients with chronic obstructive pulmonary disease.[151] Regarding asthma exacerbations, current evidence is too slim to allow definite conclusions.[152] For patients suffering from sickle cell anemia, current evidence suggests that pneumococcal vaccines are useful to prevent infections.[153]

Meningococcal and Haemophilus Influenzae Vaccines

N meningitidis is the leading cause of bacterial meningitis and continues to represent a major health problem worldwide. Meningococcal infections are most commonly attributed to N meningitidis serogroups A, B, C, Y, and W-135. While no vaccine is yet available for serogroup B, two quadrivalent vaccines for serogroups A, C, Y, and W-135 are currently licensed: the meningococcal conjugate vaccine (MCV4) and the meningococcal polysaccharide vaccine (MPSV4). MPSV4 was the first to be developed and, although it was highly protective against meningococcal meningitis in a number of clinical trials,[154] it was gradually abandoned in favor of the conjugate vaccine. Currently, MCV4 is recommended for all individuals aged 2 to 55 years at higher risk for meningococcal infections.

Conjugation limits the decreased immunogenicity in children less than 2 years old by linking the meningococcal polysaccharide to various immunogenic carrier proteins. This has been shown to be very effective for N meningitidis serogroup C, and a conjugate vaccine against this serogroup (MCC vaccine) is on the market in several countries, but not in the United States. Indeed, in a number of clinical trials, MCC has proven to be both safe and immunogenic in preventing meningococcal C meningitis and septicemia.[155,156]

Infection with Haemophilus influenzae type b (Hib) was the leading cause of bacterial meningitis and septicemia in young children before the widespread introduction of infant and childhood immunization against Hib in 1985.

The development of conjugate vaccines has been a major advance in the fight against Hib infections, and has allowed the vaccination of children under 2 years of age. Hib conjugate vaccines are now used in the routine immunization schedule of over 100 countries, and the World Health Organization recommends their use for all nations. Two meta-analyses confirm that these vaccines are effective in preventing Hib-related meningitis and pneumonia in children, without any serious adverse effects.[157,158] A recent Cochrane systematic review further suggests that oral whole-cell Hib vaccines can be effective for patients with chronic bronchitis by reducing the rates of acute Hib-related exacerbations.[159]

Hepatitis B Vaccines

More than one third of the world's population is currently infected with hepatitis B, making it a serious global health problem. Acute infection due to hepatitis B virus (HBV) can lead to chronic liver inflammation in 10% of immunocompetent adults and as many as 90% of infected infants. Chronic hepatitis is a major risk factor for the development of progressive liver disease, cirrhosis, and hepatocellular carcinoma.

Vaccines for the prevention of HBV infections have been available since 1982, and most national guidelines around the world recommend anti-HBV vaccination for all infants. Despite this widespread acceptance, questions regarding the vaccine's ability to prevent infection still remain. A recent Cochrane review was unable to come up with enough evidence to support the use of the hepatitis B vaccine in persons not previously exposed to HBV (**Table 5**).[160] For infants born to HBV-positive mothers, hepatitis B vaccination does reduce infection rates.[161] A third meta-analysis performed by the Cochrane collaboration supports the use of hepatitis B vaccines to prevent HBV infections in health care workers, a high-risk group for this infection.[162]

Due to their increased exposure to blood products, patients with chronic renal failure represent another high-risk group for HBV infection. According to some reports, these patients have the additional disadvantage of responding poorly to hepatitis B vaccinations. A meta-analysis of clinical trials of end-stage renal disease patients suggested that this poor response could in fact be due to the older age of the individuals studied.[163] A similar meta-analysis performed on healthy subjects supports this view.[164] Contrasting the above findings, a recent Cochrane review showed that hepatitis B vaccination can induce the production of protective antibodies in patients with chronic renal failure.[165]

Despite this controversy, several strategies have been proposed to increase seroconversion rates in chronic renal failure patients. Among these, the use of intradermal vaccine administration routes, instead of intramuscular vaccine administration routes, has been proved to be effective, at least in the short term.[166] The use of adjuvants, such as thymopentin and granulocyte-macrophage colony-stimulating factor, to increase the immunogenicity of hepatitis B vaccines, also appear to be helpful, as shown by three meta-analyses.[167–169] In contrast, the use of peritoneal dialysis, in place of maintenance, does not seem to significantly affect seroconversion rates in these patients.[170]

BCG Vaccine

Tuberculosis, primarily caused by *Mycobacterium tuberculosis*, continues to represent a major health problem worldwide, particularly in the developing world. Most infected individuals present with latent infection, a subclinical form of infection that progresses to active tuberculosis in less than 10% to 15% of those infected. To diagnose these patients, tuberculin skin tests are commonly applied, although cautious interpretation and experience is required.[171]

First developed in 1908, BCG vaccine (from bacille Calmette-Guérin) is the only vaccine currently available for the prevention of tuberculosis. The World Health Organization recommends the administration of one dose of this vaccine to all infants in those areas of the world where tuberculosis is endemic. Although the efficacy of BCG vaccination remains controversial, most previous trials report high protection rates from miliary and meningeal disease, but lower rates for pulmonary disease.[172–174]

Table 5
Meta-analyses on HBV vaccines

Author, Year	Intervention/Parameter Studied	Outcomes/Conclusions	Number of Trials, Population Analyzed
Mathew et al, 2008[160,a]	HBV vaccine for persons who are HBsAg negative	Unclear effect	12 trials, HBsAg negative persons
Lee et al, 2006[161]	HBV vaccine for newborn infants of HBsAg-positive mothers	Effective	29 trials, newborn infants
Chen et al, 2005[162,a]	HBV vaccine for health care workers	Effective	21 trials, health care workers
Schroth et al, 2004[165,a]	HBV vaccine for CRF patients	Can induce hepatitis B antibodies	7 trials, CRF patients
Fabrizi et al, 2004[163]	Relationship between age and immune response to HBV vaccine in ESRD patients	Older age is associated with an impaired immune response	17 trials, 1800 ESRD patients
Fisman et al, 2002[164]	Relationship between age and immune response to HBV vaccine	Older age is associated with an impaired immune response	24 trials
Cruciani et al, 2007[167]	GM-CSF adjuvant to HBV vaccine	Improves seroprotection rates in both healthy and CRF individuals	13 trials, 734 subjects
Fabrizi et al, 2006[169]	GM-CSF adjuvant to HBV vaccine in ESRD patients	Improves seroprotection rates	17 trials, 187 ESRD patients
Fabrizi et al, 2006[168]	Thymopentin adjuvant to HBV vaccine in ESRD patients	Improves seroprotection rates	11 trials, 272 ESRD patients
Fabrizi et al, 2006[170]	Maintenance vs peritoneal dialysis and immune response to HBV vaccine	No link between dialysis mode and seroprotection rates	14 trials, 1211 dialysis patients
Fabrizi et al, 2006[166]	Intradermal vs intramuscular administration of HBV vaccine to CRF patients	Intradermal route achieves higher seroprotection rates	12 trials, 640 CRF patients

Abbreviations: CRF, chronic renal failure; ESRD, end-stage renal disease; GM-CSF, granulocyte-macrophage colony-stimulating factor; HBsAg, hepatitis B surface antigen.
[a] Cochrane systematic review.

Several lines of evidence indicate that BCG vaccination, in addition to offering protection against *M tuberculosis*, can also protect against other types of mycobacteria, such as *Mycobacterium leprae*, the causative agent of leprosy.[175,176] Furthermore, BCG has been applied as an adjuvant treatment in immunotherapeutic protocols against bladder cancer. More specifically, BCG is infused intravesically after transurethral resection of superficial bladder cancer to prevent recurrence of this aggressive tumor. A number of previous meta-analyses confirm that this strategy can be more effective than chemotherapy in reducing recurrences and in preventing progression in patients with papillary tumors and carcinoma in situ.[177-181] Nevertheless, some researchers argue that chemotherapy can perform equally well in these cases, and attribute the above findings to inadequate patient inclusion and eligibility criteria.[182]

Human Papilloma Virus Vaccines

Human papilloma virus (HPV) infection represents the commonest sexually transmitted disease in the Western world. Infections with HPV can result in anogenital warts, juvenile recurrent respiratory papillomatosis, low-grade cervical neoplasia, and cervical cancer. The realization that HPV is associated with the development of cervical cancer led to the recent development of two highly effective vaccines against HPV.

In 2006, the Europen Union and the United States approved a quadrivalent vaccine against HPV serotypes 6, 11, 16, and 18. In 2007, the European Union approved a bivalent vaccine against HPV 16 and 18. Approval of that vaccine in the United States is still pending. HPV 16 and 18 are associated with approximately 80% of cervical cancer cases, while types 6 and 11 are associated with anogenital warts. Many countries have incorporated these vaccines into their national immunization schedules, targeting women 11 to 26 years old. A number of meta-analyses have summarized the available evidence showing excellent efficacy rates.[183-185] HPV types 31, 33, 35, 45, 52, and 58 are also frequently associated with the development of cervical cancer in various parts of the world and should be the focus of future vaccine development efforts.[184-190]

SUMMARY

In pediatric infections, meta-analyses have helped clarify several controversial management issues. Unfortunately, many more aspects remain to be elucidated. This is particularly true in the field of UTIs, the most common serious bacterial infections in children, where prospective, well-designed, randomized clinical trials are urgently needed.

Regarding vaccines, it is generally acknowledged that, although meta-analyses can provide useful information on their value, people who make decisions and set policies should not rely on that information alone, but rather use it alongside other sources of information. The fact that government policies do not always coincide with conclusions produced by meta-analyses in the field of vaccinations should not be regarded as a failure of the statistical methodology, but rather as a result of the complex societal and financial (cost versus benefit) decisions.

REFERENCES

1. Ten great public health achievements—United States, 1900–1999. MMWR Morb Mortal Wkly Rep 1999;48:241–3.
2. Falagas ME, Giannopoulou KP, Vardakas KZ, et al. Comparison of antibiotics with placebo for treatment of acute sinusitis: a meta-analysis of randomised controlled trials. Lancet Infect Dis 2008;8:543–52.
3. Bellemare S, Hartling L, Wiebe N, et al. Oral rehydration versus intravenous therapy for treating dehydration due to gastroenteritis in children: a meta-analysis of randomised controlled trials. BMC Med 2004;2:11.
4. Fonseca BK, Holdgate A, Craig JC. Enteral vs intravenous rehydration therapy for children with gastroenteritis: a meta-analysis of randomized controlled trials. Arch Pediatr Adolesc Med 2004;158:483–90.

5. Hartling L, Bellemare S, Wiebe N, et al. Oral versus intravenous rehydration for treating dehydration due to gastroenteritis in children. Cochrane Database Syst Rev 2006;3:CD004390.
6. Fontaine O, Gore SM, Pierce NF. Rice-based oral rehydration solution for treating diarrhoea. Cochrane Database Syst Rev 2000:CD001264.
7. Hahn S, Kim S, Garner P. Reduced osmolarity oral rehydration solution for treating dehydration caused by acute diarrhoea in children. Cochrane Database Syst Rev 2002:CD002847.
8. King CK, Glass R, Bresee JS, et al. Managing acute gastroenteritis among children: oral rehydration, maintenance, and nutritional therapy. MMWR Recomm Rep 2003;52:1–16.
9. Brown KH, Peerson JM, Fontaine O. Use of nonhuman milks in the dietary management of young children with acute diarrhea: a meta-analysis of clinical trials. Pediatrics 1994;93:17–27.
10. Lukacik M, Thomas RL, Aranda JV. A meta-analysis of the effects of oral zinc in the treatment of acute and persistent diarrhea. Pediatrics 2008;121:326–36.
11. Patro B, Golicki D, Szajewska H. Meta-analysis: zinc supplementation for acute gastroenteritis in children. Aliment Pharmacol Ther 2008;28:713–23.
12. Aggarwal R, Sentz J, Miller MA. Role of zinc administration in prevention of childhood diarrhea and respiratory illnesses: a meta-analysis. Pediatrics 2007;119: 1120–30.
13. Grotto I, Mimouni M, Gdalevich M, et al. Vitamin A supplementation and childhood morbidity from diarrhea and respiratory infections: a meta-analysis. J Pediatr 2003;142:297–304.
14. Sazawal S, Hiremath G, Dhingra U, et al. Efficacy of probiotics in prevention of acute diarrhoea: a meta-analysis of masked, randomised, placebo-controlled trials. Lancet Infect Dis 2006;6:374–82.
15. Johnston BC, Supina AL, Ospina M, et al. Probiotics for the prevention of pediatric antibiotic-associated diarrhea. Cochrane Database Syst Rev 2007;CD004827.
16. Allen SJ, Okoko B, Martinez E, et al. Probiotics for treating infectious diarrhoea. Cochrane Database Syst Rev 2004:CD003048.
17. Huang JS, Bousvaros A, Lee JW, et al. Efficacy of probiotic use in acute diarrhea in children: a meta-analysis. Dig Dis Sci 2002;47:2625–34.
18. Johnston BC, Supina AL, Vohra S. Probiotics for pediatric antibiotic-associated diarrhea: a meta-analysis of randomized placebo-controlled trials. CMAJ 2006; 175:377–83.
19. Van Niel CW, Feudtner C, Garrison MM, et al. Lactobacillus therapy for acute infectious diarrhea in children: a meta-analysis. Pediatrics 2002; 109:678–84.
20. Szajewska H, Skorka A, Dylag M. Meta-analysis: Saccharomyces boulardii for treating acute diarrhoea in children. Aliment Pharmacol Ther 2007;25:257–64.
21. Szajewska H, Skorka A, Ruszczynski M, et al. Meta-analysis: Lactobacillus GG for treating acute diarrhoea in children. Aliment Pharmacol Ther 2007;25: 871–81.
22. Szajewska H, Ruszczynski M, Radzikowski A. Probiotics in the prevention of antibiotic-associated diarrhea in children: a meta-analysis of randomized controlled trials. J Pediatr 2006;149:367–72.
23. Alhashimi D, Alhashimi H, Fedorowicz Z. Antiemetics for reducing vomiting related to acute gastroenteritis in children and adolescents. Cochrane Database Syst Rev 2006:CD005506.

24. Szajewska H, Gieruszczak-Bialek D, Dylag M. Meta-analysis: ondansetron for vomiting in acute gastroenteritis in children. Aliment Pharmacol Ther 2007;25: 393–400.
25. Szajewska H, Dziechciarz P, Mrukowicz J. Meta-analysis: smectite in the treatment of acute infectious diarrhoea in children. Aliment Pharmacol Ther 2006; 23:217–27.
26. DeCamp LR, Byerley JS, Doshi N, et al. Use of antiemetic agents in acute gastroenteritis: a systematic review and meta-analysis. Arch Pediatr Adolesc Med 2008;162:858–65.
27. Jacobs J, Jonas WB, Jimenez-Perez M, et al. Homeopathy for childhood diarrhea: combined results and metaanalysis from three randomized, controlled clinical trials. Pediatr Infect Dis J 2003;22:229–34.
28. Soares-Weiser K, Goldberg E, Tamimi G, et al. Rotavirus vaccine for preventing diarrhoea. Cochrane Database Syst Rev 2004:CD002848.
29. Gadomski AM, Bhasale AL. Bronchodilators for bronchiolitis. Cochrane Database Syst Rev 2006;3:CD001266.
30. Kellner JD, Ohlsson A, Gadomski AM, et al. Efficacy of bronchodilator therapy in bronchiolitis. A meta-analysis. Arch Pediatr Adolesc Med 1996;150:1166–72.
31. Hartling L, Wiebe N, Russell K, et al. Epinephrine for bronchiolitis. Cochrane Database Syst Rev 2004:CD003123.
32. Smucny J, Becker L, Glazier R. Beta2-agonists for acute bronchitis. Cochrane Database Syst Rev 2006:CD001726.
33. Flores G, Horwitz RI. Efficacy of beta2-agonists in bronchiolitis: a reappraisal and meta-analysis. Pediatrics 1997;100:233–9.
34. Spurling GK, Fonseka K, Doust J, et al. Antibiotics for bronchiolitis in children. Cochrane Database Syst Rev 2007;CD005189.
35. Ventre K, Haroon M, Davison C. Surfactant therapy for bronchiolitis in critically ill infants. Cochrane Database Syst Rev 2006;3:CD005150.
36. Ventre K, Randolph AG. Ribavirin for respiratory syncytial virus infection of the lower respiratory tract in infants and young children. Cochrane Database Syst Rev 2007:CD000181.
37. Garrison MM, Christakis DA, Harvey E, et al. Systemic corticosteroids in infant bronchiolitis: a meta-analysis. Pediatrics 2000;105:E44.
38. Blom D, Ermers M, Bont L, et al. Inhaled corticosteroids during acute bronchiolitis in the prevention of post-bronchiolitic wheezing. Cochrane Database Syst Rev 2007:CD004881.
39. Patel H, Platt R, Lozano JM, et al. Glucocorticoids for acute viral bronchiolitis in infants and young children. Cochrane Database Syst Rev 2004: CD004878.
40. Davison C, Ventre KM, Luchetti M, et al. Efficacy of interventions for bronchiolitis in critically ill infants: a systematic review and meta-analysis. Pediatr Crit Care Med 2004;5:482–9.
41. Perrotta C, Ortiz Z, Roque M. Chest physiotherapy for acute bronchiolitis in paediatric patients between 0 and 24 months old. Cochrane Database Syst Rev 2007:CD004873.
42. Dherani M, Pope D, Mascarenhas M, et al. Indoor air pollution from unprocessed solid fuel use and pneumonia risk in children aged under five years: a systematic review and meta-analysis. Bull World Health Organ 2008;86:390–8C.
43. Flood RG, Badik J, Aronoff SC. The utility of serum C-reactive protein in differentiating bacterial from nonbacterial pneumonia in children: a meta-analysis of 1230 children. Pediatr Infect Dis J 2008;27:95–9.

44. Sazawal S, Black RE. Effect of pneumonia case management on mortality in neonates, infants, and preschool children: a meta-analysis of community-based trials. Lancet Infect Dis 2003;3:547–56.
45. Kabra SK, Lodha R, Pandey RM. Antibiotics for community acquired pneumonia in children. Cochrane Database Syst Rev 2006;3:CD004874.
46. Haider BA, Saeed MA, Bhutta ZA. Short-course versus long-course antibiotic therapy for non-severe community-acquired pneumonia in children aged 2 months to 59 months. Cochrane Database Syst Rev 2008:CD005976.
47. Rojas MX, Granados C. Oral antibiotics versus parenteral antibiotics for severe pneumonia in children. Cochrane Database Syst Rev 2006:CD004979.
48. Gavranich JB, Chang AB. Antibiotics for community acquired lower respiratory tract infections (LRTI) secondary to mycoplasma pneumoniae in children. Cochrane Database Syst Rev 2005:CD004875.
49. Chen H, Zhuo Q, Yuan W, et al. Vitamin A for preventing acute lower respiratory tract infections in children up to seven years of age. Cochrane Database Syst Rev 2008:CD006090.
50. Ni J, Wei J, Wu T. Vitamin a for non-measles pneumonia in children. Cochrane Database Syst Rev 2005:CD003700.
51. Smith SM, Schroeder K, Fahey T. Over-the-counter medications for acute cough in children and adults in ambulatory settings. Cochrane Database Syst Rev 2008:CD001831.
52. Marchant JM, Morris P, Gaffney JT, et al. Antibiotics for prolonged moist cough in children. Cochrane Database Syst Rev 2005:CD004822.
53. American Academy of Pediatrics Subcommittee on Management of Acute Otitis Media. Diagnosis and management of acute otitis media. Pediatrics 2004;113:1451–65.
54. Segal N, Leibovitz E, Dagan R, et al. Acute otitis media—diagnosis and treatment in the era of antibiotic resistant organisms: updated clinical practice guidelines. Int J Pediatr Otorhinolaryngol 2005;69:1311–9.
55. Koopman L, Hoes AW, Glasziou PP, et al. Antibiotic therapy to prevent the development of asymptomatic middle ear effusion in children with acute otitis media: a meta-analysis of individual patient data. Arch Otolaryngol Head Neck Surg 2008;134:128–32.
56. Rovers MM, Glasziou P, Appelman CL, et al. Antibiotics for acute otitis media: a meta-analysis with individual patient data. Lancet 2006;368:1429–35.
57. Glasziou PP, Del Mar CB, Sanders SL, et al. Antibiotics for acute otitis media in children. Cochrane Database Syst Rev 2004:CD000219.
58. Damoiseaux RA, van Balen FA, Hoes AW, et al. Antibiotic treatment of acute otitis media in children under two years of age: evidence based? Br J Gen Pract 1998;48:1861–4.
59. Rosenfeld RM, Vertrees JE, Carr J, et al. Clinical efficacy of antimicrobial drugs for acute otitis media: metaanalysis of 5400 children from thirty-three randomized trials. J Pediatr 1994;124:355–67.
60. Del Mar C, Glasziou P, Hayem M. Are antibiotics indicated as initial treatment for children with acute otitis media? A meta-analysis. BMJ 1997;314:1526–9.
61. Kozyrskyj AL, Hildes-Ripstein GE, Longstaffe SE, et al. Short course antibiotics for acute otitis media. Cochrane Database Syst Rev 2000:CD001095.
62. Kozyrskyj AL, Hildes-Ripstein GE, Longstaffe SE, et al. Treatment of acute otitis media with a shortened course of antibiotics: a meta-analysis. JAMA 1998;279:1736–42.

63. Leach AJ, Morris PS. Antibiotics for the prevention of acute and chronic suppurative otitis media in children. Cochrane Database Syst Rev 2006: CD004401.
64. Coleman C, Moore M. Decongestants and antihistamines for acute otitis media in children. Cochrane Database Syst Rev 2008:CD001727.
65. Foxlee R, Johansson A, Wejfalk J, et al. Topical analgesia for acute otitis media. Cochrane Database Syst Rev 2006;3:CD005657.
66. Corbeel L. What is new in otitis media? Eur J Pediatr 2007;166:511–9.
67. Roberts JE, Rosenfeld RM, Zeisel SA. Otitis media and speech and language: a meta-analysis of prospective studies. Pediatrics 2004;113:e238–48.
68. Simpson SA, Thomas CL, van der Linden MK, et al. Identification of children in the first four years of life for early treatment for otitis media with effusion. Cochrane Database Syst Rev 2007:CD004163.
69. Griffin GH, Flynn C, Bailey RE, et al. Antihistamines and/or decongestants for otitis media with effusion (OME) in children. Cochrane Database Syst Rev 2006:CD003423.
70. Thomas CL, Simpson S, Butler CC, et al. Oral or topical nasal steroids for hearing loss associated with otitis media with effusion in children. Cochrane Database Syst Rev 2006;3:CD001935.
71. Berman S, Roark R, Luckey D. Theoretical cost effectiveness of management options for children with persisting middle ear effusions. Pediatrics 1994;93:353–63.
72. Rovers MM, Black N, Browning GG, et al. Grommets in otitis media with effusion: an individual patient data meta-analysis. Arch Dis Child 2005;90:480–5.
73. Lous J, Burton MJ, Felding JU, et al. Grommets (ventilation tubes) for hearing loss associated with otitis media with effusion in children. Cochrane Database Syst Rev 2005:CD001801.
74. Perera R, Haynes J, Glasziou P, et al. Autoinflation for hearing loss associated with otitis media with effusion. Cochrane Database Syst Rev 2006:CD006285.
75. Russell K, Wiebe N, Saenz A, et al. Glucocorticoids for croup. Cochrane Database Syst Rev 2004:CD001955.
76. Ausejo M, Saenz A, Pham B, et al. The effectiveness of glucocorticoids in treating croup: meta-analysis. BMJ 1999;319:595–600.
77. Kairys SW, Olmstead EM, O'Connor GT. Steroid treatment of laryngotracheitis: a meta-analysis of the evidence from randomized trials. Pediatrics 1989;83: 683–93.
78. Moore M, Little P. Humidified air inhalation for treating croup. Cochrane Database Syst Rev 2006;3:CD002870.
79. Brook I. A pooled comparison of cefdinir and penicillin in the treatment of group A beta-hemolytic streptococcal pharyngotonsillitis. Clin Ther 2005;27: 1266–73.
80. Deeter RG, Kalman DL, Rogan MP, et al. Therapy for pharyngitis and tonsillitis caused by group a beta-hemolytic streptococci: a meta-analysis comparing the efficacy and safety of cefadroxil monohydrate versus oral penicillin V. Clin Ther 1992;14:740–54.
81. Pichichero ME, Margolis PA. A comparison of cephalosporins and penicillins in the treatment of group A beta-hemolytic streptococcal pharyngitis: a meta-analysis supporting the concept of microbial copathogenicity. Pediatr Infect Dis J 1991;10:275–81.
82. Casey JR, Pichichero ME. Meta-analysis of cephalosporin versus penicillin treatment of group A streptococcal tonsillopharyngitis in children. Pediatrics 2004; 113:866–82.

83. Lan AJ, Colford JM, Colford JM Jr. The impact of dosing frequency on the efficacy of 10-day penicillin or amoxicillin therapy for streptococcal tonsillopharyngitis: a meta-analysis. Pediatrics 2000;105:E19.

84. Falagas ME, Vouloumanou EK, Matthaiou DK, et al. Effectiveness and safety of short-course vs long-course antibiotic therapy for group A beta hemolytic streptococcal tonsillopharyngitis: a meta-analysis of randomized trials. Mayo Clin Proc 2008;83:880–9.

85. Wu YP, Roberts MC. A meta-analysis of interventions to increase adherence to medication regimens for pediatric otitis media and streptococcal pharyngitis. J Pediatr Psychol 2008;33:789–96.

86. Dhiwakar M, Clement WA, Supriya M, et al. Antibiotics to reduce post-tonsillectomy morbidity. Cochrane Database Syst Rev 2008:CD005607.

87. Del Mar CB, Glasziou PP, Spinks AB. Antibiotics for sore throat. Cochrane Database Syst Rev 2004:CD000023.

88. Shaikh N, Morone NE, Bost JE, et al. Prevalence of urinary tract infection in childhood: a meta-analysis. Pediatr Infect Dis J 2008;27:302–8.

89. Gorelick MH, Shaw KN. Screening tests for urinary tract infection in children: a meta-analysis. Pediatrics 1999;104:e54.

90. Huicho L, Campos-Sanchez M, Alamo C. Metaanalysis of urine screening tests for determining the risk of urinary tract infection in children. Pediatr Infect Dis J 2002;21:1–11, 88.

91. Hodson EM, Willis NS, Craig JC. Antibiotics for acute pyelonephritis in children. Cochrane Database Syst Rev 2007:CD003772.

92. Keren R, Chan E. A meta-analysis of randomized, controlled trials comparing short- and long-course antibiotic therapy for urinary tract infections in children. Pediatrics 2002;109:E70.

93. Michael M, Hodson EM, Craig JC, et al. Short versus standard duration oral antibiotic therapy for acute urinary tract infection in children. Cochrane Database Syst Rev 2003:CD003966.

94. Tran D, Muchant DG, Aronoff SC. Short-course versus conventional length antimicrobial therapy for uncomplicated lower urinary tract infections in children: a meta-analysis of 1279 patients. J Pediatr 2001;139:93–9.

95. Williams GJ, Wei L, Lee A, et al. Long-term antibiotics for preventing recurrent urinary tract infection in children. Cochrane Database Syst Rev 2006;3:CD001534.

96. Sudarsanam T, Rupali P, Tharyan P, et al. Pre-admission antibiotics for suspected cases of meningococcal disease. Cochrane Database Syst Rev 2008: CD005437.

97. Prasad K, Kumar A, Gupta PK, et al. Third generation cephalosporins versus conventional antibiotics for treating acute bacterial meningitis. Cochrane Database Syst Rev 2007:CD001832.

98. Shah S, Ohlsson A, Shah V. Intraventricular antibiotics for bacterial meningitis in neonates. Cochrane Database Syst Rev 2004:CD004496.

99. Fraser A, Gafter-Gvili A, Paul M, et al. Antibiotics for preventing meningococcal infections. Cochrane Database Syst Rev 2006:CD004785.

100. Baraff LJ, Oslund S, Prather M. Effect of antibiotic therapy and etiologic microorganism on the risk of bacterial meningitis in children with occult bacteremia. Pediatrics 1993;92:140–3.

101. Rothrock SG, Harper MB, Green SM, et al. Do oral antibiotics prevent meningitis and serious bacterial infections in children with streptococcus pneumoniae occult bacteremia? A meta-analysis. Pediatrics 1997;99:438–44.

102. Bulloch B, Craig WR, Klassen TP. The use of antibiotics to prevent serious sequelae in children at risk for occult bacteremia: a meta-analysis. Acad Emerg Med 1997;4:679–83.
103. Rothrock SG, Green SM, Harper MB, et al. Parenteral vs oral antibiotics in the prevention of serious bacterial infections in children with streptococcus pneumoniae occult bacteremia: a meta-analysis. Acad Emerg Med 1998;5:599–606.
104. van de Beek D, de Gans J, McIntyre P, et al. Corticosteroids for acute bacterial meningitis. Cochrane Database Syst Rev 2007:CD004405.
105. McIntyre PB, Berkey CS, King SM, et al. Dexamethasone as adjunctive therapy in bacterial meningitis. A meta-analysis of randomized clinical trials since 1988. JAMA 1997;278:925–31.
106. Yurkowski PJ, Plaisance KI. Prevention of auditory sequelae in pediatric bacterial meningitis: a meta-analysis. Pharmacotherapy 1993;13:494–9.
107. Geiman BJ, Smith AL. Dexamethasone and bacterial meningitis. A meta-analysis of randomized controlled trials. West J Med 1992;157:27–31.
108. Havens PL, Wendelberger KJ, Hoffman GM, et al. Corticosteroids as adjunctive therapy in bacterial meningitis. A meta-analysis of clinical trials. Am J Dis Child 1989;143:1051–5.
109. Maconochie I, Baumer H, Stewart ME. Fluid therapy for acute bacterial meningitis. Cochrane Database Syst Rev 2008:CD004786.
110. Waters V, Ratjen F. Combination antimicrobial susceptibility testing for acute exacerbations in chronic infection of pseudomonas aeruginosa in cystic fibrosis. Cochrane Database Syst Rev 2008:CD006961.
111. Southern KW, Barker PM, Solis A. Macrolide antibiotics for cystic fibrosis. Cochrane Database Syst Rev 2004:CD002203.
112. Elphick HE, Tan A. Single versus combination intravenous antibiotic therapy for people with cystic fibrosis. Cochrane Database Syst Rev 2005:CD002007.
113. Smyth AR, Tan KH. Once-daily versus multiple-daily dosing with intravenous aminoglycosides for cystic fibrosis. Cochrane Database Syst Rev 2006;3: CD002009.
114. Balaguer A, Gonzalez de Dios J. Home intravenous antibiotics for cystic fibrosis. Cochrane Database Syst Rev 2008:CD001917.
115. Remmington T, Jahnke N, Harkensee C. Oral anti-pseudomonal antibiotics for cystic fibrosis. Cochrane Database Syst Rev 2007:CD005405.
116. Fernandes B, Plummer A, Wildman M. Duration of intravenous antibiotic therapy in people with cystic fibrosis. Cochrane Database Syst Rev 2008:CD006682.
117. Ryan G, Mukhopadhyay S, Singh M. Nebulised anti-pseudomonal antibiotics for cystic fibrosis. Cochrane Database Syst Rev 2003:CD001021.
118. Breen L, Aswani N. Elective versus symptomatic intravenous antibiotic therapy for cystic fibrosis. Cochrane Database Syst Rev 2001:CD002767.
119. Wood DM, Smyth AR. Antibiotic strategies for eradicating pseudomonas aeruginosa in people with cystic fibrosis. Cochrane Database Syst Rev 2006: CD004197.
120. Smyth A, Walters S. Prophylactic antibiotics for cystic fibrosis. Cochrane Database Syst Rev 2003:CD001912.
121. Keogan MT, Johansen HK. Vaccines for preventing infection with pseudomonas aeruginosa in people with cystic fibrosis. Cochrane Database Syst Rev 2000: CD001399.
122. Tan A, Bhalla P, Smyth R. Vaccines for preventing influenza in people with cystic fibrosis. Cochrane Database Syst Rev 2000:CD001753.

123. Beyer WE, Palache AM, de Jong JC, et al. Cold-adapted live influenza vaccine versus inactivated vaccine: systemic vaccine reactions, local and systemic antibody response, and vaccine efficacy. A meta-analysis. Vaccine 2002;20: 1340–53.

124. Beyer WE, Palache AM, Osterhaus AD. Comparison of serology and reactogenicity between influenza subunit vaccines and whole virus or split vaccines: a review and meta-analysis of the literature. Clin Drug Investig 1998;15:1–12.

125. Beyer WE, Palache AM, Kerstens R, et al. Gender differences in local and systemic reactions to inactivated influenza vaccine, established by a meta-analysis of fourteen independent studies. Eur J Clin Microbiol Infect Dis 1996;15:65–70.

126. Jefferson T, Rivetti A, Harnden A, et al. Vaccines for preventing influenza in healthy children. Cochrane Database Syst Rev 2008:CD004879.

127. Manzoli L, Schioppa F, Boccia A, et al. The efficacy of influenza vaccine for healthy children: a meta-analysis evaluating potential sources of variation in efficacy estimates including study quality. Pediatr Infect Dis J 2007;26:97–106.

128. Negri E, Colombo C, Giordano L, et al. Influenza vaccine in healthy children: a meta-analysis. Vaccine 2005;23:2851–61.

129. Jefferson TO, Rivetti D, Di Pietrantonj C, et al. Vaccines for preventing influenza in healthy adults. Cochrane Database Syst Rev 2007:CD001269.

130. Villari P, Manzoli L, Boccia A. Methodological quality of studies and patient age as major sources of variation in efficacy estimates of influenza vaccination in healthy adults: a meta-analysis. Vaccine 2004;22:3475–86.

131. Poole PJ, Chacko E, Wood-Baker RW, et al. Influenza vaccine for patients with chronic obstructive pulmonary disease. Cochrane Database Syst Rev 2006: CD002733.

132. Atashili J, Kalilani L, Adimora AA. Efficacy and clinical effectiveness of influenza vaccines in HIV-infected individuals: a meta-analysis. BMC Infect Dis 2006;6:138.

133. Keller T, Weeda VB, van Dongen CJ, et al. Influenza vaccines for preventing coronary heart disease. Cochrane Database Syst Rev 2008:CD005050.

134. Cates CJ, Jefferson TO, Rowe BH. Vaccines for preventing influenza in people with asthma. Cochrane Database Syst Rev 2008:CD000364.

135. Chang CC, Morris PS, Chang AB. Influenza vaccine for children and adults with bronchiectasis. Cochrane Database Syst Rev 2007:CD006218.

136. Anema A, Mills E, Montaner J, et al. Efficacy of influenza vaccination in HIV-positive patients: a systematic review and meta-analysis. HIV Med 2008;9: 57–61.

137. Rivetti D, Jefferson T, Thomas R, et al. Vaccines for preventing influenza in the elderly. Cochrane Database Syst Rev 2006;3:CD004876.

138. Vu T, Farish S, Jenkins M, et al. A meta-analysis of effectiveness of influenza vaccine in persons aged 65 years and over living in the community. Vaccine 2002;20:1831–6.

139. Gross PA, Hermogenes AW, Sacks HS, et al. The efficacy of influenza vaccine in elderly persons. A meta-analysis and review of the literature. Ann Intern Med 1995;123:518–27.

140. Puig Barbera J, Marquez Calderon S. Effectiveness of influenza vaccine in the elderly. A critical review of the bibliography. Med Clin (Barc) 1995;105:645–8.

141. Thomas RE, Jefferson T, Demicheli V, et al. Influenza vaccination for healthcare workers who work with the elderly. Cochrane Database Syst Rev 2006;3: CD005187.

142. Lucero MG, Dulalia VE, Parreno RN, et al. Pneumococcal conjugate vaccines for preventing vaccine-type invasive pneumococcal disease and pneumonia with

consolidation on x-ray in children under two years of age. Cochrane Database Syst Rev 2004:CD004977.

143. Straetemans M, Sanders EA, Veenhoven RH, et al. Pneumococcal vaccines for preventing otitis media. Cochrane Database Syst Rev 2004:CD001480.

144. Chaithongwongwatthana S, Yamasmit W, Limpongsanurak S, et al. Pneumococcal vaccination during pregnancy for preventing infant infection. Cochrane Database Syst Rev 2006:CD004903.

145. Moberley SA, Holden J, Tatham DP, et al. Vaccines for preventing pneumococcal infection in adults. Cochrane Database Syst Rev 2008:CD000422.

146. Cornu C, Yzebe D, Leophonte P, et al. Efficacy of pneumococcal polysaccharide vaccine in immunocompetent adults: a meta-analysis of randomized trials. Vaccine 2001;19:4780–90.

147. Moore RA, Wiffen PJ, Lipsky BA. Are the pneumococcal polysaccharide vaccines effective? Meta-analysis of the prospective trials. BMC Fam Pract 2000;1:1.

148. Fine MJ, Smith MA, Carson CA, et al. Efficacy of pneumococcal vaccination in adults. A meta-analysis of randomized controlled trials. Arch Intern Med 1994; 154:2666–77.

149. Hutchison BG, Oxman AD, Shannon HS, et al. Clinical effectiveness of pneumococcal vaccine. Meta-analysis. Can Fam Physician 1999;45:2381–93.

150. Melegaro A, Edmunds WJ. The 23-valent pneumococcal polysaccharide vaccine. Part I. Efficacy of PPV in the elderly: a comparison of meta-analyses. Eur J Epidemiol 2004;19:353–63.

151. Granger R, Walters J, Poole PJ, et al. Injectable vaccines for preventing pneumococcal infection in patients with chronic obstructive pulmonary disease. Cochrane Database Syst Rev 2006:CD001390.

152. Sheikh A, Alves B, Dhami S. Pneumococcal vaccine for asthma. Cochrane Database Syst Rev 2002:CD002165.

153. Davies EG, Riddington C, Lottenberg R, et al. Pneumococcal vaccines for sickle cell disease. Cochrane Database Syst Rev 2004:CD003885.

154. Patel M, Lee CK. Polysaccharide vaccines for preventing serogroup A meningococcal meningitis. Cochrane Database Syst Rev 2005:CD001093.

155. Conterno LO, Silva Filho CR, Ruggeberg JU, et al. Conjugate vaccines for preventing meningococcal C meningitis and septicaemia. Cochrane Database Syst Rev 2006;3:CD001834.

156. Pollabauer EM, Petermann R, Ehrlich HJ. Group C meningococcal polysaccharide-tetanus toxoid conjugate vaccine: a meta-analysis of immunogenicity, safety and posology. Hum Vaccin 2005;1:131–9.

157. Swingler G, Fransman D, Hussey G. Conjugate vaccines for preventing Haemophilus influenzae type b infections. Cochrane Database Syst Rev 2007: CD001729.

158. Obonyo CO, Lau J. Efficacy of Haemophilus influenzae type b vaccination of children: a meta-analysis. Eur J Clin Microbiol Infect Dis 2006;25:90–7.

159. Foxwell AR, Cripps AW, Dear KB. Haemophilus influenzae oral whole cell vaccination for preventing acute exacerbations of chronic bronchitis. Cochrane Database Syst Rev 2006:CD001958.

160. Mathew JL, El Dib R, Mathew PJ, et al. Hepatitis B immunisation in persons not previously exposed to hepatitis B or with unknown exposure status. Cochrane Database Syst Rev 2008:CD006481.

161. Lee C, Gong Y, Brok J, et al. Hepatitis B immunisation for newborn infants of hepatitis B surface antigen-positive mothers. Cochrane Database Syst Rev 2006:CD004790.

162. Chen W, Gluud C. Vaccines for preventing hepatitis B in health-care workers. Cochrane Database Syst Rev 2005:CD000100.
163. Fabrizi F, Martin P, Dixit V, et al. Meta-analysis: the effect of age on immunological response to hepatitis B vaccine in end-stage renal disease. Aliment Pharmacol Ther 2004;20:1053–62.
164. Fisman DN, Agrawal D, Leder K. The effect of age on immunologic response to recombinant hepatitis B vaccine: a meta-analysis. Clin Infect Dis 2002;35: 1368–75.
165. Schroth RJ, Hitchon CA, Uhanova J, et al. Hepatitis B vaccination for patients with chronic renal failure. Cochrane Database Syst Rev 2004: CD003775.
166. Fabrizi F, Dixit V, Magnini M, et al. Meta-analysis: intradermal vs. intramuscular vaccination against hepatitis B virus in patients with chronic kidney disease. Aliment Pharmacol Ther 2006;24:497–506.
167. Cruciani M, Mengoli C, Serpelloni G, et al. Granulocyte macrophage colony-stimulating factor as an adjuvant for hepatitis B vaccination: a meta-analysis. Vaccine 2007;25:709–18.
168. Fabrizi F, Dixit V, Martin P. Meta-analysis: the adjuvant role of thymopentin on immunological response to hepatitis B virus vaccine in end-stage renal disease. Aliment Pharmacol Ther 2006;23:1559–66.
169. Fabrizi F, Ganeshan SV, Dixit V, et al. Meta-analysis: the adjuvant role of granulocyte macrophage-colony stimulating factor on immunological response to hepatitis B virus vaccine in end-stage renal disease. Aliment Pharmacol Ther 2006;24:789–96.
170. Fabrizi F, Dixit V, Bunnapradist S, et al. Meta-analysis: the dialysis mode and immunological response to hepatitis B virus vaccine in dialysis population. Aliment Pharmacol Ther 2006;23:1105–12.
171. Wang L, Turner MO, Elwood RK, et al. A meta-analysis of the effect of bacille Calmette Guerin vaccination on tuberculin skin test measurements. Thorax 2002;57:804–9.
172. Rodrigues LC, Diwan VK, Wheeler JG. Protective effect of BCG against tuberculous meningitis and miliary tuberculosis: a meta-analysis. Int J Epidemiol 1993; 22:1154–8.
173. Colditz GA, Berkey CS, Mosteller F, et al. The efficacy of bacillus Calmette-Guerin vaccination of newborns and infants in the prevention of tuberculosis: meta-analyses of the published literature. Pediatrics 1995;96:29–35.
174. Trunz BB, Fine P, Dye C. Effect of BCG vaccination on childhood tuberculous meningitis and miliary tuberculosis worldwide: a meta-analysis and assessment of cost-effectiveness. Lancet 2006;367:1173–80.
175. Setia MS, Steinmaus C, Ho CS, et al. The role of BCG in prevention of leprosy: a meta-analysis. Lancet Infect Dis 2006;6:162–70.
176. Zodpey SP. Protective effect of bacillus Calmette Guerin (BCG) vaccine in the prevention of leprosy: a meta-analysis. Indian J Dermatol Venereol Leprol 2007;73:86–93.
177. Han RF, Pan JG. Can intravesical bacillus Calmette-Guerin reduce recurrence in patients with superficial bladder cancer? A meta-analysis of randomized trials. Urology 2006;67:1216–23.
178. Sylvester RJ, van der Meijden AP, Witjes JA, et al. Bacillus Calmette-Guerin versus chemotherapy for the intravesical treatment of patients with carcinoma in situ of the bladder: a meta-analysis of the published results of randomized clinical trials. J Urol 2005;174:86–91 [discussion, 91–2].

179. Shelley MD, Wilt TJ, Court J, et al. Intravesical bacillus Calmette-Guerin is superior to mitomycin C in reducing tumour recurrence in high-risk superficial bladder cancer: a meta-analysis of randomized trials. BJU Int 2004;93:485–90.
180. Sylvester RJ, van der MA, Lamm DL. Intravesical bacillus Calmette-Guerin reduces the risk of progression in patients with superficial bladder cancer: a meta-analysis of the published results of randomized clinical trials. J Urol 2002;168:1964–70.
181. Bohle A, Bock PR. Intravesical bacille Calmette-Guerin versus mitomycin C in superficial bladder cancer: formal meta-analysis of comparative studies on tumor progression. Urology 2004;63:682–6 [discussion, 86–7].
182. Huncharek M, Kupelnick B. The influence of intravesical therapy on progression of superficial transitional cell carcinoma of the bladder: a metaanalytic comparison of chemotherapy versus bacilli Calmette-Guerin immunotherapy. Am J Clin Oncol 2004;27:522–8.
183. La Torre G, de Waure C, Chiaradia G, et al. HPV vaccine efficacy in preventing persistent cervical HPV infection: a systematic review, meta-analysis. Vaccine 2007;25:8352–8.
184. Bhatla N, Lal N, Bao YP, et al. A meta-analysis of human papillomavirus type-distribution in women from South Asia: implications for vaccination. Vaccine 2008;26:2811–7.
185. Bao YP, Li N, Wang H, et al. [Study on the distribution of human papillomavirus types in cervix among Chinese women: a meta-analysis]. Zhonghua Liu Xing Bing Xue Za Zhi 2007;28:941–6.
186. Bae JH, Lee SJ, Kim CJ, et al. Human papillomavirus (HPV) type distribution in Korean women: a meta-analysis. J Microbiol Biotechnol 2008;18:788–94.
187. Bao YP, Li N, Smith JS, et al. Human papillomavirus type-distribution in the cervix of chinese women: a meta-analysis. Int J STD AIDS 2008;19:106–11.
188. Smith JS, Lindsay L, Hoots B, et al. Human papillomavirus type distribution in invasive cervical cancer and high-grade cervical lesions: a meta-analysis update. Int J Cancer 2007;121:621–32.
189. Clifford GM, Smith JS, Aguado T, et al. Comparison of HPV type distribution in high-grade cervical lesions and cervical cancer: a meta-analysis. Br J Cancer 2003;89:101–5.
190. Brotherton JM. How much cervical cancer in Australia is vaccine preventable? A meta-analysis. Vaccine 2008;26:250–6.

Index

Note: Page numbers of article titles are in **boldface** type.

A

Abdominal infections, combination therapy for, 286–287
Abdominal surgery
  antimicrobial agents for, meta-analysis on, 408–409
  meta-analyses focusing on, 416–417
Acute otitis externa
  ciprofloxacin-based otic suspension for, 333
  quinolones for, 333
Acute otitis media, azithromycin for, 334
Acute suppurative otitis media, ofloxacin for, 334
Adefovir, for hepatitis B, 322
Amodiaquine, for malaria, 396
Amoxicillin, for sinusitis, 334
Amoxicillin/clavulanic acid, for COPD, 337
Antibiotic(s). See *Antimicrobial agents.*
Antibiotic-resistant infections, risk factors for, identification of, meta-analyses
  on, 218–219
Antimicrobial agents
  for community-acquired pneumonia, 339–340
  for COPD, 336–337
  for infections
    optimization of duration of, meta-analyses on, **269–276**
      acute bacterial meningitis, 270–271
      acute bacterial sinusitis, 271
      acute otitis media, 271
      acute pyelonephritis, 273
      brucellosis, 273–274
      chronic bronchitis, 272
      community-acquired pneumonia, 272–273
      cystitis in women, 273
      described, 269–270
      discussion of, 274–275
      literature review of, 270
      streptococcal tonsillopharyngitis, 271–272
    surgical, meta-analysis on, 408–416. See also *Antimicrobial agents, for surgical*
    infections.
  for nosocomial pneumonia/ventilator-associated pneumonia, 343–344
  for surgical infections, meta-analysis on, 408–416
    abdominal surgery, 408–409
    breast surgery, 409, 416
    neurosurgery, 409, 416

Infect Dis Clin N Am 23 (2009) 459–470
doi:10.1016/S0891-5520(09)00025-7
0891-5520/09/$ – see front matter © 2009 Elsevier Inc. All rights reserved.

id.theclinics.com

Antimicrobial (*continued*)
    obstetrics and gynecology, 409, 416
    orthopedics, 416
    peri-operative prophylaxis in surgery, 409
    thoracic surgery, 409
    vascular surgery, 409
  inhaled, for nosocomial pneumonia/ventilator-associated pneumonia, 343
  meta-analyses focusing on, 410–415
Antiretroviral resistance testing, in HIV-infected persons, 302–303
Antiretroviral therapy, for HIV infections, adverse effects of, 304
Artemisin combinations, for malaria, 397–400
Azithromycin
    for acute otitis media, 334
    for community-acquired pneumonia, 339
    for COPD, 337
    for sinusitis, 334
    for tonsillitis/tonsillopharyngitis, 335

B

Bacterial infections
    diagnostic accuracy of tests for, evaluation of, meta-analyses in, 232–233
    risk factors for, identification of, meta-analyses on, 215–218
Bacterial meningitis
    acute, meta-analyses on optimization of duration of antimicrobial agents for, 270–271
    in children, meta-analyses on, 441
Bacterial sinusitis, acute, meta-analyses on optimization of duration of antimicrobial agents
    for, 271
BCG (bacille Calmette-Guérin) vaccine, in children, meta-analyses on, 447–449
Bed therapy, rotational, for nosocomial pneumonia/ventilator-associated pneumonia, 341
Behavioral interventions, in HIV infection transmission reduction, meta-analyses on,
    309–314. See also *HIV infection, transmission of, behavioral interventions in reducing
    risk of, meta-analyses on.*
Bias
    avoidance of, in systematic review, 185–187
    in meta-analyses of diagnostic tests in infectious diseases, 241
    misclassification of, in meta-analyses in identification of risk factors for infections, 220
    publication, in meta-analyses in identification of risk factors for infections, 221
Breast surgery, antimicrobial agents for, meta-analysis on, 409, 416
Bronchiolitis, in children, meta-analyses on, 435–438
Bronchitis, chronic, meta-analyses on optimization of duration of antimicrobial agents for,
    272
Bronchodilator(s), inhaled, for COPD, 337
Brucellosis, meta-analyses on optimization of duration of antimicrobial agents for, 273–274

C

Carbapenem(s), for nosocomial pneumonia/ventilator-associated pneumonia, 344
Cardiothoracic surgery, meta-analyses focusing on, 417
Cephalosporin(s), for tonsillitis/tonsillopharyngitis, 335
Children

infections in, meta-analyses on, **433–442**
    acute gastroenteritis and diarrhea, 434–435
    bacterial meningitis, 441
    bronchiolitis, 435–438
    croup, 439
    cystic fibrosis, 441–442
    otitis media, 438
    pneumonia, 435–438
    tonsillitis, 439
    UTIs, 439–441
  UTIs in, prevention and treatment of, 368–373
  vaccines for, meta-analyses on, **442–449**
    BCG vaccine, 447–449
      meta-analyses on, 447–449
    Haemophilus influenzae vaccines, 446–447
    hepatitis B vaccines, 447
    HPV vaccines, 449
    influenza vaccines, 442–443
    meningococcal vaccines, 446–447
    pneumonoccocal vaccines, 443–446
Chronic obstructive pulmonary disease (COPD), meta-analyses on, 335–338
Ciprofloxacin-based otic suspension, for acute otitis externa, 333
Circumcision, male, HIV infection reduction due to, 296–297
Clinical questions
  in combination therapy vs. monotherapy for hospital-based infections, 279–280
  in systematic review, 183–185
Cochrane Collaboration, in systematic reviews, 192
Cochrane Handbook, 192
Cochrane Infectious Diseases Group, on malaria, 389–390
Combination therapy
  for abdominal infections, 286–287
  for endocarditis, 285
  for fungal infections, 287–288
  for hospital-based infections, vs. monotherapy, **277–293**
    clinical proof in, 278–279
    clinical questions in, 279–280
    reasons for, 277–278
Community-acquired pneumonia
  meta-analyses on, 338–340
  meta-analyses on optimization of duration of antimicrobial agents for, 272–273
Confounding factors, in meta-analyses in identification of risk factors for infections,
  219–220
COPD. See *Chronic obstructive pulmonary disease (COPD).*
Corticosteroid(s)
  for community-acquired pneumonia, 340
  for sinusitis, 334
  systemic, inhaled, 338
Croup, in children, meta-analyses on, 439
Cystic fibrosis, in children, meta-analyses on, 441–442
Cystitis, in women, meta-analyses on optimization of duration of antimicrobial agents for,
  273

D

Diagnostic and prognostic test meta-analysis, 206
Diagnostic tests, in infectious diseases, meta-analyses of, **225–267**
    bacterial infections, 232–233
    bias in, 241
    clinical setting in, 227, 228, 230
    discussion of, 247, 251, 262
    findings from, 241, 247
    fungal infections, 242–243
    graphic presentation of, 229, 231
    heterogeneity in, 241
    inclusion criteria in, 227, 228
    index and reference tests in, 229–231
    infectious disease syndromes, 252–261
    materials and methods in, 226
    methods of, 241
    mycobacterial infections, 234–240
    objectives of, 227, 228
    patient population in, 227, 228, 230
    protozoan infections, 248–250
    quality and methods of, 229–231, 241
    results of, 226–247
    study design in, 228, 230
    study results of, 229, 231
    target condition description in, 227, 230
    viral infections, 244–246
Diarrhea, in children, meta-analyses on, 434–435
Diet(s), enriched, for nosocomial pneumonia/ventilator-associated pneumonia, 343
Drug(s). See specific agents.

E

Effect metrics, in primary studies, 198–199
Elderly, UTIs in, prevention and treatment of, 365–368
Endocarditis, combination therapy for, 285

F

Fixed-effects, in meta-analysis, 199–202
Forest plots, in meta-analysis, 202–203
Fungal infections
    combination therapy for, 287–288
    diagnostic accuracy of tests for, meta-analyses in evaluation of, 242–243

G

Gastroenteritis, acute, in children, meta-analyses on, 434–435
Gram-negative infections, β-lactams–aminoglycosides combination therapy for, 282–285
Gram-positive infections, combination therapy for, 285
Graph(s), in meta-analysis, 202–203
Gynecology, obstetrics and, antimicrobial agents for, meta-analysis on, 409, 416

H

Haemophilus influenzae vaccines, in children, meta-analyses on, 446–447
Hepatitis
  A
    prevention of
      immunoglobulins in, 316–317
      vaccine in, 316–317
    viral hepatitis due to, 316–317
  B, 317–324
    chronic
      definitions related to, 318
      diagnostic criteria for, 318
    described, 317–318
    prevention of
      immunoglobulins in, 318–319
      vaccine in, 318–319
    treatment of, 319–324
      adefovir in, 322
      combination therapy in, 323
      interferon in, 319–321
      lamivudine in, 321–322
      recommendations for, 323–324
    vaccines for, in children, meta-analyses on, 447
  C, 324–326
    transmission of, risk factors for, meta-analyses on, 214–215
    treatment of, 325–326
  viral, meta-analyses on, **315–330**
Herbal medicines, for sinusitis, 335
Heterogeneity
  in meta-analyses in identification of risk factors for infections, 220
  in meta-analyses of diagnostic tests in infectious diseases, 241
  statistical, reasons for, 203–205
HIV infection
  antiretroviral resistance testing in, 302–303
  antiretroviral therapy for
    adherence to, 303–304
    efficacy of, 300–302
      in resource-limited settings, 302
      in treatment-naïve persons, 300–301
      switching regimen because of side effects and, 301
  in men who have sex with men, epidemiology of, 298
  meta-analyses on, **295–308**
  prognostic markers for, 299–300
  risk factors for, 296–298
    heterosexual infectivity, 296
    male circumcision and, 296–297
    STIs, 297–298
  transmission of
    behavioral interventions in reducing risk of, meta-analyses on, **309–314**
      in heterosexuals, 309–310

HIV infection (*continued*)
       in HIV-infected persons, 312
       in injection drug users, 311–312
       in men who have sex with men, 310–311
       in minority populations, 310
       synthesis of, 312
     mother-to-child, 298–299
     risk factors for, meta-analyses on, 214–215
   vaccines for, efficacy of, 304–305
Hospital-based infections, combination therapy vs. monotherapy for, **277–293.** See also *Combination therapy, for hospital-based infections, vs. monotherapy.*
HPV vaccines. See *Human papilloma virus (HPV) vaccines.*
Human immunodeficiency virus (HIV) infection. See *HIV infection.*
Human papilloma virus (HPV) vaccines, in children, meta-analyses on, 449
Humidifiers, passive vs. active, for nosocomial pneumonia/ventilator-associated
   pneumonia, 341

   I

Immunoglobulin(s)
   in hepatitis A prevention, 316–317
   in hepatitis B prevention, 318–319
Infection(s). See also specific infections.
   abdominal, combination therapy for, 286–287
   antimicrobial agents for, optimization of duration of, meta-analyses on, **269–276.** See also *Antimicrobial agents, for infections, optimization of duration of, meta-analyses on.*
   gram-negative, ß-lactams–aminoglycosides combination therapy for, 282–285
   gram-positive, combination therapy for, 285
   hospital-based, combination therapy vs. monotherapy for, **277–293.** See also *Combination therapy, for hospital-based infections, vs. monotherapy.*
   in children, meta-analyses on, **433–442**
   risk factors for, identification of, meta-analyses on, **211–224**
      analysis of quality in, 221
      antibiotic-resistant infections, 218–219
      bacterial infections, 215–218
      confounding factors in, 219–220
      examples of, 214–219
      hepatitis C, 214–215
      heterogeneity in, 220
      HIV infection transmission, 214–215
      justification for, 219–221
      limits of, 211–214
      misclassification bias in, 220
      publication bias in, 221
   surgical, meta-analysis on, **407–432.** See also *Surgical infections, meta-analysis on.*
Infectious disease(s) classical, narrative, and systematic reviews of, comparison among,
   182
Infectious disease syndromes, diagnostic accuracy of tests for, evaluation of,
   meta-analyses in, 252–261
Infectious diseases, systematic reviews and meta-analyses in, **181–194**
   avoiding bias in, 185–187

clinical question in, 183–185
combining studies in, 187–188
heterogeneity in, 188–190
Infectious diseases, 190
limitations of, 191
problems related to, 190
results interpretation of, 191–192
strengths of, 190
Influenza, vaccines for, in children, meta-analyses on, 442–443
Insecticide-treated nets, in malaria prevention, 393–395
Interferon, for hepatitis B, 319–321

L

ß-Lactam(s), for community-acquired pneumonia, 339
ß-Lactam(s)–aminoglycosides combination therapy, for *Pseudomonas aeruginosa*
    infections, 282–285
Lamivudine, for hepatitis B, 321–322
Linezolid, for nosocomial pneumonia/ventilator-associated pneumonia, 344
Liver disease, hepatitis and, 315

M

Macrolide(s), for COPD, 337
Malaria
    Cochrane Infectious Diseases Group on, 389–390
    during pregnancy, prevention of, insecticide-treated nets in, 394–395
    incidence of, 387–389
    prevention of, 390–396
        drugs in, 390–392
        insecticide-treated nets in, 393–395
        vaccines in, 395–396
    systemic reviews in, **387–404**
    treatment of, 396–400
        amodiaquine in, 396
        artemisin combinations in, 397–400
        primaquine in, 400
Mechanical ventilation, noninvasive
    for COPD, 338
    for nosocomial pneumonia/ventilator-associated pneumonia, 342
Meningitis, bacterial, in children, meta-analyses on, 441
Meningococcal vaccines, in children, meta-analyses on, 446–447
Meta-analysis(es). See also specific topics, e.g., *Urinary tract infections (UTIs), prevention
    of, meta-analyses in.*
    cumulative, forest plots and, 202–203
    defined, 187, 433
    in identification of risk factors for infections, **211–224**
    in infectious diseases, **181–194**
        in combination therapy vs. monotherapy for hospital-based infections, general
            concepts, 280–282
    in UTIs prevention and treatment, **355–385**

Meta-analysis(es) (*continued*)
    network, 205
    of diagnostic tests, 206
        in infectious diseases, **225–267**
    of prognositc tests, 206
    on abdominal surgery, 416–417
    on antimicrobial agents, 410–415
    on behavioral interventions in reducing risk of HIV infection transmission, **309–314**
    on cardiothoracic surgery, 417
    on effects of interventions for surgical infections, 418–423
    on HIV infections, **295–308**
    on obstetrics, 424
    on optimization of duration of antimicrobial agents for infections, **269–276**
    on orthopedics, 424
    on pediatric infections and vaccines, **433–459**
    on respiratory tract infections prevention and treatment, **331–353**
    on surgical infections, **407–432**
    on vascular surgery, 417
    on viral hepatitis, **315–330**
    statistical considerations in, **195–210**
        effect metrics in primary studies, 198–199
        fixed-effects, 199–202
        graphs, 202–203
        heterogeneity in, reasons for, 203–205
        quantitative synthesis, 199
        random-effects, 199–202
    systematic review and, 196–198
    types of, 205–207
Methylxanthine(s), inhaled, 337
Metrics, effect, in primary studies, 198–199
Mycobacterial infections, diagnostic accuracy of tests for, evaluation of, meta-analyses of, 234–240
Mycolytic(s), systemic, 338

N

Net(s), insecticide-treated, in malaria prevention, 393–395
Network meta-analysis, 205
Neurosurgery, antimicrobial agents for, meta-analysis on, 409, 416
NIMV. See *Noninvasive mechanical ventilation (NIMV)*.
Noninvasive mechanical ventilation (NIMV)
    for nosocomial pneumonia/ventilator-associated pneumonia, 342
    systemic, 338
Nosocomial pneumonia/ventilator-associated pneumonia
    meta-analyses on, 340–343
    NIMV for, 342

O

Obstetrics and gynecology
    antimicrobial agents for, meta-analysis on, 409, 416

meta-analyses focusing on, 424
Ofloxacin, for acute suppurative otitis media, 334
Oral rehydration therapy, for acute gastroenteritis in children, 434–435
Orthopedics
    antimicrobial agents for, meta-analysis on, 416
    meta-analyses on, 424
Otic suspension, ciprofloxacin-based, for acute otitis externa, 333
Otitis, meta-analyses on, 333–334
Otitis media
    acute
        azithromycin for, 334
        meta-analyses on optimization of duration of antimicrobial agents for, 271
    acute suppurative, ofloxacin for, 334
    in children, meta-analyses on, 438

P

Pharmaco-nutrients, for nosocomial pneumonia/ventilator-associated pneumonia, 343
Pneumonia(s)
    community-acquired
        meta-analyses on, 338–340
        meta-analyses on optimization of duration of antimicrobial agents for, 272–273
    in children, meta-analyses on, 435–438
    nosocomial, meta-analyses on, 340–343
    ventilator-associated, meta-analyses on, 340–343
Pneumonoccocal vaccines, in children, meta-analyses on, 443–446
Postpyloric feeding, for nosocomial pneumonia/ventilator-associated pneumonia, 342
Pregnancy
    malaria prevention during, insecticide-treated nets in, 394–395
    UTIs during, prevention and treatment of, 363–364
Primaquine, for malaria, 400
Probiotics, for nosocomial pneumonia/ventilator-associated pneumonia, 343
Prone positioning, for nosocomial pneumonia/ventilator-associated pneumonia, 341
Protozoan infections, diagnostic accuracy of tests for, evaluation of, meta-analyses in,
    248–250
Pseudomonas aeruginosa infections, ß-lactams–aminoglycosides combination therapy for,
    282–285
Publication bias, in meta-analyses in identification of risk factors for infections, 221
Pyelonephritis, acute, meta-analyses on optimization of duration of antimicrobial agents
    for, 273

Q

Quality, analysis of, in meta-analyses in identification of risk factors for infections, 221
Quantitative synthesis, 199
Quinolone(s)
    for acute otitis externa, 333
    for community-acquired pneumonia, 339
    for COPD, 337
    for nosocomial pneumonia/ventilator-associated pneumonia, 344
    for sinusitis, 334

R

Random-effects, 199–202
Respiratory tract infections
  described, 331
  prevention and treatment of, meta-analyses on, **331–353**
    COPD, 335–338
    methods in, 332
    otitis, 333–334
    sinusitis, 334–335
    tonsillitis/tonsillopharyngitis, 335
Rotational bed therapy, for nosocomial pneumonia/ventilator-associated pneumonia, 341

S

Sexually transmitted infections (STIs), HIV infection related to, 297–298
Sinusitis
  bacterial, acute, meta-analyses on optimization of duration of antimicrobial agents for, 271
  meta-analyses on, 334–335
Statistical considerations, in meta-analysis, **195–210**. See also *Meta-analysis(es), statistical considerations in.*
STIs. See *Sexually transmitted infections (STIs).*
Streptococcal tonsillopharyngitis, meta-analyses on optimization of duration of antimicrobial agents for, 271–272
Subglottic secretion drainage, for nosocomial pneumonia/ventilator-associated pneumonia, 342
Surgical infections
  interventions for, meta-analyses on effect of, 418–423
  meta-analyses on, **407–432**
    antimicrobial agents, 408–416
      in abdominal surgery, 408–409
      in breast surgery, 409, 416
      in neurosurgery, 409, 416
      in obstetrics and gynecology, 409, 416
      in orthopedics, 416
      in peri-operative prophylaxis in surgery, 409
      in thoracic surgery, 409
      in vascular surgery, 409
    literature search related to, 408
    study selection and extraction in, 408
Systematic review(s)
  in infectious diseases, **181–194**. See also *Infectious disease(s), systematic reviews and meta-analyses in.*
  in malaria, **387–404**
  meta-analysis and, 196–198
  steps in conducting, 196–198

T

The Cochrane Collaboration, 389–390
Thoracic surgery, antimicrobial agents for, meta-analysis on, 409

Tonsillitis, in children, meta-analyses on, 439
Tonsillitis/tonsillopharyngitis, meta-analyses on, 335
Tonsillopharyngitis, streptococcal, meta-analyses on optimization of duration of
    antimicrobial agents for, 271–272
Tracheal suction systems, closed vs. open, for nosocomial pneumonia/
    ventilator-associated pneumonia, 341
Tracheostomy, for nosocomial pneumonia/ventilator-associated pneumonia, 340–341

U

Urinary tract infections (UTIs)
    complications of, 355
        hospital admissions resulting from, 355
    defining characteristics of, 356
    in children, meta-analyses on, 439–441
    prevention of
        from evidence to treatment recommendations, 373–374
        in children, 368–373
        in pregnant women, 363–364
        in special populations, 365–368
        in the elderly, 365
        in women, 357–362
        interventions in, 356
        literature review of, methods of, 357
        meta-analyses in, **355–385**
        research in, future directions in, 384
    treatment of
        from evidence to treatment recommendations, 384
        in children, 368–373
        in pregnant women, 364
        in special populations, 365–368
        in the elderly, 365
        in women, 362–363
        interventions in, 356
        literature review of, methods of, 357
        meta-analyses in, **355–385**
        research in, future directions in, 384
UTIs. See *Urinary tract infections (UTIs)*.

V

Vaccine(s)
    against influenza, in COPD prevention, 336
    against pneumococcus, in COPD prevention, 335–336
    BCG, in children, meta-analyses on, 447–448
    for HIV infection, efficacy of, 304–305
    Haemophilus influenzae, in children, meta-analyses on, 446–447
    hepatitis B, in children, meta-analyses on, 447
    HPV, in children, meta-analyses on, 449
    in hepatitis A prevention, 316–317
    in hepatitis B prevention, 318–319

Vaccine(s) (*continued*)
   in malaria prevention, 395–396
   influenza, vaccines for, meta-analyses on, 442–443
   meningococcal, in children, meta-analyses on, 446–447
   pediatric, meta-analyses on, **442–449**
   pneumococcal, in children, meta-analyses on, 443–446
Vascular surgery
   antimicrobial agents for, meta-analysis on, 409
   meta-analyses focusing on, 417
Viral hepatitis
   liver disease due to, 315
   meta-analyses on, **315–330**
Viral infections, diagnostic accuracy of tests for, evaluation of, meta-analyses
   in, 244–246

Printed and bound by CPI Group (UK) Ltd, Croydon, CR0 4YY

03/10/2024

01040462-0009